Clinical Handbook of Psychotropic Drugs for Children and Adolescents

Kalyna Z. Bezchlibnyk-Butler, BSc (Pharm), FCSHP
and
Adil S. Virani, BSc (Pharm), PharmD[A], FCSHP

The Editors wish to acknowledge contributions from the following chapter co-editors:

E. Jane Garland, MD, FRCPC[B] (Antidepressants)
Barry A. Martin, MD, FRCPC[C] (Electroconvulsive Therapy)
Herb Orlik MD, FRCP (C)[D] (Antipsychotics)
Lukas Propper, MD[D] (Anxiolytics, Hypnotics)
Aiden Stokes, MD, PhD[D] (Mood Stabilizers)
Margaret Weiss MD, PhD[E] (Drugs for ADHD)

[A] Fraser Health Authority and Faculty of Pharmaceutical Sciences, University of British Columbia, Vancouver, BC, Canada
[B] BC's Childrens's Hospital and University of British Columbia, Vancouver, BC
[C] Centre for Addiction and Mental Health and Department of Psychiatry, University of Toronto, Toronto, Canada
[D] IWK Health Centre and Department of Psychiatry, Dalhousie University, Halifax, Nova Scotia, Canada
[E] ADHD Program Children's and Women's Health Centre, Vancouver, BC

CINCINNATI STATE WITHDRAWN

D1262785

JOHNNIE MAE BERRY LIBRARY
ATI STATE
ITRAL PARKWAY
TI, OHIO 45223-2690

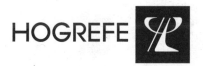

HOGREFE

The primary editors wish to dedicate the *Clinical Handbook of Psychotropic Drugs for Children and Adolescents* to their respective family members for their love, support, as well as patience during the hours spent reviewing and editing this publication.

Kalyna Z. Bezchlibnyk-Butler:
to my husband Douglas and sons Jeremy and Michael

Adil S. Virani:
to my wife Ashifa, daughter Sophia-Iman, and son Keyan-Aman.

Library of Congress Cataloging-in-Publication Data

is available via the Library of Congress Marc Database under the
LC Control Number 2006938378

National Library of Canada Cataloguing in Publication

Clinical handbook of psychotropic drugs for children and adolescents / Kalyna Z. Bezchlibnyk-Butler, Adil S. Virani, eds. —2nd rev. ed.
Includes bibliographical references and index.

ISBN–13: 978-0-88937-309-9
ISBN–10: 0-88937-309-4

1. Psychotropic drugs—Handbooks, manuals, etc. 2. Pediatric psychopharmacology—Handbooks, manuals, etc. I. Bezchlibnyk-Butler, Kalyna Z., 1947– II. Virani, Adil S., 1969– III. Title: Psychotropic drugs.

RM 315.C56 2007 615'.788083 C2006-906449-0

The authors and publisher have made every effort to ensure that drug selections and dosages suggested in this text are in accord with current recommendations and practice at the time of publication. Given that changes may occur in a medication's indications and differences are seen among countries, specific "indications" listed in this text as "approved" should be viewed in conjunction with product monographs approved in your jurisdiction of interest. Due to changing government regulations, continuing research, and changing information concerning drug therapy and reactions, the reader is urged to check the package insert for each drug for any change in indications and dosage, or for added precautions. The authors and publisher disclaim any responsibility for any consequences which may follow from the use of information presented in this book.

© 2007 by Hogrefe & Huber Publishers

PUBLISHING OFFICES

USA:	Hogrefe & Huber Publishers, 875 Massachusetts Avenue, 7th Floor, Cambridge, MA 02139 Phone (866) 823-4726, Fax (617) 354-6875 E-mail info@hhpub.com
EUROPE:	Hogrefe & Huber Publishers, Rohnsweg 25, 37085 Götringen Germany, Phone +49 551 49609-0, Fax +49 551 49609-88 E-mail hh@hhpub.com

SALES & DISTRIBUTION

USA:	Hogrefe & Huber Publishers, Cust. Services Department, 30 Amberwood Parkway, Ashland, OH 44805 Phone (800) 228-3749, Fax (419) 281-6883 E-mail custserv@hhpub.com
EUROPE:	Hogrefe & Huber Publishers, Rohnsweg 25, 37085 Götringen Germany, Phone +49 551 49609-0, Fax +49 551 49609-88 E-mail hh@hhpub.com

OTHER OFFICES

CANADA:	Hogrefe & Huber Publishers, 1543 Bayview Avenue, Toronto, Ontario M4G 3B5
SWITZERLAND:	Hogrefe & Huber Publishers, Länggass-Strasse 76, CH-3000 Bern 9

Hogrefe & Huber Publishers
Incorporated and registered in the State of Washington, USA,
and in Göttingen, Lower Saxony, Germany

No part of this book may be reproduced, stored in a retrieval system or transmitted, in any form or by any means, electronic, mechanical, photocopying, microfilming, recording or otherwise, without written permission from the publisher.

Printed and bound in the USA
ISBN 978-0-88937-309-9

TABLE OF CONTENTS

INTRODUCTION

The *Clinical Handbook* is a user-friendly and practical resource guide on the use of psychotropic drugs in children and adolescents. Its content is based on published literature (including basic science data, controlled clinical trials, and anecdotal case reports) as well as clinical experience.

Many classes of psychotropic drugs are used to treat childhood and adolescent mental illness on the basis of efficacy in adults, despite not being currently approved for use in these populations. The lack of approval does not necessarily reflect lack of safety or efficacy, but it does reflect a lack of controlled studies in these age groups. Many product monographs include a statement stating their drug has not been adequately studied in children and the safety of the drug has not been established under a specific age.

In the Product Availability section of each chapter, the *Clinical Handbook* includes monograph statements regarding the recommendations for the use of each drug in children and adolescents. Approved indications (usually for adults) are stated; also included are nonapproved indications for these drugs. Each chapter includes data from open and double-blind studies, where available, regarding doses, adverse effects, and other considerations in children and adolescents.

Because of a lack of comparative data in children and adolescents for most drug classes, Adverse Reaction tables and Drug Interaction charts reflect information that pertains to heterogeneous age groups (young, adult, and elderly).

Patient and Caregiver Information Sheets have been included for all drugs categories, to facilitate education/counseling of patients receiving these medications.

Most youths with a diagnosable psychiatric disorder require multi-modal interventions to address the symptoms of the disorder, the comorbid conditions, and the psychological, social, and developmental sequelae. Individual and family psychoeducation are essential, and psychosocial interventions should be considered for most psychiatric disorders.

Until systematic double-blind studies of various psychotropic drugs have been conducted to determine the efficacy, the pharmacokinetics, as well as the relative and absolute risks of each drug in this population, physicians who choose to use specific psychotropic drugs in children and adolescents should review all available studies and monitor their patients on a regular basis. Consideration should be given to obtaining informed consent from the caregiver or youth (depending on the age) for use in unapproved indications.

The purpose of this handbook is to provide quick access to relevant, practical, and important information clinicians should be aware of when considering pharmacological options available in the treatment of childhood and adolescent psychiatric disorders. It provides an overview of the plausible alternatives, dosing guidelines, as well as information on drug interactions and potential side effects. It is meant to be a resource to both those in training and experienced clinicians.

As the *Clinical Handbook* is intended to be a clinical summary of current information, the authors welcome input from readers as to the content or format. Please write to:

Mrs. K.Z. Butler
E-Mail Kalyna@sympatico.ca

PSYCHIATRIC DISORDERS IN CHILDREN AND ADOLESCENTS

Significant psychiatric illnesses affect approximately 10–15% of North American children and adolescents. These consist of conditions such as mood and anxiety disorders, bipolar disorder, attention-deficit hyperactivity disorder (ADHD), schizophrenia, Tourette's syndrome, and pervasive developmental disorders. Symptoms of these disorders are often serious and have an enormous impact on the lives of the patients and their families. Many factors complicate the recognition, management, and treatment of psychiatric disorders in children and adolescents. These include a high variance in symptom presentation and interpretation, diagnostic difficulties, scarcity of resources, research limitations, environmental influences, societal attitudes, and medication issues.

Attention Deficit Hyperactivity Disorder (ADHD)

ADHD is a heterogeneous behavioral disorder first evident in children before the age of 7.

Incidence
- 3–7% (4–12% in USA)

Onset
- Symptoms begin as early as age 3
- 3–6 times more common in male than female children (but may be underreported in females); some individuals with inattentive subtype may mask symptoms by being quiet

Risk Factors
- Genetic link suggested
- Complications during pregnancy or delivery
- Adverse family environment

Comorbidity
- Mood and anxiety disorders, bipolar disorder, Tourette's syndrome, conduct disorder, oppositional defiant disorder, and learning disorders
- Rule out vision and learning deficits, developmental delays, neurological abnormalities, endocrine disorders, and sleep disorders

Presentation and Symptoms
- Subtypes include: (1) Impulsive/hyperactive; (2) inattentive; (3) combined – most common
- Ages 6–12: easily distracted, hyperactive, disorganized, impulsive, interrupts others in class, bursts out answers, has difficulties in peer relationships, has difficulty communicating (10–54% have speech problems), and displays aggressive behavior
- Ages 13–18: has sense of inner restlessness, poor concentration, daydreaming, forgetful, schoolwork disorganized, fails to work independently and follow through, poor self-esteem and poor peer relationships, difficulty with authority figures, engages in "risky" behavior

Course of Illness
- Hyperactive/impulsive behaviors tend to diminish as the child ages; inattention and restlessness often continue
- About 70% of children who are diagnosed with ADHD continue to have some symptoms in mid-adolescence and about 40% continue into adulthood

Consequences of ADHD
- Can result in poor academic performance, self-esteem, social and interpersonal relationships
- High risk of injuries (4 times that of norm) and 3 times as many motor vehicle accidents (50% vs 19%)

Attention Deficit Hyperactivity Disorder (ADHD) (cont.)

- If inadequately treated, these children and adolescents are at increased risk for abusing substances (50% vs 30% in normal population) and developing antisocial personality disorder
- Educational and employment difficulties, problems with driving and with sexual relationships
- Risk of teen pregnancy is 50% (vs 4% in normal population)
- 20% risk of incarceration (vs 1% in normal population)
- Minor involuntary movements, or tics, occur in 8–11% of school-age children with ADHD

Treatment
- Multimodal treatment approach recommended, including psychoeducation, pharmacotherapy, and behavioral interventions
- See chapters on Drugs for ADHD (p. 19) and Antidepressants (p. 40)

Major Depressive Disorder (MDD)

Incidence
- Preschoolers: rare
- Children: 1–2%; males = females
- Adolescents: up to 15%; twice as frequent in females than males. Atypical depression reported in 15% of youths (age 6–19) diagnosed with MDD

Onset
- Most often starts in adolescence
- There is evidence that depression is becoming more prevalent in children < 10 years old

Risk Factors
- Risk is 3 times higher in children who have a parent diagnosed with MDD
- Previous depressive episodes
- Anxiety disorders, chronic medical illness, substance abuse
- Strong association of childhood trauma and abuse with depression and suicidality in adulthood

Comorbidity
- Seen in about 40% of children and adolescents
- Separation anxiety and ADHD common in children
- Generalized anxiety disorder, social phobias, ADHD, conduct disorder, and substance abuse more common in adolescents
- Depression common in persons with mental retardation (may be manifest by aggressive behavior)

Presentation and Symptoms
- Vary with age
- Ages 3–4: disruptive behaviors (acting out, aggression, temper tantrums, hyperactivity, and oppositional behaviors), somatic symptoms (e.g., headache, stomach pains), enuresis and encopresis, social withdrawal, eating or sleeping difficulties, and separation problems
- Ages 5–8: sadness, social withdrawal, low self-esteem, excessive guilt, self-blame, unexplainable somatic symptoms, enuresis and encopresis, being accident prone, carelessness, lying, oppositional, and aggressive behaviors
- Ages 9–12: sadness, somatic complaints, difficulty concentrating, school problems, separation anxiety, isolation, apathy, anhedonia, hopelessness, irritability, and suicidal ideation

- **Adolescent:** decreased school performance, irritability, anxiety, and anger are common; other symptoms are similar to those seen in adults, e.g., sleep and appetite changes, social withdrawal, somatic symptoms, anhedonia, antisocial behavior, and substance abuse. High risk of suicide in this population (up to 32% will make a suicide attempt and 2.5–7% will die as a result of suicide)

Course of Illness	• Variable with some individuals experiencing multiple exacerbations and remissions • Recurrence rates are up to 70% within 5 years • 20–40% develop bipolar disorder over time
Diagnosis	• Criteria for diagnosing depression in children are not well defined • Children may have greater mood lability, which can hamper diagnosis • The clinician cannot ask complicated questions of young children, which makes it difficult to assess depressive symptoms; multiple informants often needed to corroborate diagnosis
Consequences of Depression	• MDD in associated with increased suicide risk • Can impair age-dependent social and cognitive skills and result in social dysfunction and academic underachievement, tobacco use, substance/ alcohol abuse and teen pregnancy • Childhood depression strongly increases the risk for future mood disorders (4-fold increase in the risk of depression in adulthood for those who have experienced significant depressed mood as a child or adolescent) • A depressive episode in childhood may represent an early stage of bipolar disorder
Treatment	• Consider nonpharmacological treatment strategies for mild to moderate depression (extensive evidence supports the use of cognitive behavior therapy = CBT in children and adolescents or interpersonal therapy = IPT) • For chronic or refractory depression, a multimodal treatment approach is recommended including psychoeducation, pharmacotherapy, and psychosocial interventions • See chapter on Antidepressants (p. 40) • There is a high placebo response rate (up to 50%) in children, which makes it difficult to detect a therapeutic effect of the treatment • Lower dosages of antidepressants, often based on body weight, are commonly used in children; however, children often have faster drug metabolism rates which may lead to lower therapeutic drug levels (which may account for the perception of poor drug response in clinical trials)

Bipolar Disorder (BD)

Incidence	• Prevalence in adolescents is about 1% • Rarely can occur in very young children; children may have atypical presentations
Onset	• Median age of onset is about age 18, however, some parents report symptoms beginning during preschool years
Risk Factors	• Family history of mood disorder (concordance rate of 50–70% in monozygotic twins vs 13–30% in dizygotic twins) • Substance abuse
Comorbidity	• Concurrent ADHD seen in 73–98% of prepubescent patients with BD, vs 54–74% of adolescents • High rates of conduct disorder, oppositional defiant disorder, tic disorders, anxiety disorders, substance use disorder • High risk of suicide

Psychiatric Disorders

Bipolar Disorder (BD) (cont.)

Presentation and Symptoms	• BD is often not recognized until late adolescence • Depression is usually the first affective episode in females, while males usually first present with mania; 1/3 of children first experience depression, 1/3 have mania, and 1/3 present with a mixed state • Mania is often misdiagnosed in children and young adolescents because of an atypical presentation. It is usually characterized by short periods of mood lability with irritability, impulsivity, recklessness, aggressiveness, self-injury or hypersexuality • Mania is frequently misdiagnosed as schizophrenia (severe cases) or ADHD, a behavior disorder (e.g., oppositional defiant disorder or conduct disorder) or personality disorder (e.g., borderline personality disorder)
Course of Illness	• Chronic, remitting-relapsing • Early onset BD patients have a more severe illness course • Childhood BD does not necessarily evolve into adult BD

Diagnosis	• Criteria for diagnosing mood disorders in children are not well defined; can use acronym FIND when assessing mania symptoms in pediatric patients:
	  – F: Frequency – symptoms occur most days in a week
	  – I: Intensity – symptoms are severe enough to cause dysfunction/disturbance
	  – N: Number – symptoms occur 3–4 times/day
	  – D: Duration – symptoms occur for 4 h or more/day
	• Family history of BD often an important finding (in 40–50% of children)
	• Children may have greater mood lability, which can hamper diagnosis, e.g., rage episode followed by lassitude, remorse, or depression
	• Children often present with persistent mood, behavioral, and possibly cognitive difficulties
	• The clinician cannot ask complicated questions of young children, which makes it difficult to assess depressive symptoms; multiple informants often needed to corroborate diagnosis

Treatment	• Long-term multimodal treatment approach recommended, including psychoeducation, pharmacotherapy, and psychosocial interventions • Comorbid conditions (e.g., ADHD, anxiety disorders) should be treated once BD is stabilized • Children may experience a worsening of their clinical picture if treated with psychostimulants or antidepressants • Life-style modification strategies include: stress reduction, regular sleep habits, accomodation at school, and avoidance of caffeine, alcohol and illicit drugs • Guidelines recommend initial therapy include mood stabilizer (lithium, valproate, carbamazepine) and/or atypical (novel) antipsychotic (olanzapine, quetiapine, risperidone) for manic or mixed episodes • See chapters on Mood Stabilizers (Lithium and Anticonvulsants) (p. 199), Second-Generation Antipsychotics (p. 115), and Antidepressants (p. 40) • ECT is regarded as a treatment of last resort (p. 103)

Schizophrenia

Psychotic episodes can occur in children with a number of diagnoses, including schizophrenia, complex developmental disorders, and pervasive developmental disorders (e.g., autism).

In adolescents, symptoms must be distinguished from those of bipolar disorder (e.g., mania), Axis II disorders (e.g., schizotypal and borderline personality disorders) and those resulting from substance abuse.

Incidence
- Rare in children; < 0.2% incidence under age 13
- Occurs twice as often in males as in females

Onset
- Onset occurs typically in late adolescence or early adulthood (ages 15 to 30) – lifetime prevalence of 1%
- Mean age of onset in children is 8.6 years and mean age of diagnosis is 10.6 years

Risk Factors
- Increased risk if first-degree relative has a diagnosis of schizophrenia (48% for identical twins, 13% for fraternal twins, 13% for offspring, and 9% for siblings)
- Substance abuse

Comorbidity
- Mood disorders, OCD, ADHD, oppositional defiant disorder, conduct disorder, substance use disorder
- Rule out schizoid personality disorders, developmental disorders, nonpsychotic behavioral disorders, as well as medical causes of psychotic symptoms including CNS lesions, tumors or infections, metabolic disorders and seizure disorders

Presentation and Symptoms
- Children
  - Onset of psychotic symptoms before age 12 is considered a severe form of schizophrenia. Prodromal signs seen before age 7 include: developmental delays, learning disabilities, behavioral problems, solitary play, excessive anxiety, neurological problems, speech and language difficulties and social withdrawal
  - Symptoms occur insidiously rather than acutely; auditory hallucinations and delusions are the most common presenting symptoms
  - Children show 3 characteristic communication deficits: loose associations, illogical thinking, and impaired language skills
  - There appears to be a high rate of genetic abnormalities in childhood-onset schizophrenia and progressive changes in brain morphology (ventricular enlargement and reduced total brain volume)
- Adolescents
  - The onset may occur insidiously after months of prodromal symptoms
  - Some patients may experience negative symptoms that overshadow the presence of positive symptoms or the onset may appear suddenly with an acute psychotic episode (e.g., precipitated by drug abuse)
- Both positive and negative symptoms can occur:
  - Positive symptoms in children and adolescents include delusions, hallucinations, paranoia, speech and thought disruptions (e.g., word salad, thought broadcasting, and loose associations), unusual or bizarre behaviors (e.g., waxy or stuporous posture), echolalia, or echopraxia
  - Negative symptoms include affective flattening or blunting, alogia, avolition, anhedonia, inattention, amotivation, anergia, and poor grooming and hygiene

Course of Illness
- Childhood and adolescent-onset schizophrenia is generally more severe and treatment-refractory, and has a poorer prognosis than adult-onset illness
- The earlier the diagnosis and treatment, the better the prognosis; early treatment can delay the onset of psychosis but may not prevent it, however, it may have benefits on cognition

Psychiatric Disorders

Schizophrenia (cont.)

Consequences of Schizophrenia

- Variable, with some individuals experiencing multiple exacerbations and remissions, while others (about 50%) remain chronically ill with minimal improvement
- Can impair age-dependent social and cognitive skills and result in social dysfunction and academic underachievement
- Associated with cognitive and neurobiological deficits that produce long-term functional impairment
- Risk of suicide is 5% in this population

Treatment

- Multimodal treatment approach recommended, including psychoeducation, pharmacotherapy, and psychosocial interventions. Hospitalization may also be needed
- See chapter on Antipsychotics (p. 109)

Anxiety Disorders

There is a relatively strong relationship between anxiety disorders in children and their parents (risk is 2- to 4-fold if a parent has an anxiety disorder; risk for anxiety also high if a parent has a depressive disorder). Traumatic events during childhood reported to markedly increase risk for anxiety disorders later in life

It is important to rule out medical conditions that could contribute to or aggravate the anxiety disorder (e.g., asthma). 30–50% of children with anxiety disorders also have a depressive disorder, either unipolar or bipolar

SEPARATION ANXIETY DISORDER

Incidence

- 3–5%; most common anxiety disorder in children
- May be slightly more common in females than males

Onset

- Ages 5–12 years. Typically a diagnosis may not be made until the age of 8–9 years, as separation anxiety disorder is considered a normal early sign of adjustment in those aged 6 months to 4 years of age

Risk Factors

- May be associated with parental anxiety or depressive disorders
- 50–75% of children with separation anxiety disorder are from homes associated with low socioeconomic status
- Reported to occur in up to 80% of children with school refusal

Comorbidity

- MDD, posttraumatic stress disorder, pervasive developmental disorders

Presentation and Symptoms

- Characterized by developmentally inappropriate and excessive anxiety or recurrent fear of separation from home or a loved one, e.g., may manifest as refusal to attend school (75% of cases) or repeated complaints of physical symptoms (e.g., headaches, stomach aches) when separation occurs or is anticipated; some children develop signs of a panic attack

- Boys and girls manifest similar symptoms
- Children aged 5–8 most commonly report unrealistic worry about harm to parents or attachment figures and school refusal
- Children aged 9–12 usually manifest excessive distress at times of separation
- Adolescents manifest somatic complaints and school refusal
- May require parental assistance to complete simple tasks (e.g., getting dressed, brushing teeth)

Course of Illness
- The duration of the disorder reflects its severity
- Longitudinal studies suggest that childhood separation anxiety disorder may be a risk factor for other anxiety disorders

Treatment
- The majority of mild cases are treated with behavior therapy or other forms of psychotherapy
- Pharmacological therapy is generally reserved for severe cases or in the presence of serious psychiatric complications such as depression or suicidality
- See chapters on SSRIs (p. 41) and Benzodiazepines (p. 169)

OBSESSIVE COMPULSIVE DISORDER (OCD)

Incidence
- Up to 3%

Onset
- May be difficult to distinguish in children from mild rituals that are normal in early childhood
- Can begin as early as age 3

Comorbidity
- Depression, BD, ADHD, anxiety disorders (panic disorder, social phobia), schizophrenia, disruptive behaviors, and Tourette's syndrome

Presentation and Symptoms
- Similar to those seen in adults
- Obsession: persistent ideas, thoughts, impulses, or images that are experienced as intrusive, inappropriate, and cause marked anxiety or distress
- Compulsions: repetitive behaviors (e.g., handwashing, checking) or mental acts (e.g., counting, repeating) performed to prevent or reduce anxiety or distress.
- Children can be secretive about their symptoms fearing what others may think

Course of Illness
- Can severely impact functioning and academic performance
- Untreated OCD can become chronic and incapacitating to the individual

Treatment
- Pharmacotherapy and behavioral therapies, including cognitive behavior therapy
- See chapters on SSRIs (p. 41), and Nonselective Cyclic Antidepressants (p. 72)

GENERALIZED ANXIETY DISORDER (GAD)

Incidence
- Lifetime prevalence rate of 8%

Onset
- Often begins in childhood or adolescence

Psychiatric Disorders

Anxiety Disorders (cont.)

Risk Factors	• Family history of anxiety or depression
Comorbidity	• Depressive disorders, social phobia, ADHD, substance abuse disorder
Presentation and Symptoms	• Frequent, persistent, and intense fear incongruent with the circumstances or developmental age • Symptoms include refusal to attend school, somatic complaints such as feelings of restlessness, fatigue, muscle tension, and insomnia
Course of Illness	• Fluctuates, worsening at times (especially during times of stress), and persists for many years
Treatment	• The majority of mild cases are treated with behavior therapy or other forms of psychotherapy (e.g., CBT or IPT) • Pharmacological therapy is generally reserved for moderate to severe cases • See chapters on SSRIs (p. 41) and Buspirone (p. 184)

SOCIAL PHOBIA

Incidence	• 1–2%
Onset	• Seen in preschool and school-aged children, but usually begins between ages 13 and 20; more than 50% of patients are affected before adolescence
Risk Factors	• Family history of social phobia • Early childhood trauma or abuse (up to 50%) • May be influenced by parental modeling of childhood social fears
Comorbidity	• Depressive disorders, panic disorder, and generalized anxiety disorder
Presentation and Symptoms	• Intense anxiety upon exposure to situations in which the individual may be scrutinized and possibly embarrassed; may involve specific fears related to a situation or close social contact
Treatment	• The majority of mild cases are treated with behavior therapy or other forms of psychotherapy (such as CBT or IPT) • There are limited data on effective pharmacological treatments in children • Pharmacological therapy is generally reserved for moderate to severe cases • See chapters on SSRIs (p. 41) and Buspirone (p. 184)

PANIC DISORDER

Incidence	• 2–3.3%
Onset	• Often begins during adolescence; although it may start during childhood, it is often difficult to diagnose at an early age
Risk Factors	• Tends to run in families; risk high if both parents have an anxiety disorder (especially social phobia) or a BD • Exposure to childhood sexual or physical abuse

Comorbidity	• 19% of children also have BD
	• MDD, dysthymia, hypomania, other anxiety disorder (especially GAD, social phobia, separation anxiety), or conduct disorder
	• Asthma (6.5–24% in adults)
Presentation and Symptoms	• Panic attacks refer to unexpected and repeated periods of intense fear or discomfort, along with symptoms (below) which can last minutes to hours. Panic attacks frequently develop without warning.
	• Racing or pounding heartbeat
	• Intense fearfulness (a sense that something terrible is happening)
	• Dizziness or lightheadedness, faintness
	• Shortness of breath or a feeling of being smothered
	• Trembling or shaking
	• Fear of dying, losing control, or losing your mind
	• Sense of unreality
Course of Illness	• Panic attacks can interfere with a child's or adolescent's relationships, schoolwork, and normal development. Children and adolescents with panic disorder may begin to feel anxious most of the time, even when they are not having panic attacks. Some begin to avoid situations where they fear a panic attack may occur, or situations where help may not be available; e.g. a child may be reluctant to go to school or be separated from his or her parents. In severe cases, the child or adolescent may be afraid to leave home – agoraphobia.
	• Some children and adolescents with panic disorder can develop severe depression and may be at risk of suicidal behavior.
	• As an attempt to decrease anxiety, some adolescents with panic disorder will use alcohol or drugs
	• Panic attacks during adolescence are associated with an increased risk of development of personality disorders during young adulthood
Treatment	• Many children and adolescents with panic disorder respond well to the combination of medication and psychotherapy. With treatment, the panic attacks can usually be stopped. Early treatment can prevent the complications of panic disorder such as agoraphobia, depression and substance abuse
	• Psychotherapy may also help the child and family learn ways to reduce stress or conflict that could otherwise cause a panic attack. With techniques taught in cognitive behavioral therapy, the child may also learn new ways to control anxiety or panic attacks when they occur
	• See chapters on SSRI's and Benzodiazepines

POSTTRAUMATIC STRESS DISORDER (PTSD)

Incidence	• 15–43% of girls and 14–43% of boys have experienced at least one traumatic event in their lifetime. Of those children and adolescents who have experienced a trauma, 3–15% of girls and 1–6% of boys could be diagnosed with PTSD
Onset	• PTSD is diagnosed when a child or adolescent who experiences a catastrophic event develops ongoing difficulties (see symptoms, below). The stressful or traumatic event involves a situation where someone's life has been threatened or severe injury has occurred (e.g., they may be the victim or a witness of physical abuse, sexual abuse, violence in the home or in the community, automobile accidents, natural disasters (such as flood, fire, earthquakes), and being diagnosed with a life-threatening illness)
Risk Factors	• Severity of the traumatic event; whether the trauma is repeated
	• The child's proximity to the trauma; interpersonal trauma (e.g., rape, assault) poses higher risk
	• His/her relationship to the victim(s)
	• Parental reaction to the event; less distress lowers levels of PTSD symptoms

Anxiety Disorders (cont.)

Comorbidity	• Commonly co-occurring disorder is major depression
	• Other disorders include other anxiety disorders such as separation anxiety, panic disorder, and generalized anxiety disorder, ADHD, oppositional defiant disorder, conduct disorder, and substance use disorder
Presentation and Symptoms	• The three symptom clusters of PTSD include: (A) Re-experiencing, (B) Avoidance and numbing, and (C) Hyperarousal
	• Following a trauma, children may initially show agitated or confused behavior with intense fear, helplessness, anger, sadness, horror or denial. Children who experience repeated trauma might develop a dissociation (emotional numbing to deaden or block the pain and trauma). Children with PTSD avoid situations or places that remind them of the trauma. They may also become less responsive emotionally, depressed, withdrawn, and more detached from their feelings
	• **Very young children** may present with few PTSD symptoms. This may be because eight of the PTSD symptoms require a verbal description of one's feelings and experiences. Instead, young children may report more generalized fears (such as to strangers) or separation anxiety, avoidance of situations that may or may not be related to the trauma, sleep disturbances, and a preoccupation with words or symbols that may or may not be related to the trauma. These children may also display posttraumatic play in which they repeat themes of the trauma. In addition, children may lose an acquired developmental skill (such as toilet training) as a result of experiencing a traumatic event
	• **Elementary school-aged children** may not experience visual flashbacks or amnesia for aspects of the trauma. However, they do experience missequencing trauma-related events when recalling the memory. In addition, they may have a belief that there were warning signs that predicted the trauma; as a result, children often believe that if they are alert enough, they will recognize warning signs and avoid future traumas. School-aged children also reportedly exhibit compulsive repetition of some aspect of the trauma, or reenactment of the trauma in play, drawings, or verbalizations
	• In **adolescents,** symptoms may begin to more closely resemble PTSD in adults. Adolescents are more likely to engage in traumatic reenactment, in which they incorporate aspects of the trauma into their daily lives. In addition, adolescents are more likely than younger children or adults to exhibit impulsive and aggressive behaviors
	• Children with PTSD may also show the following symptoms:
	– Worry about dying at an early age
	– Losing interest in activities
	– Having physical symptoms such as headaches and stomachaches
	– Showing more sudden and extreme emotional reactions
	– Having problems falling or staying asleep
	– Showing irritability or angry outbursts
	– Having problems concentrating
	– Acting younger than their age (for example, clingy or whiny behavior, thumb sucking)
	– Showing increased alertness to the environment
	– Repeating behavior that reminds them of the trauma
Course of Illness	• Although some children show a natural remission in PTSD symptoms over a period of a few months, a significant number of children continue to exhibit symptoms for years if untreated
Treatment	• Once the trauma has occurred, early intervention is essential. Education and support from parents, the school, and peers is important

Emphasis needs to be placed upon establishing a feeling of safety
- A multimodal treatment approach is usually required:
  - a) Cognitive-Behavioral Therapy (CBT) is most effective and generally includes the child directly discussing the traumatic event (exposure), anxiety management techniques such as relaxation and assertiveness training, and correction of inaccurate or distorted trauma-related thoughts. Psychotherapy (individual, group, or family), which allows the child to speak, draw, play, or write about the event is helpful
  - b) Medication may be useful to deal with agitation, anxiety, hyperarousal, impulsivity, self-injurious behavior, aggression, or with comorbid conditions such as depression, ADHD or psychosis – see chapters on SSRIs (p. 41), Antipsychotics (p. 109), Clonidine (p. 33) and Benzodiazepines (p. 169), buspirone (p. 184), anticonvulsants (p. 208)

Tic Spectrum Disorders

A tic is a sudden rapid, recurrent, nonrhythmic, stereotypic movement or vocalization (e.g., blinking, neck jerks, coughing, swearing)

Types: 1) chronic motor or vocal tic disorder (2–5% of children); 2) transient tic disorder (19% of children); 3) Tourette's syndrome; 4) Tic disorder not otherwise specified

TOURETTE'S SYNDROME

Incidence	• Males: 0.1%, females: 0.01%
Onset	• One or more transient symptoms appear insidiously between ages 2 and 15 and are followed by more persistent motor and vocal tics • Average age for motor tics is 7 years • Average age for vocal tics is 11 years
Risk Factors	• Considered a hereditary disorder with an autosomal dominant pattern of inheritance; thought to be an abnormality in the dopamine system • May develop secondary to idiopathic or hereditary disorders, e.g., Huntington's disease, infections, developmental disorders, or drugs
Comorbidity	• Most frequently OCD (50–74%) and ADHD (50%); also oppositional defiant disorder, major depressive disorder, anxiety disorders, and aggression
Presentation and Symptoms	• Diagnosed when multiple motor tics and at least one vocal tic occur frequently over a period of at least 1 year • Simple motor tics seen in about 90% • Vocal tics and grunts seen in about 98% • Coprolalia (foul language) occurs in 10–30%
Course of Illness	• Tics show a fluctuating course and tend to decline by adulthood. Patients are able to suppress tics for short periods of time, but experience urges to perform tics and a sense of relief when they do occur • Frequency and severity of tics can increase with stress, excitement, or caffeine use; mental or physical activities, alcohol, nicotine, and cannabinoids appear to decrease the incidence of tics • Cause social embarrassment and decrease self-esteem, which can impair academic, social and occupational functioning • Repetitive or violent movements may result in self-injury (e.g., falls, fractures) or pain to muscles and joints. Vocal tics can affect breathing, speech, and swallowing

Psychiatric Disorders

Tic Spectrum Disorders (cont.)

Treatment	• See chapters on Antipsychotics (p. 109) and Clonidine (p. 33) • Minor benefit seen with benzodiazepines (clonazepam), botulinum toxin IM, and flutamide (antiandrogen) • Behavioral approaches (minor benefit)

Pervasive Developmental Disorders (PDD)

Neurodevelopmental disorders usually affect children before age 5; characterized by impairments in social interactions and communication and behavior, with repetitive interests and activities; majority of patients have mental retardation. Incidence of PDD = 0.6%

Problematic behaviors, rather than the core symptoms of PDD, are the major targets of pharmacotherapy

Types: 1) Autistic disorder; 2) Retts; 3) Childhood disintegrative disorder; 4) Asperger's; 5) PDD not otherwise specified

AUTISTIC DISORDER

Incidence	• Up to 0.13% • Up to 75% of cases involve significant mental retardation (IQ < 70) • 4–5 times higher in males than females
Onset	• Symptoms are usually recognized in the first year of life, but it is difficult to make a reliable diagnosis in children younger than 2 years • 94% of cases are seen before the age of 3
Risk Factors	• Unknown; may be genetic or related to a viral infection or inherited enzyme deficiency; concordance in monozygotic twins is 36–100% and is < 24% in dizygotic twins • CNS shown to be altered in several brain regions, specifically medial prefrontal cortex and amygdala • Evenly distributed among socioeconomic classes and ethnic groups
Comorbidity	• Frequently associated with mental retardation (70–80%), ADHD • High incidence of EEG abnormalities and seizure disorders (about 25%) • Blindness, deafness, tuberous sclerosis, cerebral palsy, congenital rubella and neurofibromatosis
Presentation and Symptoms	• Symptoms diverse across and within individuals and changes over course of development • Qualitative impairment in social interactions, communication, and presence of repetitive and stereotypic activities or behavior. *Maladaptive behaviors* include hyperactivity, anxiety, anger, as well as stereotypies and other repetitive behaviors; about 20–30% of children exhibit serious behavior problems such as temper tantrums, aggression and self-injury (particularly those with severe mental retardation) As the person ages, depression, obsessive-compulsive symptoms, inappropriate social interactions, and occasionally psychotic symptoms may become more prominent
Course of Illness	• Onset in first years of life disrupts diverse developmental processes • Tends to be a lifelong condition with impact on academic, cognitive, and social functioning • Early diagnosis and treatment can improve long-term outcomes • Up to 30% of children develop epilepsy during early adolescence • Life expectancy is reduced

Treatment	• Family, psychiatric, and medical history as well as occupational and psychological assessment important to determine treatment – including audilogical, visual, neurological examinations and laboratory screening
	• Goals: to improve social response and communication and reduce unusual and maladaptive behaviors
	• Multimodal treatment approach recommended: primarily educational and behavioral interventions; drugs reserved for severe cases
	• Pharmacological treatment may be effective for various behavioral symptoms, especially aggression, temper tantrums, self-injurious behavior and repetitive and impulsive behavior. See chapters on Antipsychotics (p. 109), Antidepressants (p. 40), and Anticonvulsants (p. 208)
	• 8 double-blind studies suggest naltrexone has minor benefit for self-injurious behavior
	• No major benefit seen with fenfluramine
	• Contradictory data as to efficacy of psychostimulants (p. 19) and clonidine (p. 33)

ASPERGER'S DISORDER

Incidence	• 0.026%
Onset	• Later than autism; usually around the age of 2 or 3 years; early development in language and cognition appears normal, then child begins to pursue unusual interests with intensity and social deficits become prominent when interacting with peers
Risk Factors	• Unknown
Comorbidity	• Depression may first appear in adolescence
Presentation and Symptoms	• Behaviors are similar to those seen in Autistic Disorder; however, Asperger's cases show higher intellectual skills and almost normal expressive language skills. Relative to those with autistic conditions of similar mental age, individuals with Asperger's are more aware of appropriate social skills. They tend to have a lesser degree of motor deficits than those with autism and may be overly focused on a particular topic or special interest. Their nonverbal communication skills are usually poor
Course of Illness	• Tends to be a lifelong condition with impact on academic, cognitive, and social functioning
Treatment	• Multimodal, including psychosocial, educational, and pharmacological
	• Need to establish target symptoms for intervention, treat comorbid conditions, establish goals for educational intervention, and monitor efficacy of treatment and changes in functioning
	• See chapters on Antipsychotics (p. 109), Antidepressants (p. 40), and Anticonvulsants (p. 208)
	• Contradictory data as to efficacy of psychostimulants
	• Early data suggests a role for guanfacine (p. 36) and cholinesterase inhibitors (p. 272)

Disruptive Behavior Disorders

CONDUCT DISORDER (CD)

Incidence	• 1–10%

Psychiatric
Disorders

Disruptive Behavior Disorders (cont.)

Onset	• Usually in early adolescence, but impairments can be seen by age 5 in early-onset conduct disorder
Risk Factors	• Dysfunctional family • Oppositional defiant disorder (2.7–40% of children develop conduct disorder)
Comorbidity	• ADHD, BD
Presentation and Symptoms	• Early onset: impairment in reading, language and motor development. Show signs of impulsivity, aggression and hyperactivity by age 5 • Adolescent: – repetitive and persistent pattern of disruptive behavior and violation of rights of others or of societal norms – includes: aggression towards people and animals, theft, destruction of property, deceitfulness, and serious violation of rules • 2 types: impulsive-affective; controlling-predatory
Course of Illness	• Early onset: delinquent behavior and violent crimes often begin at an early age and increase in seriousness; continues into adulthood • Adolescent: only 25% continue delinquent behavior into adulthood; precursor to adult antisocial personality disorder
Treatment	• Behavioral therapies (including individual therapy, parent management training, and group therapy), interventions at school and with peer group • Pharmacological treatments – See chapters on Antipsychotics (p. 109), Antidepressants (p. 40), Lithium (p. 199), Anticonvulsants (p. 208), Stimulants (p. 19), and Anxiolytics (p. 169)

OPPOSITIONAL DEFIANT DISORDER (ODD)

Incidence	• 6–7%
Onset	• Recognized at an early age
Risk Factors	• Genetics • Dysfunctional family
Comorbidity	• ADHD, BD
Presentation and Symptoms	• Persistent negativistic, irrational, hostile, and noncompliant behavior, misbehaving • Frequent loss of temper, defiance, tendency to be argumentative, easily annoyed by others and deliberately try to annoy others, spiteful, blame others for their mistakes
Course of Illness	• 57% of patients with ODD and ADHD continue to have ODD symptoms after 4 years
Treatment	• Behavioral, including parent management training (response rate 40–50%) • Pharmacological – See Chapters on Antipsychotics (p. 109), Antidepressants (p. 40), Stimulants (p. 19), and Mood Stabilizers (p. 198).

- AACAP official action. Practice parameters in the assessment and treatment of children and adolescents with bipolar disorder (1997). *Journal of the American Academy of Child and Adolescent Psychiatry 36(1),* 138–157.
- Adler-Nevo, G., Manassis, K. (2005). Pharmacotherapy for acute stress disorder (ASD) and posttraumatic stress disorder (PTSD) in children and adolescents. *Child and Adolescent Psychopharmacology News 10(5),* 1–7.
- Aman, M.G., Gharabawi, G.M. (2004). Treatment of behavior disorders in mental retardation: report on transitioning to atypical antipsychotics with an emphasis on risperidone. *J Clin Psychiat 65(9),* 1197–1210.
- American Academy of Child and Adolescent PsychiatryOfficial Action (1997). Practice parameters for the assessment and treatment of children and adolescents with anxiety disorders. *Journal of the American Academy of Child and Adolescent Psychiatry 36(10),* 695–845.
- American Psychiatric Association (1997). Practice guidelines for the treatment of patients with schizophrenia. *American Journal of Psychiatry 154(4) (Apr. Suppl.),* 1–63.
- Ballenger, J.C. (2001). Overview of different pharmacotherapies for attaining remission in Generalized Anxiety Disorder. *Journal of Clinical Psychiatry 62(Suppl. 19),* 11–19.
- Bukhari, L., Anand, A., McDougle, C.S. (2003). Psychopharmacology of pediatric depression. *International Drug Therapy Newsletter 38(10),* 73–80.
- Carrey, N. (2001). Developmental neurobiology: Implication for pediatric psychopharmacology. *Canadian Journal of Psychiatry 46,* 810–818.
- Clinical Guidelines for the Treatment of Depressive Disorders; Ca. Psychiatr. Assoc. (CANMAT) (2001). *Canadian Journal of Psychiatry 46(Suppl.),* 1S–47S.
- Connor, D.F., Carlson, G.A., Chang, K.D. et al. (2006). Juvenile maladaptive aggression. A review of prevention, treatment and service configuration and a proposed research agenda. *Journal of Clinical Psychiatry 67(5),* 808–820.
- DelBello, M. Grcevich S. (2004). Phenomenology and epidemiology of childhood psychiatric disorders that may necessitate treatment with atypical antipsychotics. *J Clin Psychiat 65(Suppl. 6),* 12–19.
- Emslie, G.J., Ryan, N.D., Wagner, K.D. (2005). Major depressive disorder in children and adolescents: Clinical trial design and antidepressant efficacy. *Journal of Clinical Psychiatry 66(Suppl. 7),* 14–20.
- Expert Consensus Guideline Series (2003). Optimizing pharmacologic treatment of psychotic disorders. *Journal of Clinical Psychiatry 64 (Suppl. 12),,* 1–100.
- Findling R.L. (2003). Treatment of aggression in children. Primary Care Companion, *Journal of Clinical Psychiatry 5(Suppl. 6),* 5–9.
- Goddard, A.W., Shekhar, A., Anand, A. et al. (2002). Psychopharmacology of pediatric anxiety disorders. *International Drug Therapy Newsletter 37(12),* 89– 94.
- Goodwin, R.D., Gotlib, I.H. (2004). Panic attacks and psychopathology among youth. *Acta Psychiatr Scand. 109(3),* 216–221.
- Greenhill L.L., Pliszka, S., Dulcan, M.K. et al. (2002). Summary of the practice paramenters for the use of stimulant medications in the treatment of children, adolescents and adults. *Journal of the American Academy of Child and Adolescent Psychiatry 41(Suppl.)* Feb. www.aacap.org.
- Hollander, E., Bienstock, C.A., Koran, L.M. et al. (2002). Refractory obsessivecompulsive disorder: State-of-the-art treatment. *Journal of Clinical Psychiatry 63(Suppl. 6),* 20–29.
- James, A.C.D., Javaloyes, A.M. (2002). Practitioner Reviews: The treatment of bipolar disorder in children and adolescents. *Journal of Child Psychology and Psychiatry 42(4),* 439–449.
- Jellinek, M.S., Snyder, J.B. (1998). Depression and suicide in children and adolescents. *Pediatric Review 19,* 255.

Psychiatric Disorders

Psychiatric Disorders in Children and Adolescents – References and Selected Readings (cont.)

- Ketter, T.A., Wang, P.W. (2002). Predictors of treatment response in bipolar disorders: Evidence from clinical and brain imaging studies. *Journal of Clinical Psychiatry 63(Suppl. 3),* 21–25.
- Kolmen, B.K. et al. (1995). Naltrexone in young autistic children: A double blind, placebo-controlled crossover study. *Journal of the American Academy of Child and Adolescent Psychiatry 34,* 223–231.
- Kowatch R.A., Fristad, M., Birmaher, B. (2005) Treatment guidelines for children and adolescents with bipolar disorder. *JAACAP 44(3),* 213–235
- Masi, G., Mucci, M., Millepiedi, S. (2001) Separation anxiety disorder in children and adolescents: epidemiology, diagnosis and management. *CNS Drugs 15(2),* 93–104.
- McDougle, C.J., Stigler, K.A., Posey, D.J. (2003). Treatment of aggression in children. *Journal of Clinical Psychiatry 64(Suppl. 4),* 16–25.
- McDougle, C.J., Stigler, K.A., Posey, D.J. (2003) Treatment of aggression in children and adolescents with autism and conduct disorder. *J Clin Psychiat 64(Suppl 4),* 16–25.
- Panic disorder in children and adolescents #50 AACAP Facts for Families www.aacap.org/publications/factsfam/panic.htm
- Pavuluri, M.N., Naylor, M.W., Janicak, P.G. (2002). Recognition and treatment of pediatric bipolar disorder. *Contemporary Psychiatry 1(1),* 1–9.
- Pies, R. et al. (2002). Pharmacological treatment of self-injurious behavior. *International Drug Therapy Newsletter 37(2),* 9–12.
- Posey, D.J. (2002). Practical pharmacotherapeutic management of autism: A review and update ofcommonly prescribed drugs. *International Drug Therapy Newsletter 37(1),* 1–6.
- Posttraumatic stress disorder (PTSD) #70, AACAP Facts for Families www.aacap.org/publications/factsfam/ptsd70.htm
- Scahill, L., Chappell, P.B., King, R. et al. (2000). Pharmacologic treatment of tic disorders. *Child and Adolescent Psychiatric Clinics of North America 9(1),* 99–117.
- Spence, T.S., Biederman, J., Wilens, T.E. et al. (2002). Overview and neurobiology of Attention-Deficit/Hyperactivity Disorder. *Journal of Clinical Psychiatry 63(Suppl. 12),* 3–9.
- Stigler K.A. (2004) Pharmacotherapy of hyperactivity and inattention in pervasive developmental disorders. *Int. Drug Ther Newsletter 39(8),* 57–60.
- Suppes, T., Dennehy, E.B., Swann, A.C. et al. (2002). Report of the Texas Consensus Conference Panel on medication treatment of bipolar disorder 2000.
- Toichi, M., Findling, R.L. (2002). Age, severity, and pharmacotherapy in Autism/Pervasive Developmental Disorders. *International Drug TherapyNewsletter 37(11),* 81–87.
- Volkmar, F., Cook Jr., E., Pomeroy, J. et al (1999) Summary of the practice parameters for the assessment and treatment of children, adolescents and adults with autism and other pervasive developmental disorders 38 (Suppl.) Dec. www.aacap.org.
- Wagner, K.D. (2004) Diagnosis and treatment of bipolar disorder in children and adolescents. *J Clin Psychiat 65(Suppl. 15),* 30–35.
- Weller, E. (2004) Pharmacotherapy of adolescents with bipolar disorder. *Int. Drug Therapy Newsletter 39(11),* 81–87.
- Weller, E. (2004) Pharmacotherapy of children with bipolar disorder. *Int. Drug Therapy Newsletter 39(10),* 73–80.
- Wilens, T.E, Dodson, W. (2004) A clinical perspective in Attention-Deficit/Hyperactivity Disorder into adulthood. *J Clin Psychiat 36(10),* 1301–1313.
- Working Group on Bipolar Disorder (2002). Practice guidelines for the treatment of patients with bipolar disorder. *American Journal of Psychiatry 159(4, Suppl.),* 1–50.
- Wozniak, J. (2005) Recognizing and managing bipolar disorder in children. *J Clin Psychiat 66 (Suppl. 1),* 18–23.
- Younus, M., Labellarte, M.J. (2002). Insomnia in children: When are hypnotics indicated? *Pediatric Drugs 4(6),* 391–403.

DRUGS FOR ATTENTION DEFICIT HYPERACTIVITY DISORDER

CLASSIFICATION

• Drugs for ADHD can be classified as follows:

Chemical Class	Agent	Page
Psychostimulant	▲ Amphetamines and related drugs ▲ Methylphenidate, dexmethylphenidate	See p. 19 See p. 19
Selective Norepinephrine Reuptake Inhibitor	▲ Atomoxetine	See p. 27
Adrenergic agent	Clonidine Guanfacine [B]	See p. 33 See p. 36
Antidepressant	Bupropion Venlafaxine Tricyclic agents Monoamine oxidase inhibitors	See p. 53 See p. 58 See p. 72 See p. 82
Dopaminergic agent	Modafinil	See p. 273

▲ Approved indication [B]Not available in Canada

Psychostimulants

PRODUCT AVAILABILITY

Generic Name	Trade Name[A]	Dosage Forms and Strengths	Monograph Statement
Dextroamphetamine	Dexedrine, Dextrostat Dexedrine Spansules	Tablets: 5 mg, 10 mg[B] Elixir: 5 mg/5 ml Spansules: 5 mg[B], 10 mg, 15 mg	Not recommended for children under age 3
Methamphetamine[B] (Desoxyephedrine)	Desoxyn	Tablets: 5 mg, 10 mg Sustained-release gradumet tablets: 5 mg, 10 mg, 15 mg	Not recommended for children under age 6
Dextroamphetamine/ Amphetamine salts	Adderall[B] Adderall XR	Tablets[B]: 5 mg, 7.5 mg, 10 mg, 12.5 mg, 15 mg, 20 mg, 30 mg Capsules: 5 mg, 10 mg, 15 mg, 20 mg, 25 mg, 30 mg	Not recommended for children under age 3

Psychostimulants (cont.)

Generic Name	Trade Name[A]	Dosage Forms and Strengths	Monograph Statement
Methylphenidate	Ritalin Methylin[B] Ritalin SR, Metadate ER[B], Methylin ER[B] Metadate CD[B] Ritalin LA[B] Concerta Biphentin[C]	Tablets: 5 mg, 10 mg, 20 mg Chewable tablets[B]: 2.5 mg, 5 mg, 10 mg Oral solution[B]: 5 mg/5 ml, 10 mg/5 ml Sustained-release tablets: 10 mg[B], 20 mg Extended-release capsules[B]: 10 mg, 20 mg, 30 mg Extended-release capsules[B]: 10 mg, 20 mg, 30 mg, 40 mg Osmotic-controlled-release tablets: 18 mg, 27 mg, 36 mg, 54 mg Controlled-release capsules[C]: 10 mg, 15 mg, 20 mg, 30 mg, 40 mg, 50 mg	Not recommended for children under age 6
Methylphenidate transdermal system[B]	Daytrana	Transdermal patch: 27.5 mg, 41.3 mg, 55 mg, 82.5 mg	Safety and efficacy not established in children under age 6
Dexmethylphenidate[B]	Focalin Focalin XR	Tablets: 2.5 mg, 5 mg, 10 mg Extended-release capsules 5 mg, 10 mg, 20 mg	Safety and efficacy not established in children under age 6

[A] Generic preparations may be available, [B] Not marketed in Canada, [C] Not marketed in USA

INDICATIONS

Approved in Children and Adolescents	• ADHD • Narcolepsy
Approved (for Adults)	• Attention-deficit/hyperactivity disorder (ADHD), primarily inattentive, combined or hyperactive-impulsive subtypes • Parkinson's disease • Narcolepsy • Obesity (dextroamphetamine – USA only)
Other Uses in children and Adolescents	• Augmentation of cyclic antidepressants, SSRIs, and RIMA • Chronic fatigue and neurasthenia • Positive results with methylphenidate in decreasing anger, irritability and aggression in brain-injured patients, oppositional defiant disorder, conduct disorder, and ADHD • Methylphenidate reported to have a modest effect on inattention, hyperactivity, irritability, and social withdrawal in autism and mental retardation (paradoxical overactivity and agitation can occur); contradictory data as to be benefit in autism

GENERAL COMMENTS

- All psychostimulants have been found to be equally efficacious; limited data supporting long-acting methylphenidate and increased remission rates
- Decrease interrupting, impulsive responses, fidgeting, finger-tapping; increase attention, focus, short-term memory, reaction time, problem solving, and improve interpersonal interactions

- General response occurs within the first week; response seen in up to 75% of children; effect not as robust in adolescents; in preschoolers, clinical effects are more variable and adverse effects more common – reserve for more serious cases
- Psychostimulants suggested to decrease physical and verbal aggression and reduce negative or antisocial interactions
- An untreated comorbid psychiatric disorder (e.g., mood or anxiety disorder) may diminish stimulant response or may decrease the patient's tolerance of the medication – data contradictory
- Psychostimulants can be abused or diverted for street purposes; use with caution and careful monitoring in patients with current abuse of drugs or alcohol. Children with ADHD being effectively treated with stimulants are significantly less likely to abuse substances than those with untreated ADHD

PHARMACOLOGY

- See chart p. 30
- Mechanism of action in treating ADHD is not well understood
- Sympathomimetic amines act as dopamine agonists (increase striatal dopamine)

LONG-ACTING FORMULATIONS

Drug	Drug	Formulation	Duration of Effect	Usual dosing
Methylphenidate biphasic release	Biphentin	40% immediate-release + 60% delayed-release	10–12 hours	Once daily; can open and sprinkle on food
	Concerta	22% immediate-release coating + 78% delayed-release osmotic mechanism	12 hours	Once daily
	Metadate CD	30% immediate-release beads + 70% delayed-release beads in a capsule	8 hours	Once daily
	Ritalin LA	50% immediate-release beads + 50% delayed-release beads in a capsule	8 hours	Once daily; can sprinkle on food
Methylphenidate sustained/slow release	Ritalin SR	Provides a slow continual release of drug from a wax matrix	4–6 hours	Multiple daily dosing
	Methylin ER	Provides a slow continual release of drug due to diffusion and erosion from a hydrophilic polymer for a effect	4–8 hours	Multiple daily dosing
	Metadate ER	Provides a slow continual release of drug from a wax matrix	4–8 hours	Multiple daily dosing
Methylphenidate transdermal patch	Daytrana	Drug dispersed in an acrylic adhesive which is dispersed in a silicone adhesive. Total dose delivered is dependent on patch size and wear time (see Dosing p. 22)	9 hours	On in AM, off after 9 hours
Dexmethylphenidate extended-release	Focalin XR	50% immediate-release beads + 50% enteric-coated delayed-release beads in a capsule	12 hours	Once daily; can sprinkle on food
Dextroamphetamine/ Amphetamines salts	Adderall XR	50% immediate-release beads + 50% delayed-release beads in a capsule	12 hours	Once daily; can sprinkle on food
Dextroamphetamine	Dexedrine Spansules	Bead system contains both immediate-release and sustained-release drug	6–9 hours	Multiple daily dosing; can sprinkle on food
Methamphetamine	Desoxyn Gradunet	Slow-release tablet	8 hours	Once daily

Psychostimulants (cont.)

DOSING

- See chart p. 30
- Treatment is started at low doses and gradually increased over several days; initial improvement noted may plateau after three weeks of continuous use (i.e., a decreased "energizing" feeling) – this does not imply tolerance. Patients should compare the plateau to their baseline, not to the peak effect seen in the first week, as otherwise there will be an urge to increase the dose
- To minimize anorexia, give drug with or after meals; with Metadate CD food delays C_{max} by 1 h and a high-fat meal increases C_{max} by 30% and AUC by 17%
- Divided doses required with regular preparations of methylphenidate (dose every 2–6 h)
- Though controversial, as some data suggest continued activation, administration of a small dose (e.g., 5 mg) ½ h before bedtime can sometimes help to calm the child to permit sleep
- Methylphenidate SR has a smoother onset, but little advantage in duration and no advantage in efficacy over regular tablets; compliance may be improved with long-acting formulations
- Patients who have problems swallowing pills may use one of several medications formulated as beads (see table p. 21) by opening the capsules, sprinkling the beads on apple sauce, and swallowing the mixture without chewing
- The sustained-release, controlled-release, and extended-release formulations may decrease inter-dose dysphoria or rebound hyperactivity. Supplementation with short-acting preparations occasionally needed in the morning (to speed up onset) or in the afternoon (to extend duration of action)
- When converting from methylphenidate to dexmethylphenidate use half the daily dose (e.g., give 2.5 mg bid dexmethylphenidate for 5 mg bid methylphenidate)
- Transdermal patch (Daytrana): total dose delivered is dependent on patch size and wear time. Dose delivered over 9 h: 10 mg for 27.5 mg patch, 15 mg for 41.3 mg patch, 20 mg for 55 mg patch, and 30 mg for 82.5 mg patch; dose titration recommended on a weekly basis (9 h wear period/day), as required. Patch can be removed earlier than 9 h for shorter duration of effect or if late-day side effects are problematic

PHARMACOKINETICS

- See chart p. 30–31
- Large interindividual variation in absorption and bioavailability; high-fat meal may delay C_{max} of methylphenidate and dexmethylphenidate
- Low protein binding
- Osmotic-controlled and extended-release methylphenidate tablets are formulated with different cores which release the active drug at different times, into the body (see Extended-Release Products)
- Excretion of amphetamines is pH-dependent and is enhanced in acidic urine
- Transdermal patch releases methylphenidate at a steady rate per hour, related to dose. Absorption and C_{max} may increase with chronic dosing; rate and extent of absorption increase if patch is applied to inflamed skin or if heat is applied over patch.

Dosage Conversion from Immediate to Extended-Release Products

It is generally recommended to start treatment with a low dose of a long-acting preparation and titrate the dose slowly to a therapeutic level

Conversion between dosage formulations are approximations and dependent on several factors:
- The pharmacokinetics of each preparation, including the duration of action of each product
- The patient's age and weight (dosing recommendations usually are based on weight)
- The patient's response may vary between preparations of the same drug

It is always important to monitor both response and adverse effects at each dosage level

IMMEDIATE-RELEASE PRODUCTS	EXTENDED-RELEASE PRODUCTS (daily dose)
Immediate-release Methylphenidate	
5 mg bid-tid	Metadate/Methylin ER, Biphentin, or Ritalin LA 10–20 mg, or Metadate CD 10–20 mg or Concerta 18 mg
10 mg bid-tid	Metadate/Methylin ER, Biphentin, or Ritalin LA 20–30 mg or Ritalin SR 20mg, or Metadate CD 30 mg or Concerta 27–36 mg
15 mg bid-tid	Metadate/Methylin ER, Biphentin, or Ritalin LA 30–40 mg or Ritalin SR 40 mg or Metadate CD 30–40 mg or Concerta 36–54 mg
20 mg bid-tid	Metadate/Methylin ER, Biphentin, or Ritalin LA 40–50 mg or Ritalin SR 40–60 mg or Concerta 54 mg-72 mg
30 mg bid	Metadate/Methylin ER, Biphentin, or Ritalin LA 50–60 mg, or Ritalin SR 60 mg, or Concerta 72 mg
Immediate-release Dexmethylphenidate Focalin 2.5 mg bid	Focalin XR 5 mg daily
Immediate-release Dextroamphetamine-amphetamine salts Adderall 5 mg bid	Adderall XR 10 mg daily
Immediate-release Dextroamphetamine 5 mg bid	Dexedrine Spansules 10 mg daily (large inter-patient variance noted in conversion, from 1:1 to about 1:1.5)

Note: Conversion to Daytrana transdermal patch is currently unknown; titration recommended (see Dosing)

ONSET AND DURATION OF ACTION

- See charts p. 21, 31

ADVERSE EFFECTS

- See chart p. 31
- Heart rate and blood pressure should be monitored after every dose increase in patients with cardiac risk factors (e.g., hypertension, heart failure, MI or ventricular arrhythmia); stroke MI and sudden death reported with all stimulants in children and adults
- Controlled studies suggest that adverse effects in preschoolers (aged 3–7) are comparable to those seen in school-age children (dose-dependent)
- Adverse effects may be more problematic in children and adolescents with autism – symptoms may be exacerbated
- Effects on growth and weight appear to be small and related to dose and duration of drug use [drug holidays used to minimize this – evidence is contradictory]
- Reports of exacerbation of OCD symptoms in children on high doses
- Drug-induced insomnia can be managed by changing the timing of the stimulant dose [clonidine (0.05–0.4 mg), melatonin (data contradictory), l-tryptophan, antihistamines, or trazodone (25–50 mg) at bedtime may be useful]; rebound insomnia reported as effects of afternoon stimulant wears off
- Anorexia common, GI distress and weight loss [can be minimized by taking medication with meals, eating smaller meals more frequently or drinking high-calorie fluids]; if loss of weight exceeds 10% of body weight, consider switching to another agent
- Hyperactive rebound can occur in the afternoon or evening [an earlier second dose, more frequent dosing, or the use of slow-release preparation can be tried]
- Common adverse effects include sadness, irritability, anxiety, clinging behavior, insomnia
- Dysphoria or sadness reported – may be related to withdrawal effects; use of sustained-release product or addition of a noradrenergic antidepressant may be helpful

Psychostimulants (cont.)

	• Rare hepatotoxic effects have been associated with use of pemoline, sometimes occurring months after drug initiation; deaths have been reported. Stop drug if liver enzymes are elevated. Risk increased in patients with pre-existing hepatic disease and in patients receiving concomitant methylphenidate
	• May exacerbate psychotic symptoms in children with a genetic predisposition or prior history of psychosis; risk for inducing mixed/manic episode in patients with BAD
DISCONTINUATION SYNDROME	• Tolerance to effects occurs in about 15% of patients (may occur rapidly); dose increases may be required to produce similar effects
	• Abrupt withdrawal after prolonged (months) use may result in dysphoria, rebound insomnia, or a rebound in symptoms of ADHD
	• Case of priapism reported in 16-year-old each time he forgot to take his dose of extended-release methylphenidate (Concerta) 54 mg
PRECAUTIONS	• Do a cardiac history and physical assessment prior to prescribing stimulants; increased risk of serious cardiovascular problems, including heart attacks and sudden death; use with caution in patients with cardiovascular disease, including hypertension, tachyarrhythmias, and hardening of the arteries. DO NOT USE in patients with structural cardiac abnormalities
	• Use cautiously in patients with anxiety, tension, agitation, restlessness
	• May exacerbate thought disorder in psychotic patients
	• May precipitate manic or hypomanic symptoms in a patient with undiagnosed bipolar disorder, and can exacerbate psychotic symptoms
	• Use cautiously in hyperthyroidism as psychostimulants may cause hypothyroidism
	• May lower the seizure threshold
	• May cause an idiopathic hypothyroidism, though patient euthyroid
	• Do periodic CBC (methylphenidate, dextroamphetamine) due to rare reports of leukopenia and nutrition-based anemia
	• Chronic abuse in patients can lead to tolerance and psychic dependence; drug dependence in children is rare; however, it may be of concern in adolescents with comorbid antisocial personality disorder or severe conduct disorder. Stimulants can be abused orally, intravenously, or nasally
	• Tics or dyskinesias can be unmasked in children with ADHD with a genetic predisposition
	• In patients with Tourette's syndrome there may be an initial worsening of tics; dose may need to be adjusted [clonidine or guanfacine may be effective]
	• Use with caution and with careful monitoring in patients with a recent history of alcohol and/or drug abuse. Some adolescents, or parents, may divert psychostimulants for illegal purposes
	• Application of external heat over Daytrana patch results in temperature-dependent increases in release of methylphenidate (greater than 2-fold)
CONTRAINDICATIONS	• Patients with structural cardiac abnormalities or tachyarrhythmias, severe angina pectoris, severe hypertension
	• Do not use in patients with a history of functional psychosis
	• Use cautiously if there is a positive family history of Tourette's syndrome (tic incidence 20–50% in this population)
	• Anorexia nervosa
	• Anxiety, tension, agitation
	• Thyrotoxicosis, glaucoma
	• Patients taking MAOIs

- Baseline physical and psychiatric assessment including cardiac history, BP, pulse, height, and weight; repeat at least annually. Patients with cardiac disease should be further evaluated via EKG and echocardiograph
- Cardiac evaluation recommended if patient experiences excessive increase in blood pressure and heart rate, exertional chest pain or unexplained syncope
- Do periodic CBC (methylphenidate, dextroamphetamine) due to rare reports of leukopenia and nutrition-based anemia

TOXICITY

- See p. 32

USE IN PREGNANCY

- See p. 32

NURSING IMPLICATIONS

- While medication has demonstrated superiority, a multimodal approach to ADHD treatment increases the probability of a positive outcome; some non-pharmacological approaches include behavior modification strategies, individual and family psychotherapy, as well as special education for the child
- Monitor therapy by watching for adverse effects, and changes in mood and activity level, concentration, and impulsiveness
- Monitor height and weight (children); if constitutional small stature, drug holidays may help minimize growth suppression
- Ensure that spansules, sustained/extended-release, or osmotic-controlled release preparations are not chewed, but are swallowed whole
- Patients who have problems swallowing pills can use the preparations formulated as beads (i.e., Dexedrine spansules, Metadate CD, Biphentin, Ritalin LA, or Adderall XR), by opening the capsule, sprinkling the beads on apple sauce, and swallowing the mixture without chewing
- Caution patients not to stop drug abruptly
- Doses in latter part of day may cause insomnia
- To minimize anorexia, give drug with or after meals
- Heart rate and blood pressure should be monitored after every dose increase
- The Concerta tablet shell does not dissolve; inform the patient that he/she may see the shell in the toilet sometimes, after a bowel movement
- Daytrana patch should be applied (immediately upon removal of protective pouch) to clean, dry skin on the hip, 2 h before desired effect, and taken off about 9 h later; advise patient not to apply patch to inflamed skin, and to avoid exposure of patch to applied heat (e.g., electric or heating pads, blankets). Dispose of patch by folding together the adhesive side – can be flushed down the toilet.

PATIENT INSTRUCTIONS

- Detailed instructions for patients and caregivers are provided in the Information Sheet on p. 285.

DRUG INTERACTIONS

- Clinically significant interactions are listed below

DRUGS INTERACTING WITH METHYLPHENIDATE AND DEXMETHYLPHENIDATE

Class of Drug	Example	Interaction Effects
Antibacterial	Linezolid	AVOID combination as linezolid inhibits MAO enzymes (discontinue stimulant while linezolid used)
Anticoagulant	Warfarin	Decreased metabolism of anticoagulant Increased PT ratio or INR response
Anticonvulsant	Carbamazepine	Decreased plasma level of methylphenidate and its metabolite, and of dexmethylphenidate
	Phenytoin, phenobarbital, primidone	Increased phenytoin and phenobarbital levels due to inhibited metabolism
Antidepressant MAOI (Irreversible)	Phenelzine, tranylcypromine, pargyline	Release of large amount of norepinephrine with hypertensive reaction; combination used RARELY to augment antidepressant therapy with strict monitoring
RIMA	Moclobemide	Increased blood pressure and enhanced effect if used over prolonged period or in high doses

Psychostimulants (cont.)

Class of Drug	Example	Interaction Effects
Tricyclic	Amitriptyline, etc.	Used together to augment antidepressant effect Plasma level of antidepressant may be increased Cardiovascular effects increased, with combination, in children; monitor BP and EKG Case reports of neurotoxic effects with imipramine, but considered rare; monitor
SSRI		Additive effects in depression, dysthymia, and OCD in patients with ADHD Plasma level of antidepressant may be increased
SNRI	Venlafaxine	Case of serotonin syndrome after one dose of venlafaxine added to methylphenidate
Antihistamine	Diphenhydramine	Antagonism of sedative effects
Antipsychotics		Antipsychotics may block the central stimulant effect through dopamine blockade Early data suggest that methylphenidate may exacerbate or prolong withdrawal dyskinesia following Antipsychotics discontinuation
Clonidine		Additive effect on sleep, hyperactivity and aggression associated with ADHD – use caution due to case reports of sudden death [monitor EKG]
Guanethidine		Decreased hypotensive effect; may be dose dependent
Herbal preparation	Ephedra, yohimbine, St. John's Wort	May cause hypertension, arrhythmias, and/or CNS stimulation
Theophylline		Reports of increased tachycardia, palpitations, dizziness, weakness, and agitation with combination

DRUGS INTERACTING WITH DEXTROAMPHETAMINE

Class of Drug	Example	Interaction Effects
Acidifying agent	Ammonium chloride, fruit juices, ascorbic acid	Decreased absorption, increased elimination and decreased plasma level of dextroamphetamine
Alkalinizing agent	Potassium citrate, sodium bicarbonate	Increased absorption, prolonged half-life and decreased elimination of amphetamines
Antidepressant		
MAOI (Irreversible)	Phenelzine, tranylcypromine	Hypertensive crisis due to increased norepinephrine release; AVOID
RIMA	Moclobemide	Slightly enhanced effect if used over prolonged period or in high doses
SSRIs	Sertraline, paroxetine	Additive effects in depression, dysthymia and OCD in patients with ADHD Paroxetine may increase plasma level of dextroamphetamine due to inhibited metabolism via CYP2D6
Trycyclic		May result in increased level of either the antidepressent or amphetamine
Antihistamine	Diphenhydramine	Antagonism of sedative effects
Antipsychotics		Antagonize stimulant and toxic effects of dextroamphetamine through dopamine blockade
Barbiturate	Phenobarbital, amobarbital	Antagonize pharmacological effects of amphetamines
Guanethidine		Decreased hypotensive effect; may be dose-dependent
Sibutramine		Potential hypertension and tachycardia – use with caution

Atomoxetine

Generic Name	Trade Name	Dosage Forms and Strengths	Monograph Statements
Atomoxetine	Strattera	Capsules: 10 mg, 18 mg, 25 mg, 40 mg, 60 mg	Safety and efficacy not established in children under age 6

APPROVED INDICATIONS

- Treatment of ADHD in children, adolescents, and adults

GENERAL COMMENTS

- Efficacy suggested to be comparable to that of psychostimulants; may be effective for some patients who have not responded to stimulant treatment. Benefits include a lack of euphoria, a lower risk of rebound and a lower risk of induction of tics or psychosis
- Reduces both the inattentive and hyperactive/impulsive symptoms of ADHD
- Double-blind study suggests shorter sleep latency and improved sleep with atomoxetine as compared to methylphenidate
- Full theraputic benefit may take 3–7 weeks
- Increased risk of suicidal ideation in children and adolescents (see precautions)
- Not a controlled substance

PHARMACOLOGY

- Selectively blocks the reuptake of norepinephrine; increases dopamine and norepinephrine in the frontal cortex (without increasing dopamine in subcortical areas) – leads to cognitive inhancement without abuse liability; suggested to be important in regulating attention, impulsivity and activity levels
- No stimulant or euphoriant activity

DOSING

- Dosing is based on body weight
- Children and adolescents up to 70 kg: initiate at 0.5 mg/kg/day, and increase after a minimum of 10 days to 0.8 mg/kg/day for 10 days; if clinical response is not achieved, increase to a target dose of 1.2 mg/kg/day, given once daily or bid in the morning and late afternoon. Do not exceed 1.4 mg/kg/day or 100 mg/day, whichever is less
- Over 70 kg: initiate at 40 mg/day and increase after a minimum of 10 days to 60 mg/day for 10 days; if clinical response is not achieved, increase to a target dose of 80 mg/day, given once daily or bid in the morning and late afternoon. If response is inadequate after 2–4 weeks, the dose can be increased to a maximum of 100 mg/day. Doses >100mg/day have not been found to result in additional therapeutic benefit

Atomoxetine (cont.)

- Lower doses required in those who are poor metabolizers of CYP2D6
- In patients with moderate hepatic dysfunction, reduce dose by 50%; in severe hepatic dysfunction reduce dose to 25% of the usual therapeutic range
- No dosage adjustment in patients with real insufficiency; may exacerbate hypertension in end-stage renal diseoal
- If prescribed in combination with drugs that inhibit CYP2D6 (see Drug Interactions below): initiate dose, as above, but do not increase to the usual target dose unless symptoms fail to improve *after 4 weeks* and the initial dose is well tolerated

PHARMACOKINETICS

- See p. 31
- Pharmacokinetics in children age 6 and older are similar to that in adults (plasma level proportional to dose)
- Rapidly absorbed; may be taken with or without food – high-fat meal decreases rate but not extent of absorption
- Bioavailability 63%; 94% in poor metabolizers
- Protein binding: 98% atomoxetine and 69% for OH-atomoxetine metabolite
- Peak plasma level reached in 1–2 h; 3–4 h in poor metabolizers
- Half-life = 5 h for atomoxetine and 6–8 h for hydroxyatomoxetine; in poor metabolizers the values are 21.6 h and 34–40 h, respectively; metabolized primarily by CYP2D6, also for atomoxetine and 6–8 h for by CYP2C19
- Hepatic dysfunction: 2-fold increase in AUC in moderate hepatic insufficiency and 4-fold increase in AUC in severe hepatic dysfunction

ADVERSE EFFECTS

- Common in children: headache, rhinitis, cough, upper abdominal pain, nausea, vomiting, dizziness, fatigue, emotional lability
- Severe hepatic injury has been reported in adolescents and adults who received atomoxetine for several months. Injury reversed when atomoxetine withdrawn
- Initially, decreased appetite and weight loss (average of 0.5 kg)
- Less frequent: irritability, insomnia, dry mouth, constipation, mydriasis, tremor, pruritus, depression, sexual dysfunction, urinary retention
- Small increases in blood pressure and pulse can occur at start of treatment; usually plateaus with time; no effects on QT interval reported

DISCONTINUATION SYNDROME

- There is no evidence, to date, that suggests a drug discontinuation or withdrawal syndrome exists

PRECAUTIONS

- Increased risk of suicide–related events in children and adolescents (risk from placebo conrolled trials: 6/1357 (0.44%) vs 0/851 with placebo
- Use cautiously in patients with hypertension, tachycardia, cardiovascular or cerebrovascular disease
- Due to risk of hypotension, use cautiously in any condition that may predispose patients to hypotension
- Use caution in patients with liver dysfunction – see Dosing, above

CONTRAINDICATIONS	• Patients with structural cardiac abnormities, tachyarrhythmias, severe angina pectoris or severe hypertension • Should not be administered together with an MAOI or within 2 weeks of discontinuing an MAOI • Not recommended in patients with narrow angle glaucoma due to increased risk of mydriasis
TOXICITY	• Unknown
USE IN PREGNANCY	• Pregnancy Category C – animal studies suggest teratogenic effects; effects in humans unknown
Breast Milk	• Excreted in breast milk of rats; unknown if atomoxetine is excreted in human milk
LABORATORY TESTS/ MONITORING	• Baseline physical and psychiatric assessment including cardiac history, BP and pulse; repeat at least annually. Cardiac evaluation recommended if patient experiences excessive increase in BP and heart rate, exertional chest pain or unexplained syncope • Liver function test at first symptom or sign of liver dysfunction
NURSING IMPLICATIONS	• Measure pulse and blood pressure at baseline and periodically during treatment • Monitor height and weight during treatment • Monitor for signs of liver toxicity (AST/ALT) • Monitor for increased irritability, anger, depression and suicide thoughts, especially during the first 3 weeks after drug initiation • Capsules of atomoxetine cannot be opened and sprinkled on food
PATIENT INSTRUCTIONS	• Detailed instructions for patients and caregivers are provided in the Information Sheet on p. 287
DRUG INTERACTIONS	• Clinically significant interactions are listed below

Class of Drug	Example	Interactions
Antiarrhythmic	Quinidine	Increased level of atomoxetine due to inhibited metabolism via CYP2D6
Antidepressant		
SSRI	Paroxetine, fluoxetine	Increased plasma level and T½ of atomoxetine due to inhibited metabolism via CYP2D6
MAOI	Phenelzine	Do not administer concurrently or within 2 weeks of discontinuing an MAOI
Antiviral agent	Ritonavir, delavirdine	Increased level of atomoxetine due to inhibited metabolism via CYP2D6
β-Blocker	Albuterol	Potentiation of hypertension and tachycardia with combination
Sympathomimetic	Methylphenidate, amphetamines	Possible potentiation of hypertension and tachycardia

Comparison of Psychostimulants

	Methylphenidate	Dexmethylphenidate	Dextroamphetamine/ Amphetamine salts/- Methamphetamine	Atomoxetine
Pharmacology	Selectively inhibits presynaptic transporters (i.e., reuptake) for dopamine and norepinephrine – dependent on normal neuronal activity Mildly increases levels of synaptic dopamine and NE	Selectively inhibits presynaptic transporters (i.e., reuptake) for dopamine and norepinephrine – dependent on normal neuronal activity Mildly increases levels of synaptic dopamine and NE	Cause release of dopamine, NE and 5-HT into the synapse – occurs independently of normal neuronal activity Inhibit MAO enzyme	Selectively blocks reuptake of NE and increases DA and NE in frontal cortex
Dosing ADHD	Start with 2.5 mg bid and increase by 2.5–5 mg weekly Usual dose: 5–60 mg/day or 0.25–1.0 mg/kg body weight (divided doses); up to 3 mg/kg has been used in children; little benefit with doses > 60 mg/day Extended-release: 18–20 mg qam; can increase by 18–20 mg weekly to a maximum of 54 to 60 mg/day Transdermal patch: week 1 apply 27.5 mg patch (for 9 h per day); increase in weekly intervals, as necessary	Over age 6: start with 2.5 mg bid (0.6–1 mg/kg/day) and can increase weekly by 2.5–5 mg to a maximum of 20 mg/day (divided dose, given q 4 h) Usual dose: 5–20 mg daily given q 4 h When switching from methylphenidate, the starting dose of dexmethylphenidate should be half that of methylphenidate	*Dextroamphetamine:* Age 3–5: start with 2.5 mg and increase by 2.5 mg weekly. Over age 6: start with 5 mg and increase by 5 mg weekly Usual dose: dextroamphetamine: 2.5– 40 mg/day or 0.1–0.8 mg/kg/day (divided doses); Spansules can be sprinkled on food *Adderall:* 2.5–5 mg to start and increase by 2.5–5 mg every 3–7 days up to 25 mg/day (given every 4–7 h) Adderall XR: 10–30 mg qam *Methamphetamine:* start with 5 mg odbid and increase by 5 mg/week Usual dose: 20–25 mg/day – in divided doses; Gradumet given once daily	See p. 27
Depression	10–30 mg/day		Dextroamphetamine: 5–60 mg/day in divided doses	—
Narcolepsy	10–60 mg/day (usual dose: 10 mg 2–3 times/day)		Dextroamphetamine: 5–60 mg/day in divided doses	—
Renal dysfunction	no data	no data	no data	No adjustment required; may exacerbate hypertension in end-stage renal disease
Hepatic dysfunction	no change	no change	no change	Moderate dysfunction: reduce dose by 50% Severe dysfunction: reduce dose by 75%
Pharmacokinetics				
Bioavailability	> 90%	22–25%	Dextroamphetamine: > 90% Methamphetamine: 65–70%	63–94%

	Methylphenidate	Dexmethylphenidate	Dextroamphetamine/ Amphetamine salts/- Methamphetamine	Atomoxetine
Peak plasma level	Tabs: 0.3–4 h Slow release: 1–8 h Metadate CD: 1.5 h first peak and 4.5 h second peak Concerta: 1 h first peak and 6.8 h second peak	1–1.5 h (fasting)	Dextroamphetamine: Tablets 1–4 h, Spansules: 6–10 h Adderall: Tablets 1–2 h XR: 7 h	1–2 h 3–4 h in poor metabolizers
Protein binding	8–15%	12–15%	12–15%	98% Atomoxetine and 69% OH-atomoxetine metabolite
Onset of effects	0.5–2 h (see Long-acting Formulations p. 21) Absorption from GI tract is slow and incomplete	0.5–2 h	0.5–2 h Readily absorbed from the GI tract Adderall: saccharate and aspartate salts have a delayed onset	Delayed up to 4 weeks
Food	Metadate CD: T_{max} delayed by 1 h Concerta: C_{max} delayed by 10–30% and T_{max} delayed by 1h	—	Extent of absorption decreased	—
High fat meal	T_{max} delayed	T_{max} delayed	—	Decreases rate but not extent of absorption
Plasma half-life	Regular tabs: 2.9 h mean (range: 2–4 h) SR and Concerta: 3.4 h mean Metadate CD: 6.8 h mean Daytrana: 3–4 h after removal of patch	2.2 h	Dextroamphetamine: 6–8 h in acidic pH, 18.6–33.6 h in alkaline pH Methamphetamine: 6.5–15 h Adderall: 6–8 h	5 h atomoxetine and 6–8 h metabolite Poor metabolizers: 21.6 h atomoxetine and 34–40 h metabolite
Duration of action	Regular tabs: 3–5 h Slow release – theoretically 5–8 h, but 3–5 h practically Extended release: 8–12 h	6–7 h	Dextroamphetamine: Tabs 4–5 h, Spansules: 7–8 h Adderall: Tabs 5–7 h XR: 12 h	Over 12 h
Metabolism	Metabolized by CYP2D6 Inhibits CYP2D6 and 2C9 enzymes	By de-esterification	Metabolized by CYP2D6	Metabolized primarily by CYP2D6; also by CYP2C19
Adverse Effects*				
CNS	Nervousness, anxiety, insomnia (up to 28%), restlessness, activation, irritability (up to 26%), headache (up to 14%), tearfulness, drowsiness, rebound depression; may exacerbate psychosis or mania Social withdrawal, dullness, sadness and irritability reported in children with autism Tourette's syndrome, tics (up to 10% – mostly with higher doses)	Drowsiness, headache Fever (5%) Arthralgia, dyskinesias	Nervousness, insomnia, activation, restlessness, anxiety, mania (with high doses), dysphoria, irritability, headache, confusion, delusions, rebound depression; may exacerbate psychosis or mania Headache Tremor, Tourette's syndrome, tics – usually with higher doses	Insomnia, dizziness, fatigue, headache, emotional lability Less common: drowsiness, irritability, depression, tremor Case reports of tics

Comparison of Psychostimulants (cont.)

	Methylphenidate	Dexmethylphenidate	Dextroamphetamine/ Amphetamine salts/- Methamphetamine	Atomoxetine
GI	Abdominal pain, nausea, anorexia (in up to 41% – dose-related), weight loss Potential for GI obstruction with Concerta	Abdominal pain (15%), nausea, anorexia (6%)	Abdominal pain, nausea, anorexia, weight loss	upper abdominal pain, nausea, vomiting, weight loss
Cardiovascular	Increased heart rate and blood pressure, at start of therapy, dizziness, hypotension, palpitations (see Precautions)	Increased heart rate and blood pressure at start of therapy (see Precautions)	Increased heart rate and blood pressure, at start of therapy, dizziness, palpitations (see Precautions)	Small increases in heart rate and blood pressure at start of treatment
Anticholinergic	Dry mouth, blurred vision	Blurred vision	Dry mouth, dysgeusia, blurred vision	Dry mouth, constipation, mydriasis, urinary retention
Endocrine	Growth delay (height and weight); may occur initially but tends to normalize over time (unless high chronic doses used)	Growth delay, weight loss	Growth delay (height and weight); may occur initially but tends to normalize over time (unless high chronic doses used)	Sexual dysfunction
Other	Upper respiratory infections: pharyngitis (4%), sinusitis (3%), cough (4%) Rash Leukopenia, blood dyscrasias, anemia, hair loss Contact sensitization/dermatitis with Daytrana patch; redness, itching, blistering	Cough, upper respiratory infections	Impotence, changes in libido Urticaria, anemia	Rhinitis, pruritus Cases of liver damage with elevated liver enzymes and bilirubin
Toxicity	CNS overstimulation with vomiting, agitation, tremors, hyperreflexia, convulsions, confusion, hallucinations, delirium, cardiovascular effects e.g., hypertension, tachycardia Supportive therapy should be given	CNS overstimulation with vomiting, agitation, tremors, hyperreflexia, convulsions, confusion, hallucinations, delirium, cardiovascular effects e.g., hypertension, tachycardia Supportive therapy should be given	Restlessness, dizziness, increased reflexes, tremor, insomnia, irritability, assaultiveness, hallucinations, panic, cardiovascular effects, circulatory collapse, convulsions, and coma Supportive therapy should be given	Unknown
Use in Pregnancy	No evidence of teratogenicity reported	Safety not established	High doses have embryotoxic and teratogenic potential; use of amphetamine in pregnant animals has been associated with permanent alterations in the central noradrenergic system of the neonate Increased risk of premature delivery and low birth weight; withdrawal reactions in newborn reported	Category C
Breastfeeding	No data	No data	Excreted into breast milk; recommended not to breastfeed	No data

* Dose related

Clonidine

PRODUCT AVAILABILITY

Generic Name	Trade Name(A)	Dosage Forms and Strengths	Monograph Statements
Clonidine	Catapres Catapres TTS(B)	Tablet: 0.025 mg, 0.1 mg, 0.2 mg, 0.3 mg(B) Transdermal patch(B): 0.1 mg/24 h, 0.2 mg/24 h, 0.3 mg/24 h	Safety and efficacy have not been established in children under age 12

(A) Generic praparations may be available, (B) Not marketed in Canada

INDICATIONS

Other uses in Children and Adolescents

- No approved indications in children and adolescents

- ADHD: meta-analysis of studies suggests a moderate benefit in children and adolescents; reduces hyperarousal, agitation, sleep disturbances, and aggression; useful in patients with concurrent tic disorders or conduct disorder
- Some benefit in combining with stimulants; may help decrease insomnia caused by psychostimulants (Caution – see Drug Interactions p. 26)
- Improves behavior or impulsivity when used alone or in combination with methylphenidate (Caution – see Drug Interactions p. 26); may reduce hyper-arousal behaviors in pervasive developmental disorders
- Reported to be effective for controlling some problematic behaviors in children and adults with autism
- Reported to have synergistic effect with anticonvulsant regimens in controlling aggression and impulsivity
- Of some benefit in generalized anxiety disorder, panic attacks, phobic disorders, and obsessive-compulsive disorders; may augment effects of SSRIs and cyclic antidepressants in social phobia
- Decreases startle response and hyperarousal in PTSD
- May help decrease clozapine-induced sialorrhea
- Used in heroin and nicotine withdrawal to reduce hyperactivity and increase patient comfort. Opioid antagonists (e.g., naltrexone) often given concomitantly
- Hypertension

GENERAL COMMENTS

- Reduces the hyperactive/impulsive symptoms of ADHD; less effective for inattention problems
- Considered less effective than psychostimulants, though may be beneficial for some patients who have not responded to stimulant treatment
- In anxiety disorders, psychological symptoms respond better than somatic symptoms; anxiolytic effects may be short-lived

PHARMACOLOGY

- A central and peripheral α-adrenergic agonist; acts on presynaptic neurons and inhibits noradrenergic transmission at the synapse; suggested to affect norepinephrine discharge rates in the locus ceruleus and indirectly affect dopamine firing rates

DOSING

- ADHD: 3–10 μg/kg body weight per day (0.05–0.4 mg/day) once daily or in divided doses
- Antisocial behavior/aggression: children – 0.15–0.4 mg/day as tablets or transdermal patch
- Anxiety disorders: 0.15–0.5 mg/day

Clonidine (cont.)

PHARMACOKINETICS
- Well absorbed orally and percutaneously (when applied to the arm or chest)
- Peak plasma level of oral preparation occurs in 3–5 h; therapeutic plasma concentrations of transdermal patch occur within 2–3 days
- Children metabolize clonidine faster than adults and may require more frequent dosing (4–6 times/day)
- Plasma half-life is 6–20 h; in patients with impaired renal function, half-life ranges from 18–41 h. Elimination half-life is dose-dependent

ONSET AND DURATION OF ACTION
- Oral tablets: onset of effects occurs in 30–60 minutes and lasts about 6–8 h
- Transdermal patch: therapeutic plasma concentrations are attained within 2–3 days and effects last for 7 days

ADVERSE EFFECTS
- Sedation, common on initiation
- Less common: anxiety, irritability, decreased memory, headache, dry mouth, hypotension
- Dermatological reactions reported in up to 50% of patients using the trans dermal patch

DISCONTINUATION SYNDROME
- Withdrawal reactions occur after abrupt cessation of long-term therapy (over 1–2 months); children more sensitive to rebound hypertension; taper on drug discontinuation to prevent rebound hypertension, as well as tic rebound in patients with Tourette's syndrome

PRECAUTIONS
- Use caution in combination with psychostimulants due to case reports (5 to date) of sudden death with combination
- Use with caution in patients with cerebrovascular disease, chronic renal failure, or a history of depression

TOXICITY
- Signs and symptoms of overdose occur within 60 minutes of drug ingestion and may persist for up to 48 h – children may exhibit signs of toxicity with dose of 0.1mg clonidine
- Symptoms include transient hypertension followed by hypotension, bradycardia, weakness, pallor, sedation, vomiting, hypothermia; can progress to CNS depression, diminished or absent reflexes, apnea, respiratory depression, cardiac conduction defects, seizures, and coma

Treatment
- Supportive and symptomatic

USE IN PREGNANCY
- Category C – animal studies suggest teratogenic effects; effects in humans unknown
- Clonidine crosses the placenta and may lower the heart rate of the fetus

Breast Milk
- Clonidine is distributed into breast milk; effects on infant unknown

NURSING IMPLICATIONS
- Clonidine should not be discontinued suddenly due to risk of rebound hypertension
- Handle the used transdermal patch carefully (fold in half with sticky sides together)
- Should the transdermal patch begin to loosen from the skin, apply adhesive overlay over the system to ensure good adhesion over the period of application
- Monitor for skin reactions around area where transdermal patch is applied

PATIENT INSTRUCTIONS • Detailed instructions for patients and caregivers are provided in the Information Sheet on p. 289

DRUG INTERACTIONS • Clinically significant interactions are listed below

Class of Drug	Example	Interactions
Antidepressant	Desipramine, bupropion	Clonidine withdrawal may result in excess circulating catecholamines; use caution in combination with nor-adrenergic or dopaminergic antidepressants Inhibition of antihypertensive effect of clonidine by the antidepressant
Cyclic	Imipramine, desipramine	
Antihypertensives		
General β-Blockers	 Propranolol	Additive hypotension Additive bradycardia
CNS depressants	Antihistamines, alcohol, hypnotics	Additive CNS depressant effects
Stimulant	Methylphenidate	Additive effect on sleep, hyperactivity, and aggression associated with ADHD – use caution due to case reports of sudden death [monitor EKG]

Guanfacine

PRODUCT AVAILABILITY

Generic Name	Trade Name	Dosage Forms and Strengths	Monograph Statement
Guanfacine [B]	Tenex	Tablet: 1 mg, 2 mg	Safety and efficacy in patients under 12 years of age have not been demonstrated.

[B] Not marketed in Canada

INDICATIONS

- No approved indications in children and adolescents

Other Uses in Children and Adolescents

- Double blind and open studies suggest efficacy in treatment-refractory patients with ADHD non-responsive to other medications or in patients with comorbid tic disorders; improves arousal, hyperactivity, inattention, and immature behavior
- A retrospective analysis of 80 patients with PDD suggested a role for guanfacine in treating hyperactivity, inattention, insomnia, and tics in this population. Patients with Asperger disorder responded better than those with autism.
- Reported beneficial in decreasing nightmares of PTSD

GENERAL COMMENTS

- Approved for use in hypertension in USA
- Less sedation and hypotension than clonidine

PHARMACOLOGY

- Alpha 2A agonist

DOSING

- 0.5–3 mg/day given bid (0.03–0.1 mg/kg/day) as an oral tablet or transdermal patch
- Children metabolize guanfacine faster than adults and may require more frequent dosing (2–3 times a day)

PHARMACOKINETICS

- Peak plasma concentrations occur from 1 to 4 hours after single oral doses
- 70% bound to plasma proteins
- Younger patients tend to have shorter elimination half-lives (13–14 hr); guanfacine and its metabolites are excreted primarily in the urine; The clearance of guanfacine in patients with varying degrees of renal insufficiency is reduced, but plasma levels of drug are only slightly increased compared to patients with normal renal function

ADVERSE EFFECTS
- Sedation, hypotension (with cases of syncope), and bradycardia common
- Headache, stomach-ache, insomnia, fatigue, irritability and anorexia reported
- Case reports of induced mania

WITHDRAWAL
- If stopped abruptly increases in plasma and urinary catecholamines occur which can result in symptoms of nervousness and anxiety
- Rebound hypertension also reported

PRECAUTIONS
- Use cautiously in patients with renal insufficiency

CONTRAINDICATIONS
- Not recommended in patients with severe renal impairment

TOXICITY
- Drowsiness, lethargy, bradycardia and hypotension have been observed following overdose with guanfacine
- Gastric lavage and supportive therapy as appropriate. Guanfacine is not dialyzable in clinically significant amounts (2.4%)

USE IN PREGNANCY
- Category B drug

NURSING IMPLICATIONS
- Instruct patient to take medication as directed and not to stop it suddenly
- Breast Milk
- It is not known whether guanfacine is excreted in human milk

PATIENT INSTRUCTIONS
- For detailed patient instructions on guanfacine see p. 291

DRUG INTERACTIONS
- Clinically significant interactions are listed below

Class of Drug	Example	Interaction Effects
Anticonvulsant	Phenobarbital, phenytoin	Induced metabolism and decreased half-life of guanfacine
Antidepressant, tricyclic	Amiptriptyline, imipramine	Additive hypotensive effect
β-blockers	Nadolol, propranolol, timolol	Additive hypotension/bradycardia May exacerbate rebound hypertension when guanfacine is withdrawn; β-blockers should be withdrawn first
CNS drugs	Narcotics	Increased sedation when guanfacine is given with other CNS-depressant drug

Drugs for ADHD

Augmentation Strategies in ADHD

NONRESPONSE IN ADHD	• Ascertain diagnosis is correct • Ascertain if patient is compliant with therapy (speak with caregivers, check with pharmacy for late refills) • Ensure dosage prescribed is therapeutic • Consider trying an alternate stimulant if the first one was ineffective and the patient was adhering to therapy recommendations
FACTORS COMPLICATING RESPONSE	• Concurrent medical or psychiatric condition, e.g., bipolar disorder, conduct disorder, learning disability • Concurrent prescription drugs may interfere with efficacy, e.g., antipsychotics (see Drug Interactions p. 26) • Metabolic enhancers (e.g., carbamazepine) will decrease the plasma level of methylphenidate • High intake of acidifying agents (e.g., fruit juices, vitamin C) may decrease the efficacy of amphetamine preparations • Substance abuse, including alcohol, may make management difficult • Side effects to medication • Psychosocial factors may affect response; nonpharmacological treatment approaches (e.g., behavior modification, psychotherapy, and education) can increase the probability of response
DRUG COMBINATIONS IN ADHD	
Methylphenidate/ Dexmethylphenidate/ Dextroamphetamine + Clonidine	• Additive effect on hyperactivity, aggression, mood lability, and sleep problems; studies indicate efficacy in 50–80% of patients. Has been found helpful in patients with concomitant tic disorders, conduct disorder or oppositional defiant disorder. • **CAUTION:** 5 case reports of sudden death in combination with methylphenidate (monitor EKG, heart rate, and blood pressure with combination)
Psychostimulants + Antidepressants	• Tricyclics (imipramine, nortriptyline, and desipramine) useful in refractory patients or those with concomitant enuresis or bulimia; they may reduce abnormal movements in patients with tic disorders. There is an increase in the incidence of adverse effects, including cardio-vascular, GI, anticholinergic effects, and weight gain; use caution in patients at risk of overdose • SSRIs or venlafaxine may be effective in patients with concomitant mood or anxiety disorders (e.g., PTSD) • Bupropion used to augment effects of psychostimulants and in patients with concomitant mood disorder, substance abuse, or conduct disorder. May cause dermatological reactions, exacerbate tics, and increase seizure risk
Psychostimulants + Antipsychotics	• Second generation antipsychotics (risperidone, olanzapine) have been found useful in patients with comorbid symptoms of dyscontrol, aggression, hyperactivity, and tics • Low doses of haloperidol and pimozide have been used in patients with concurrent Tourette's syndrome
Psychostimulants and Mood Stabilizers	• Combination used in patients with comorbid bipolar disorder, conduct disorder, impulsivity, and aggression; case reports in children include the use of lithium, carbamazepine, valproate, and gabapentin – the possibility of drug interactions should be considered (see Drug Interactions p. 25)
Psychostimulants + Buspirone	• Open studies suggest benefit in improving hyperactivity, impulsivity, inattention, and disruptive behavior using doses of 15–30 mg daily

- American Academy of Pediatrics. (2001). Clinical Practice Guideline: Treatment of the school-aged child with attention deficit/hyperactivity disorder. *Pediatrics 108,* 1033–144.
- Biederman, J. (1998). Attention-Deficit/Hyperactivity Disorder: A life-span perspective. *Journal of Clinical Psychiatry 59(Suppl. 7),* 4–16.
- Christman, A.K. Fermo, J.D. Markowitz, J.S. (2004). Atomoxetine, a novel treatment for Attention-Deficit-Hyperactivity Disorder. *Pharmacotherapy 24(8),* 1020–1036.
- Brown, R.T., Amler, R.W., Freeman, W.S. et al. (2005). Treatment of attention-deficit hyperactivity disorder: Overview of the evidence. *Pediatrics 115(6),* e749–757.
- Gibson A.P., Bettinger, T.L., Patel, N.C. et al. (2006). Atomoxetine versus stimulants for treatment of attention deficit/hyperactivity disorder. *Annals of Pharmacotherapy 40(6),* 1134–1142.
- Greenhill, L.L, Pliszka, S., Dulcan, M.K. et al (2002) Summary of the Practice Parameter for the use of stimulant medication in the treatment of children, adolescents and adults. *JAACAP 41(Suppl.)* Feb. http://www.aacap.org
- Markowitz, J.S., Straughn, A.B., Patrick, K.S. (2003). Advances in the Pharmacotherapy of ADHD: Focus on methylphenidate formulations. *Pharmacotherapy 23(10),* 1281–1299.
- McGough, J.J., Wigal, S.B., Abikoff, H. et al. (2006). A randomized, double-blind, placebo-controlled, laboratory classroom assessment of methylphenidate transdermal system in children with ADHD. *Journal of Attention Disorders 9(3),* 476–485.
- Posey D.J., Puntney J.I., Sasher T.M., et al. (2004). Guanfacine treatment of hyperactivity and inattention in pervasive developmental disorders: a retrospective analysis of 80 cases. *J Child Adolesc Psychopharmacol 14(2)* 233-241
- Spence, T.S., Biederman, J., Wilens, T.E. et al. (2002). Novel treatments for the Attention-Deficit/Hyperactivity Disorder in Children. *Journal of Clinical Psychiatry 63(Suppl. 12),* 16–22.
- Spence, T.S., Biederman, J., Wilens, T.E. et al. (2002). Overview and neurobiology of Attention-Deficit/Hyperactivity Disorder. *Journal of Clinical Psychiatry 63(Suppl. 12),* 3–9.

ANTIDEPRESSANTS

CLASSIFICATION
- Antidepressants can be classified as follows:

Chemical Class[A]	Example	Page
Cyclic Antidepressants		
Selective Serotonin Reuptake Inhibitors (SSRI)	Example: Citalopram, fluoxetine	See p. 41
Norepinephrine Dopamine Reuptake Inhibitor (NDRI)	Bupropion	See p. 53
Selective Serotonin-Norepinephrine Reuptake Inhibitor (SNRI)	Venlafaxine	See p. 58
Serotonin-2 Antagonists/Reuptake Inhibitors (SARI)	Example: Nefazodone	See p. 63
Noradrenergic/Specific Serotonergic Agent (NaSSA)	Mirtazapine	See p. 69
Nonselective Cyclic Agents (Mixed Reuptake Inhibitor/Receptor Blockers)		See p. 72
Monoamine Oxidase Inhibitors		
Reversible MAO-A Inhibitor (RIMA)	Moclobemide	See p. 82
Irreversible MAO-A-B Inhibitors (MAOIs)	Example: Phenelzine	See p. 86

[A]Antidepressants are currently classified on the basis of their specificity for the reuptake of brain neurotransmitters. This specificity confers a pharmacologic profile on the drugs that determines their spectrum of activity and adverse effects (see Table p. 94).

GENERAL COMMENTS
- Clinical trials in children and adolescents concluded that up to 4% of youths given antidepressants experience suicidal ideation, hostility, and psychomotor agitation (twice the placebo rate of 2%)
- Antidepressants can cause restlessness or psychomotor agitation before improving core symptoms of depression; as energy levels increase, careful monitoring to prevent suicide is recommended, especially in the first weeks of antidepressant treatment
- Use of antidepressants in children with bipolar disorder (mixed episode) reported to cause increased cycling (in 79%), increased aggression (71%), and increased psychotic symptoms (23%)
- **Some antidepressants have NOT been found to be superior to placebo in the treatment of depression in clinical trials involving patients < 18 years old. SSRIs considered first line therapy for depression in youths.**
- Certain nonselective cyclic and MAOI antidepressants are toxic in overdose; limited quantities should be prescribed to patients at risk for suicide

- Only in select or severe/resistant cases can different classes of antidepressants be combined for additive efficacy in refractory cases, but caution must be exercised (see Drug Interactions p. 48)
- Prophylaxis of depression is most effective if the therapeutic dose is maintained
- Tolerance (tachyphylaxis, or "poop-out syndrome") has been reported in 10–20% of patients on various antidepressants, despite compliance with therapy. Possible explanations include adaptations in the CNS increase in disease severity or pathogenesis, loss of placebo effect, accumulation of a detrimental metabolite, unrecognized rapid cycling, or prophylactic inefficacy [Check compliance with therapy; dosage adjustment may help; switching to an alternate antidepressant (p. 98) or augmentation strategies (p. 99) have also been tried]
- Patients with resistant depression may receive augmentation therapy (see Augmentation Strategies p. 99)

THERAPEUTIC EFFECTS

- Elevation of mood, improved appetite and sleep patterns, increased physical activity, improved clarity of thinking, better memory; improved functioning, decreased feelings of guilt, worthlessness, helplessness, inadequacy, decrease in delusional preoccupation and ambivalence and related somatic complaints (such as nausea, headache)

Selective Serotonin Reuptake Inhibitors (SSRI)

PRODUCT AVAILABILITY

Chemical Class	Generic Name	Trade Name[A]	Dosage Forms and Strengths	Monograph Statement
Phthalane derivative	Citalopram	Celexa	Tablets: 10 mg, 20 mg, 40 mg Oral solution[B]: 10 mg/5 ml	Safety and efficacy not established in children under age 18
	Escitalopram	Lexapro[B], Cipralex[C]	Tablets: 5 mg[B], 10 mg, 20 mg Oral solution[B]: 5 mg/5 ml	Safety and efficacy not established in children under age 18
Bicyclic	Fluoxetine	Prozac, Sarafem[B]	Capsules: 10 mg, 20 mg, 40 mg Enteric-coated tablets: 90 mg Delayed release pellets 90 mg[B] Oral solution: 20 mg/5 ml	Approved in the USA for children over age 7
Monocyclic	Fluvoxamine [D]	Luvox	Tablets: 25 mg[B], 50 mg, 100 mg	Approved in the USA for children over age 8
Phenylpiperidine	Paroxetine hydro-chloride	Paxil	Tablets: 10 mg, 20 mg, 30 mg, 40 mg[B] Oral suspension[B]: 10 mg/5 ml	Not indicated in children under age 18 (see Precautions)
	Paroxetine mesylate [B]	Paxil CR Paxeva	Controlled-release tablets: 12.5 mg, 25 mg, 37.5 mg[B] Tablets[B]: 10 mg, 20 mg, 30 mg, 40 mg	
Tetrahydronaphthylmethylamine	Sertraline	Zoloft	Capsules/Tablets: 25 mg, 50 mg, 100 mg Oral solution: 20 mg/ml[B]	Approved in the USA for children over age 6

[A] Generic preparations may be available, [B] Not marketed in Canada, [C] Not marketed in US, [D] Not approved for depression in USA

Antidepressants

Selective Serotonin Reuptake Inhibitors (SSRI) (cont.)

INDICATIONS

Approved for Children and Adolescents	• Fluoxetine approved for depression (for ages 8–17) and for OCD (for ages 7–17) (USA) • Fluvoxamine and sertraline approved for OCD (ages > 8 years and > 7 years respectively) (USA)
Approved (for Adults)	• Major depression – double-blind and open studies (fluoxetine and sertraline) suggest moderate efficacy in children and adolescents aged 7–17 (high placebo response – 30–40%); data equivocal with most other agents (see Precautions p. 46) • Prophylaxis of recurrent major depressive disorder (unipolar affective disorder) • Treatment of secondary depression in other mental illnesses, e.g., schizophrenia • Depressed phase of bipolar disorder (see Precautions p. 46) • Bulimia nervosa (fluoxetine and sertraline) • Obsessive-compulsive disorder (OCD) (fluvoxamine, fluoxetine, paroxetine and sertraline) – double-blind and open trials suggest moderate efficacy in children aged 6–17 (evidence weak for fluvoxamine and citalopram) • Panic disorder with or without agoraphobia (paroxetine, sertraline, fluoxetine) • Social anxiety disorder (paroxetine, sertraline) – other SSRIs studied in children (fluvoxamine, fluoxetine, citalopram) • Posttraumatic stress disorder (sertraline, paroxetine – Canada and USA) • Premenstrual dysphoric disorder (fluoxetine, paroxetine, sertraline – USA) (fluoxetine – Canada) • Generalized anxiety disordered (paroxetine, escitalopram)
Other Uses in Children and Adolescents	• Dysthymia • Atypical depression – open label study with fluoxetine suggests efficacy • Separation anxiety disorder (paroxetine, fluvoxamine, sertraline); mixed results reported in elective mutism • Open label study suggests fluoxetine may decrease depression and alcohol use in adolescents with comorbid alcohol use disorder • Aggressive, impulsive behavior, self-injurious behavior • Open label studies and case reports suggest equivocal efficacy in treating core symptoms of PDD (autism) • Consensus exists that SSRIs do not treat the core symptoms of ADHD; may, however, benefit children and adolescents with concomitant mood and/or anxiety disorders • Tourette's disorder (citalopram, fluvoxamine) – early data

PHARMACOLOGY

• Exact mechanism of antidepressant action unknown; SSRIs, through inhibition of serotonin reuptake, increase concentrations of serotonin in the synapse, which causes downregulation of postsynaptic receptors. Other neurotransmitter systems may also be influenced
• Escitalopram is the S-isomer of racemic citalopram; suggested to be 2–4 times as potent a SSRI inhibitor as citalopram (studies of this agent in children and adolescents are lacking)

- Randomized double-blind studies in C&A reported a lack of efficacy over placebo for some SSRIs (sertraline, paroxetine) in the treatment of depression, though there are published trials demonstrating the efficacy of some SSRIs in pediatric patients (fluoxetine, paroxetine, sertraline, fluvoxamine) In general, SSRIs are marginally more effective in decreasing symptoms of depression in older children and adolescents
- There are few studies that evaluate the chronic (> 6 month) use of any SSRI in children; effects on growth, development and maturation are not known
- SSRIs have been associated with increased suicidal ideation, hostility, and psychomotor agitation in clinical trials involving children and adolescents. Monitor all patients for worsening of depression and suicidal thinking
- SSRIs are associated with increased agitation and non-suicidal self-harm (e.g., cutting)
- Epidemiological studies have found that suicide rates have slightly decreased from 1991–2004 while SSRI use has increased
- Fluoxetine + CBT or fluoxetine alone found to be significantly more effective at improving symptoms of adolescent depression than CBT alone or placebo
- SSRIs should be reserved for children and adolescents with moderate to severe mood or anxiety disorders.

DOSING

- See p. 92
- SSRIs are absorbed and metabolized more quickly in children than in adults; dosage requirements may be relatively higher (e.g., up to 80 mg daily of fluoxetine has been used for anxiety disorders)
- SSRIs have flat dose-response curves, i.e., most patients respond to initial doses (see p. 75)
- Dosage should be decreased (by 50%) in patients with hepatic impairment as plasma levels can increase up to 3-fold; in kidney impairment sertraline levels may increase 1.5-fold; use 50% of standard dose of paroxetine with creatinine clearance 10–50 ml/min, and 25% of the standard dose if the creatinine clearance is < 10ml/min
- Higher doses may be required in adolescents for the treatment of OCD; treatment should be continued at therapeutic doses for at least 10 weeks
- Lower starting dose may be required in panic disorder due to patient sensitivity to stimulating effects
- In adults, a dosing interval of every 2 to 7 days has been used with fluoxetine in prophylaxis of depression; once weekly dosing used in the maintenance treatment of panic disorder (no data in pediatric patients)
- Intermittent dosing (during luteal phase of menstrual cycle) found effective for the treatment of premenstrual dysphoric disorder

PHARMACOKINETICS

- See p. 92
- Rapidly absorbed; undergo little first-pass effect
- Highly bound to plasma protein; all SSRIs (least – escitalopram and fluvoxamine) will displace other drugs from protein binding and elevate their plasma level (see Drug Interactions p.)
- Metabolized primarily by the liver; all SSRIs affect cytochrome P-450 metabolizing enzyme (least – escitalopram) and will affect the metabolism of other drugs metabolized by this system (see Drug Interactions p. 48). Fluoxetine and paroxetine have been shown to decrease their own metabolism over time
- Peak plasma level of sertraline is 30% higher when drug taken with food, as first-pass metabolism is reduced
- Fluoxetine as well as its active metabolite, norfluoxetine, have the longest half-lives (up to 70 h and 330 h, respectively); this has implications for reaching steady-state drug levels as well as for drug withdrawal
- Steady-state levels reported to be higher with fluoxetine, norfluoxetine, and fluvoxamine in children (aged 6–11) than adolescents (2–3 times higher with fluvoxamine)

Selective Serotonin Reuptake Inhibitors (SSRI) (cont.)

- Children aged 6–17 metabolize sertraline more rapidly than adults (22% lower C_{max} and AUC); paroxetine is cleared more rapidly
- Clearance of fluoxetine, sertraline and fluvoxamine reduced in patients with liver cirrhosis
- Clearance of sertraline and paroxetine reduced in renal disease

ONSET AND DURATION OF ACTION	<ul><li>SSRIs are long-acting drugs and can be given in a single daily dose, usually in the morning; fluvoxamine (and sometimes sertraline) may cause sedation and can be prescribed at night</li><li>Therapeutic effect seen after 3–5 weeks; most patients with depression respond to the initial doses; increasing the dose too rapidly due to absence of therapeutic effect can result in a higher than necessary dose and side effects</li><li>Tolerance to effects seen in some patients after months of treatment ("poop-out syndrome") (see p. 41)</li><li>Recommended to continue therapy, at full effective dose, for 6–9 months after symptom remission</li></ul>
ADVERSE EFFECTS	<ul><li>The pharmacological and side effect profile of SSRIs is dependent on their *in vivo* affinity for and activity on neurotransmitters/receptors (see Table p. 94)</li><li>See accompanying chart (p. 80) for incidence of adverse effects at therapeutic doses</li><li>Adverse effects with sertraline (in 6–17-year-olds) and fluvoxamine (in 8–17-year-olds) reported to be similar to those observed in adults</li><li>Incidence may be greater in early days of treatment; patients adapt to many side effects over time</li><li>Rule out withdrawal symptoms of previous antidepressant – can be misattributed to side effects of current drug</li></ul>
CNS Effects	<ul><li>A result of antagonism at histamine H_1-receptors and μ_1-adrenoreceptors</li><li>Headache (up to 29% incidence), worsening of migraines [Management: analgesics prn]</li><li>Seizures reported, primarily in patients with underlying seizure disorder (risk low)</li></ul>
A. Cognitive Effects	<ul><li>Both activation and sedation can occur early in treatment – varies depending on SSRI used</li><li>Children are more prone to behavioral adverse effects including: agitation, restlessness (32–46%), activation, insomnia (up to 21%) [give bulk of dose in the morning], irritability, and social disinhibition (up to 25%); more frequent at higher doses – case reports that citalopram may have a lower risk of activation. CAUTION – cases of self-harm, harm to others, and suicidal urges in 2–3% children and adolescents reported with most SSRIs (except fluoxetine)</li><li>Decreased REM sleep, insomnia, and increased awakenings with all SSRIs; increased dreaming, nightmares, sexual dreams and obsessions reported with fluoxetine</li><li>Drowsiness – more common with fluvoxamine; prescribe bulk of dose at bedtime; sedation with fluoxetine may be related to high concentration of metabolite norfluoxetine</li><li>Precipitation of hypomania or mania especially where patient is experiencing the onset of bipolar disorder; increased risk in youth aged 10–14 yrs, and patients with comorbid substance abuse or Asperger disorder. Careful monitoring for "switch to mania" is necessary</li><li>Psychosis, panic reactions, anxiety, or euphoria may occur; isolated reports of antidepressants causing agitation, motor activation, aggression, impulsivity, and suicidal urges; worsening of self-injurious behavior reported</li></ul>

- Lethargy, apathy or amotivational syndrome (asthenia) reported (suggestive of frontal lobe dysfunction) – may be dose-related – rule out subthresh-old depression, hypothyroidism and parental/environmental factors [prescribe bulk of dose at bedtime; bupropion, buspirone or psychostimulant (e.g., methylphenidate 5–15 mg bid) may be helpful]
- Case reports of cognitive impairment, decreased attention and short-term memory
- Cases of serotonin syndrome with fluvoxamine, fluoxetine and paroxetine

| B. Neurological Effects |
- Increase in motor activity more common in children than adults
- Fine tremor [may respond to dose reduction or propranolol]
- Akathisia [may respond to dose reduction, propranolol or a benzodiazepine], hyperkinesia
- Exacerbation of nervous tics reported with paroxetine
- Myoclonus (e.g., periodic leg movements during sleep) [may respond to lamotrigine, gabapentin or bromocriptine]; may increase spasticity; recurrence of restless legs syndrome (paroxetine)
- May induce or worsen extrapyramidal effects when given with antipsychotics (see Drug Interactions p. 49)

| Cardiovascular Effects |
- Reports of bradycardia, tachycardia, palpitations, hypertension, and atrial fibrillation
- Dizziness and impaired balance

| GI Effects |
- A result of inhibition of 5-HT reuptake (activation of 5-HT_3 receptors)
- Nausea (up to 21%), dyspepsia (6–21%) reported; vomiting – generally decreases over time due to gradual desensitization of 5-HT_3 receptors [can minimize by starting with a low dose and taking drug with meals; cyproheptadine (2 mg) or lactobacillus acidophilus (e.g., yogurt)]; diarrhea, bloating – usually transient and dose-related
- Anorexia (up to 12% incidence) and weight loss frequently reported during early treatment – more pronounced in overweight patients and those with carbohydrate cravings – monitor weight and growth
- Reports of upper GI bleeding in adults, especially if combined with NSAIDs or ASA
- Weight gain reported with chronic use (more common with paroxetine); citalopram associated with phasic craving for carbohydrate

| Sexual Side Effects |
- A result of increased serotonergic transmission by way of the 5-HT_2 receptor (which results in reduced dopaminergic transmission), acetylcholine (ACh) blockade, and reduced nitric oxide levels – appear to be dose-related
- Reports in adolescents are considerably lower than in adults – may be due to under-reporting or lack of of questioning
- Decreased libido, impotence, ejaculatory disturbances may occur
- Anorgasmia or delayed orgasm

| Endocrine Effects |
- Can induce SIADH (syndrome of inappropriate secretion of antidiuretic hormone) with hyponatremia; risk increases with age, female sex, low body weight, smoking and concomitant diuretic or carbamazepine use
- Elevated prolactin; cases of galactorrhea reported
- Up to 30% decrease in fasting blood glucose has been reported in adults
- Gynecomastia reported in adults
- Chronic use of fluoxetine and probably other SSRIs may slightly reduce growth rate in some children and adolescents – reversible on drug discontinuation

Selective Serotonin Reuptake Inhibitors (SSRI) (cont.)

Allergic Reactions	• Rash, urticaria, psoriasis, pruritus, edema • Increased hepatic enzyme levels, bilirubinemia, jaundice, hepatitis • Rare blood dyscrasias including neutropenia and aplastic anemia • Bleeding disorders including petechiae, purpura; epistaxis, thrombocytopenia with fluoxetine; bruising reported with all SSRI drugs (case reports) – attributed to inhibition of serotonin uptake by platelets
Other Adverse Effects	• Alopecia in adults • Rhinitis common, pharyngitis, influenza-like symptoms • Sweating [Management: daily showering, talcum powder; in severe cases: Drysol solution, clonidine 0.1 mg bid, benztropine 0.5 mg hs; drug may need to be changed]
DISCONTINUATION SYNDROME	• Symptoms attributed to rapid decrease in 5HT availability • Abrupt withdrawal may cause a discontinuation syndrome consisting of *somatic symptoms:* dizziness (exacerbated by movement), lethargy, nausea, vomiting, diarrhea headache, fever, sweating, chills, malaise, incoordination, insomnia, vivid dreams; *neurological symptoms:* myalgia, paresthesias, dyskinesias, "electric-shock-like" sensations, visual discoordination; *psychological symptoms:* anxiety, agitation, crying, irritability, confusion, slowed thinking, disorientation; rarely aggression, impulsivity, hypomania, mania and depersonalization. • Most likely to occur within 1–7 days after withdrawal and typically disappear within 3 weeks • Incidence is related to half-life of antidepressant – reported most frequently with paroxetine, least with fluoxetine ☞ **THEREFORE THESE MEDICATIONS SHOULD BE WITHDRAWN GRADUALLY AFTER PROLONGED USE** • Taper antidepressant no more rapidly than 25% per week (or nearest dose possible) and monitor for recurrence of depressive symptoms
Management	• Re-institute drug or substitute a long-acting SSRI (e.g., fluoxetine) and taper more slowly • Supportive care to keep patient comfortable
PRECAUTIONS	• **Risk of self-harm and suicidal ideation reported to be higher in children and adolescents with several SSRIs (fluoxetine excluded) than with placebo. Monitor for worsening depression and suicidal thoughts especially at start of therapy and following an increase in dose** • May impair the mental and physical ability to perform hazardous tasks (e.g., driving a car or operating machinery) • May induce manic reactions in up to 30–40% of patients with bipolar disorders (BD) – reported more frequently with fluoxetine; because of risk of increased cycling, BD is a relative contraindication unless a mood stabilizer is added – adolescents whose first presentation of BD is depression account for a high incidence of switch ☞ **Use of SSRIs with other serotonergic agents may result in a Serotonin Syndrome – usually occurs within 24 h of medication initiation, overdose or change in dose. Symptoms include: nausea, diarrhea, chills, sweating, dizziness, elevated temperature, elevated blood pressure, palpitations, increased muscle tone with twitching, tremor, myoclonic jerks, hyperreflexia, unsteady gait, restlessness, agitation, excitation, disorientation, confusion and delirium; may progress to rhabdomyolysis, coma and death (see Drug**

Interactions) [**Treatment: stop medication and administer supportive care; cyproheptadine 2–8 mg (0.25 mg/kg/day) may reduce duration of symptoms**]
- Fluoxetine, paroxetine and sertraline will displace drugs from protein binding and elevate their plasma levels
- Fluoxetine, fluvoxamine, and paroxetine affect cytochrome P-450 and will inhibit the metabolism (and elevate the levels) of drugs metabolized by this system; sertraline will inhibit metabolism in higher doses (over 100 mg/day) (see Drug Interactions p. 48)
- Caution when switching from fluoxetine to another antidepressant (see Drug Interactions), or from one SSRI to another
- Lower doses should be used in patients with renal or hepatic disease

MONITORING
- Height and weight at treatment initiation and periodically throughout treatment
- For worsening depression and suicideal thoughts at start of therapy and following an increase or decrease in dose

TOXICITY
- SSRIs have a low probability of causing dose-related toxicity (one fatality reported with dose of 6000 mg of fluoxetine; seizure reported in adolescent after ingestion of 1880 mg); fatal outcome in 6 patients with citalopram 840–3920 mg (5 had also taken other sedative drugs or alcohol); fatalities reported with overdoses of citalopram and moclobemide
- Symptoms include: nausea, vomiting, tremor, myoclonus, irritability; ECG changes and seizures rarely reported with citalopram
- Case of Serotonin syndrome reported after overdose of 8 g of sertraline

Treatment
- Treatment: symptomatic and supportive

USE IN PREGNANCY
- Paroxetine may be associated with birth defects when it is taken during the first trimester; increased risk of heart defects (1.5–2%) as compared to normal (1%) – Category D drug; other SSRIs have not been demonstrated to have teratogenic effects in humans (with escitalopram teratogenic effects have been reported in animal studies)
- Possible increased risk of miscarriage
- Newborns exposed to SSRIs during second half of pregnancy seem to have a higher risk of persistent pulmonary hypertension
- If possible, avoid during first and third trimester; when stopping the SSRI, taper the dose gradually to minimize adverse fetal outcome; with fluoxetine be aware of long half-life of metabolite, norfluoxetine
- Reports of an increase in premature births and poor neonatal adaptation when drug taken in the third trimester
- Transient withdrawal effects reported in neonate include jitteriness, restlessness, irritability, tremors, acrocyanosis, tachypnea, temperature instability, and seizures (with fluoxetine is related to blood level of fluoxetine and norfluoxetine)

Breast Milk
- Fluoxetine and citalopram appear in breast milk in therapeutic levels; caution: infant can receive up to 17% of maternal dose of fluoxetine and up to 9% of dose of citalopram
- Sertraline, paroxetine and fluvoxamine are present in low concentrations in plasma of breastfed infants
- The American Academy of Pediatrics considers SSRIs as "drugs whose effect on nursing infants is unknown but may be of concern."

NURSING IMPLICATIONS
- Psychotherapy (cognitive behavior therapy and interpersonal therapy) are also important in the treatment of depression and may have minor additive effects to antidepressants
- It is important to educate the patient, family, and caregivers about symptoms, course, and treatment options for depression
- Monitor therapy by watching for adverse effects, mood, and activity level changes including thoughts of suicide or self-harm

Selective Serotonin Reuptake Inhibitors (SSRI) (cont.)

- Be aware that the medication reduces the degree of depression and may increase psychomotor activity; this may create concern about suicidal behavior
- Excessive ingestion of caffeinated foods, drugs, or beverages may increase anxiety and agitation and confuse the diagnosis
- Fluvoxamine tablets should be swallowed whole, with water, without chewing
- Sertraline should be given with food (increases peak plasma level); food will also reduce incidence of nausea with SSRIs
- Ingestion of grapefruit juice while taking fluvoxamine or sertraline may increase the plasma level of these drugs
- Monitor height and growth of children on long-term therapy

PATIENT INSTRUCTIONS

- Detailed instructions for patients and caregivers are provided in the Information Sheet on p. 292

DRUG INTERACTIONS

- Clinically significant interactions are listed below

Class of Drug	Example	Interaction Effects
Analgesic	Acetylsalicylic acid (see NSAID, p.14)	Increased risk of upper GI bleed with combined use
Anorexiant	Phentermine	Case reports of mania and psychosis in combination
Antiarrhythmic	Propafenone, flecainide, mexiletine	Increased plasma level of antiarrhythmic with fluoxetine and paroxetine due to inhibited metabolism via CYP2D6
	Quinidine, lidocaine	Increased plasma level of antiarrhythmic possible with fluoxetine, fluvoxamine, sertraline, and paroxetine due to inhibited metabolism via CYP3A4
Antibiotic	Clarithromycin	Case of delirium with fluoxetine; case of serotonin syndrome with citalopram
	Erythromycin	Increased plasma level of citalopram due to inhibited metabolism via CYP3A4 is possible but not confirmed; case of serotonin syndrome with sertraline in a 12-year-old
	Linezolid	Monitor for serotonergic effects due to linezolid's weak MAO inhibition
Anticoagulants	Warfarin	Increased risk of bleeding; increased prothrombin ratio or INR response due to decreased platelet aggregation secondary to depletion of serotonin Loss of anticoagulant control with fluoxetine – data contradictory 65% increase in plasma level of warfarin with fluvoxamine due to accumulation of R-warfarin through inhibited metabolism (via CYP1A2 and 3A4) and decreased clearance of S-isomer (via CYP2C9) and with paroxetine
Anticonvulsant	Barbiturates	Barbiturate metabolism inhibited by fluoxetine; reduced plasma level of SSRIs due to enzyme induction
	Carbamazepine, phenytion, phenobarbital	Decreased plasma level of SSRIs; half-life of paroxetine decreased by 28% Increased plasma level of carbamazepine or phenytoin due to inhibition of metabolism with fluoxetine and fluvoxamine; elevated phenytoin level with sertraline and paroxetine
	Valproate, valproic acid, divalproex	Increased nausea with fluvoxamine and carbamazepine Increased plasma level of valproate (up to 50%) with fluoxtine Valproate may increase plasma level of fluoxetine
	Topiramate	Two case reports of angle-closure glaucoma in females on combination
Antidepressant Cyclic (non-selective)	Amitriptyline, desipramine, imipramine	Elevated plasma level of cyclic antidepressant with fluoxetine, fluvoxamine and paroxetine due to release from protein binding and inhibition of oxidative metabolism; can occur with higher doses of sertraline Increased desipramine level (by 50%) with citalopram and escitalopram

Class of Drug	Example	Interaction Effects
	Clomipramine	Additive antidepressant effect in treatment-resistant patients Increased serotonergic effects
Irreversible MAOIs	Phenelzine, tranylcypromine	"Serotonin syndrome" (see p. 46) and death reported with combined use. Suggest waiting 5 weeks when switching from fluoxetine to MAOI and vice versa.
RIMA	Moclobemide	Combined therapy may have additive antidepressant effect in treatment-resistant patients; use caution and monitor for serotonergic effects; case reports of serotonin syndrome
NDRI	Bupropion	Additive antidepressant effect in refractory patients. Bupropion may reverse SSRI-induced sexual dysfunction. Case of hypersexual behavior in combination with fluoxetine Cases of anxiety, panic, delirium, tremor, myoclonus and seizure reported with fluoxetine due to inhibited metabolism of bupropion and/or fluoxetine (via CYP3A4 and 2D6), competition for protein binding, and additive pharmacological effects
NaSSA	Mirtazapine	Combination reported to alleviate insomnia and augment antidepressant response May mitigate SSRI-induced sexual dysfunction and "poop-out" syndrome Increased serotonergic effects possible Increased sedation and weight gain reported with combination Increased mirtazapine level (up to 4-fold) reported in combination with fluvoxamine due to inhibited metabolism
SARI	Trazodone, nefazodone	Elevated plasma level of SARI; increased serotonergic effects Increased level of MCPP metabolite of trazodone and nefazodone, with paroxetine (via inhibition of CYP2D6) resulting in increased anxiogenic potential Nefazodone may reverse SSRI-induced sexual dysfunction and enhance REM sleep
SNRI	Venlafaxine	Reports that combination with SSRIs that inhibit CYP2D6 (e.g., paroxetine, fluoxetine) can result in increased levels of venlafaxine with possible increase in blood pressure, anticholinergic effects, and serotonergic effects
Antiemetic (5-HT3 antagonists)	Dolasetron, granisetron, ondansetron Alosetron	Reports of serotonin syndrome with paroxetine and sertraline DO NOT USE with fluvoxamine as plasma level of alosetron increased 6-fold and half-life increased 3-fold due to inhibited metabolism via CYP3A4
Antifungal	Ketoconazole	Decreased C_{max} of ketoconazole by 21% with citalopram
Antihistamine	Diphenhydramine	Increased plasma levels of fluoxetine and paroxetine possible, due to inhibited metabolism via CYP2D6 Additive CNS effects (e.g., sedation)
Antiparkinsonian agents	Benztropine Procyclidine	Increased plasma level of benztropine with paroxetine Increased plasma level of procyclidine with paroxetine (by 40%)
Antipsychotic	General	May worsen extrapyramidal effects and akathisia, especially if antidepressant added early in the course of antipsychotic therapy May be useful for negative symptoms of schizophrenia Additive effect in treatment of OCD Case reports of dose-related mania when **risperidone** or **ziprasidone** added to SSRI
	Chlorpromazine, fluphenazine, haloperidol, perphenazine, risperidone, olanzapine	Increased serum level of antipsychotic (up to 100% increase in **haloperidol** level with fluvoxamine or fluoxetine and 4-fold increase with sertraline) (up to 21-fold increase in peak plasma level of **perphenazine** with paroxetine) (increased AUC by 119% and decreased clearance (by 50%) of **olanzapine** with fluvoxamine) (2.8-fold increase in **risperidone** level with fluoxetine as well as with paroxetine and sertraline – case of serotonin syndrome with paroxetine)

Selective Serotonin Reuptake Inhibitors (SSRI) (cont.)

Class of Drug	Example	Interaction Effects
	Thioridazine, pimozide	(40% increase in **pimozide** AUC and C_{max} with sertraline) (3-fold increase in **thioridazine** levels with fluvoxamine) **Pimozide** levels increased when combined with citalopram, sertraline, escitalopram, or fluvoxamine increasing risk of QT_C prolongation DO NOT COMBINE DO NOT COMBINE fluvoxamine, fluoxetine, or paroxetine with **thioridazine,** due to risk of cardiac conduction disturbances
	Clozapine	Fluvoxamine increases steady-state plasma clozapine levels 5–10 fold, decreases the norclozapine / clozapine ratio, and inhibits its metabolism (via multiple CYP isoenzymes); this results in a reduction of metabolic side effects (attributed to norclozapine); this results in a reduction of metabolic side effects (attributed to norclozapine) and a need to use a lower dose of clozapine to achieve therapeutic effects 76% increase in clozapine level with fluoxetine, and 40–45% increase with paroxetine and sertraline; potentially significant increases reported with citalopram
Anxiolytic Benzodiazepines	Alprazolam, diazepam, bromazepam	Increased plasma level of alprazolam (by 100%), bromazepam, triazolam and diazepam with fluvoxamine and fluoxetine, due to inhibited metabolism; small (13%) decrease in clearance of diazepam reported with sertraline Increased sedation, psychomotor and memory impairment
Buspirone		May potentiate anti-obsessional effects Anxiolytic effects of buspirone may be antagonized Increased plasma level of buspirone (3-fold) with fluvoxamine Case report of possible serotonin syndrome with fluoxetine (see p. 46)
β-Blockers	Propranolol, metoprolol	Decreased heart rate and syncope (additive effect) reported Increased side effects, lethargy, and bradycardia with fluoxetine and fluvoxamine due to decreased metabolism of the β-blocker via CYP2D6 (five-fold increase in propranolol level reported with fluvoxamine) Increased metoprolol level (100%) with citalopram and with escitalopram (by 50%)
	Pindolol	Increased concentration of serotonin at post-synaptic sites; increased onset of therapeutic response Increased half-life of pindolol (by 28%) with fluoxetine; increased plasma level with paroxetine due to inhibited metabolism via CYP2D6
Caffeine		Increased caffeine levels with fluvoxamine due to inhibited metabolism via CYP1A2; half-life increased from 5 to 31 h Increased jitteriness and insomnia
Ca-channel blocker	Nifedipine, verapamil, nicardapine	Increased side effects (headache, flushing, edema) due to inhibited clearance of Ca-channel blocker with fluoxetine, fluvoxamine, sertraline, and paroxetine via CYP3A4
	Diltiazem	Bradycardia in combination with fluvoxamine
CNS depressants	Alcohol, antihistamines Chloral hydrate	Rate of fluvoxamine absorption increased by ethanol Increased sedation and side effects with fluoxetine due to inhibited metabolism of chloral hydrate
Corticosteroid		Increased risk of GI bleed
Cyclobenzaprine		Increased side effects of cyclobenzaprine with fluoxetine, due to inhibited metabolism; observe for QT prolongation
Cyproheptadine		Report of reversal of antidepressant and antibulimic effects of fluoxetine and paroxetine

Class of Drug	Example	Interaction Effects
Digoxin		Decreased level (area under curve) of digoxin by 18% reported with paroxetine
Ergot alkaloid	Dihydroergotamine	Increased serotonergic effects with intravenous use - AVOID. Oral, rectal and subcutaneous routes can be used, with monitoring
	Ergotamine	Elevated ergotamine levels possible due to inhibited metabolism, via CYP3A4, with fluoxetine and fluvoxamine
Grapefruit juice		Decreased metabolism of fluvoxamine and sertraline resulting in increased plasma levels
H$_2$ antagonist	Cimetidine Tizanidine	Inhibited metabolism and increased plasma level of sertraline (by 25%), paroxetine (by 50%), citalopram and escitalopram Increased AUC of tizanidine (14- to 103-fold), increased C$_{max}$ (5- to 32-fold), and half-life (3-fold) with fluvoxamine due to inhibition of metabolism via CYP1A2. AVOID
Hallucinogen	LSD	Recurrence or worsening of flashbacks reported with fluoxetine, sertraline, paroxetine Grand mal seizure
Hormone	Oral contraceptive	Increased activity of combined oral contraceptive possible with fluoxetine and fluvoxamine due to inhibited metabolism
Immunosuppressant	Cyclosporin	Decreased clearance of cyclosporin with sertraline due to competition for metabolism via CYP3A4
Lithium		Increased serotonergic effects Changes in lithium level and clearance reported Caution with fluoxetine and fluvoxamine; neurotoxicity and seizures reported Increased tremor and nausea reported with sertraline and paroxetine
L-Tryptophan		May result in central and peripheral toxicity, ("serotonin syndrome" (see p. 46)
MAO-B inhibitor	Selegiline (L-deprenyl)	Case reports of serotonin syndrome, hypertension, and mania when combined with fluoxetine
Melatonin		Increased levels of melatonin with fluvoxamine due to inhibited metabolism via CYP1A2 or 2C9; endogenous melatonin secretion increased
Metoclopramide		Report of increased extrapyramidal and serotonergic effects wih sertraline
Narcotic	Codeine, oxycodone, hydrocodone	Decreased analgesic effect with fluoxetine and paroxetine due to inhibited metabolism to active moiety – morphine, oxymorphone and hydromorphone, respectively (interaction may be beneficial in the treatment of dependence by decreasing morphine and analog formation and opiate reinforcing properties)
	Pentazocine, tramadol	Report of excitatory toxicity (serotonergic) with fluoxetine and pentazocine; and with paroxetine, sertraline and tramadol
	Dextromethorphan	Visual hallucinations reported with fluoxetine
	Methadone	Elevated plasma level of methadone by 10–100% reported with fluvoxamine
	Morphine, fentanyl	Enhanced analgesia
NSAID		Increased risk of upper GI bleed with combined use (risk increased 12-fold). CAUTION
Omeprazole		Increased plasma level of citalopram due to inhibited metabolism via CYP2C19
Proguanil		Increased plasma level of proguanil with fluvoxamine due to inhibited metabolism via CYP2C19

Selective Serotonin Reuptake Inhibitors (SSRI) (cont.)

Class of Drug	Example	Interaction Effects
Protease inhibitors	Ritonavir	Increased plasma level of sertraline due to competition for metabolism; moderate increase in level of fluoxetine and paroxetine. Serotonin syndrome reported in combination with high dose of fluoxetine Cardiac and neurological side effects reported with fluoxetine, due to elevated ritonavir level (19% increase AUC)
	Fosamprenavir / ritonavir	Decreased plasma level of paroxetine
Sibutramine		Reports of serotonin syndrome (see p. 46) Case report of hypomania with citalopram
Sildenafil		Possible enhanced hypotension due to inhibited metabolism of sildenafil via CYP3A4 with fluoxetine and fluvoxamine
Smoking – cigarettes		Increased metabolism of fluvoxamine by 25% via CYP1A2
Statin	Lovastatin	Increased plasma level of statin with fluoxetine, fluvoxamine, sertraline, and paroxetine due to inhibited metabolism via CYP3A4
St. John's Wort		May augment serotonergic effects - several reports of serotonin syndrome (see p. 46)
Stimulant	Amphetamines, methylphenidate	Potentiated effect in depression, dysthymia, and OCD, in patients with comorbid ADHD; may improve response in treatment-refractory paraphilias and paraphilia-related disorders Plasma level of antidepressant may be increased
Sulfonylurea antidiabetic agent	Glyburide, tolbutamide	Increased hypoglycemia reported in diabetics Increased plasma level of tolbutamide due to reduced clearance (up to 16%) with sertraline
Tacrine		Increased plasma level of tacrine with fluvoxamine; peak plasma level increased 5-fold and clearance decreased by 88% due to inhibited metabolism via CYP1A2
Tamoxifen		Inhibitors of CYP2D6 (paroxetine, fluoxetine) appear to reduce the conversion of tamoxifen to its active metabolite (endoxifen) and may decrease the therapeutic efficacy of this drug
Theophylline		Increased plasma level of theophylline with fluvoxamine due to decreased metabolism via CYP1A2
Thyroid drug	Triiodothyronine (T_3-liothyronine)	Antidepressant effect potentiated Elevated serum thyrotropin (and reduced free thyroxine concentration) reported with sertraline
Tolterodine		Decreased oral clearance of tolterodine by up to 93% with fluoxetine due to inhibited metabolism via CYP2D6
Triptan	Sumatriptan, rizatriptan, zolmitriptan	Increased serotonergic effects possible (rare); exacerbation of migraine headache reported with combination
Zolpidem		Case reports of hallucinations and delirium when combined with sertraline, fluoxetine and paroxetine Chronic (5-night) administration of sertraline resulted in faster onset of action and increase in peak plasma concentration of zolpidem

Norepinephrine Dopamine Reuptake Inhibitor (NDRI)

PRODUCT AVAILABILITY

Chemical Class	Generic Name	Trade Name(A)	Dosage Forms and Strengths	Monograph Statement
Monocyclic agent (aminoketone)	Bupropion (amfebutamone)	Wellbutrin(B) Wellbutrin-SR, Zyban(D) Wellbutrin XL (B)	Tablets(B): 75 mg, 100 mg Sustained-release tablets: 100 mg, 150 mg, 200 mg(B) Extended-release tablets: 150 mg, 300 mg	Safety and efficacy not established in children under age 18

(A) Generic preparations may be available, (B) Not marketed in Canada, (D) Marketed as aid in smoking cessation

INDICATIONS

No approved indications in children and adolescents

Approved (for Adults)

- Major depression
- Prophylaxis of recurrent major depression
- Depressed phase of bipolar disorder
- Aid in smoking cessation (Zyban)

Other Uses in Children and Adolescents

- Open trials suggest benefit in adolescents and adults with ADHD and comorbid conduct disorder with substance use disorder
- Open trial reports benefit in 14 adolescent outpatients with ADHD, mood disorders, and substance use disorder
- Controlled studies with immediate-release preparation suggest benefit in ADHD in adults and children
- Efficacy reported in seasonal affective disorder, dysthymia and chronic fatigue syndrome; case reports of efficacy in social phobia
- Reports of efficacy in alleviating sexual dysfunction (anorgasmia, erectile problems) induced by SSRIs and SNRI
- Early data suggest bupropion reduces movements in depressed patients with periodic limb movement disorder

PHARMACOLOGY

- Inhibits the re-uptake of primarily norepinephrine (and dopamine to a lesser extent) into presynaptic neurons; limited effect on serotonergic pathways

GENERAL COMMENTS

- Monitor all patients for worsening of depression and suicidal thoughts
- Clinical trials done with immediate-release preparation in 104 children with major depressive disorders, aged 6–16, showed drug was well tolerated
- Small, unpublished open-label study found 79% of adolescents with major depressive disorders, on an average of 362 mg of bupropion, had improved

DOSING

- See p.
- Dosage in children: initiate at 1 mg/kg/day, in divided doses, and increase gradually to a maximum of 6 mg/kg/day (divided doses)
- Regular bupropion and SR preparation should be prescribed in divided doses, with a maximum of 150 mg per dose; Wellbutrin XL formulated for once daily dosing
- In adolescents with ADHD: begin at 75–100 mg/day and titrate dose by 75–100 mg per week to a maximum of 450 mg/day in divided doses (range: 3–6 mg/kg/day); up to 6 weeks may be required for maximum drug effect

Norepinephrine Dopamine Reuptake Inhibitor (NDRI) (cont.)

PHARMACOKINETICS

- Rapid absorption with peak concentration occurring within 3 h (mean = 1.5 h); peak plasma concentration of sustained-release preparation is 50–85% of the immediate-release tablets after single dosing, and 25% after chronic dosing
- Slow-release preparations appear to be better tolerated and associated with a decreased risk of seizures
- Highly bound to plasma protein (80–85%)
- Metabolized predominantly by the liver primarily via CYP2B6 and to a lesser extent by other isoenzymes – 6 metabolites; 3 are active
- Bupropion and hydroxybupropion inhibit CYP2D6 isoenzyme
- Elimination half-life: 11–14 h; with chronic dosing: 21 h (mean); C_{max}, volume of distribution and elimination half-life are greater in females than in males
- Weak inducer of its own metabolism and of other drugs
- Use cautiously in patients with hepatic impairment – reduce dose or frequency of administration

ONSET AND DURATION

- Therapeutic effect seen after 7–28 days

ADVERSE EFFECTS

- See chart on p. 96 for incidence of adverse effects

CNS Effects

- A result of antagonism at histamine H_1-receptors and α_1-adrenoreceptors

A. Cognitive Effects

- Insomnia; vivid dreams and nightmares reported; decreased REM latency and increased REM sleep
- Agitation common, anxiety, irritability, dysphoria, aggression, hostility, depersonalization coupled with urges of self-harm of harm to others (in 2–3%)
- Precipitation of hypomania or mania; may occur when patient is experiencing the onset of bipolar disorder. Increased risk in bipolar patients with comorbid substance abuse. Careful monitoring for "switch to mania" is necessary
- Can exacerbate psychotic symptoms
- Very high doses can result in CNS toxicity including confusion, impaired concentration, hallucinations, delusions, delirium, EPS
- and seizures

B. Neurological Effects

- Seizures can occur after abrupt dose increases, or use of daily doses above 300 mg; use divided doses (maximum single dose no greater than 150 mg) – anorexic and bulimic patients may be at higher risk due to possible electrolyte imbalance. Risk of seizures in adults, at doses of 100–300 mg = 0.1%; at 300–450 mg = 0.4%; above 450 mg risk increases 10-fold; risk with SR preparation = 0.15% (doses up to 300 mg)
- Disturbance in gait, fine tremor, myoclonus
- Headache common, arthralgia, neuralgias, myalgia [Management: analgesics prn]
- Exacerbation of tics reported in ADHD and Tourette's syndrome

Anticholinergic Effects

- Due to NE-reuptake inhibition
- Occur rarely
- Dry mouth
- Sweating

Cardiovascular Effects	• Modest sustained increases in blood pressure reported in adults and children (more likely in patients with pre-existing hypertension)
	• Orthostatic hypotension, dizziness occurs occasionally
	• Palpitations

Endocrine Effects	• Menstrual irregularities reported
	• Cases of hypoglycemia reported

Other Adverse Effects	• GI complaints common
	• Urticarial or pruritic rashes have been reported in up to 17% of youths; rare cases of erythema multiforme and Stevens-Johnson syndrome
	• Reports of serum sickness-like reactions (in children aged 12 and 14)
	• Rarely febrile neutropenia
	• Anorexia
	• Alopecia

DISCONTINUATION SYNDROME

• Case of mania reported 2 weeks after abrupt discontinuation of bupropion 300mg/day taken for 5 weeks to aid in smoking cessation

SPECIAL CONSIDERATIONS

• Bupropion does not potentiate the sedative effects of alcohol
• Rarely impairs sexual functioning or behavior; some improvement noted
• There is no evidence of increased abuse potential (considering bupropion is related to the sympathomimetic drug diethylpropion)

PRECAUTION

• Monitor all patients for worsening depression and suicidal thoughts at start of therapy and following an increase or decrease in dose
• May lower the seizure threshold; therefore avoid in patients with a history of convulsive disorders. Use cautiously in patients with organic brain disease and when combining with other drugs that may lower the seizure threshold. To minimize seizures with regular-release bupropion, do not exceed a dose increase of 50–100 mg in a 3-day period. No single dose should exceed 150 mg for the immediate-release or the sustained-release preparation
• Contraindicated in patients with history of anorexia, bulimia, undergoing alcohol or benzodiazepine withdrawal, or with other conditions predisposing to seizures
• Use with caution (i.e., use lower dose and monitor regularly) in patients with hepatic impairment
• Zyban, marketed for smoking cessation, contains bupropion – DO NOT COMBINE with Wellbutrin

TOXICITY

• Rare reports of death following massive overdose, preceded by uncontrolled seizures, bradycardia, cardiac failure and cardiac arrest

Management	• Induce vomiting
	• Activated charcoal given every 6–12 h
	• Supportive treatment
	• Monitor ECG and EEG

USE IN PREGNANCY

• No harm to fetus reported in animal studies; no data on effects in humans

Breast Milk	• Bupropion and metabolites are secreted in breast milk; infant can receive up to 2.7% of maternal dose – effects on infant unknown
	• Case report of probable seizure in infant

Norepinephrine Dopamine Reuptake Inhibitor (NDRI) (cont.)

NURSING IMPLICATIONS

- Risk of seizures increases if any single dose exceeds 150 mg (immediate-release or sustained-release), or if total daily dose exceeds 300 mg; doses above 150 mg daily should be given in divided doses, preferably 8 h or more apart
- Crushing or chewing the sustained-release preparation destroys the slow-release activity of the product; cutting or splitting the SR preparation in half will increase the rate of drug release in the first 15 minutes. If the tablet is split, the unused half should be discarded unless used within 24 h
- Bupropion degrades rapidly on exposure to moisture, therefore tablets should not be stored in an area of high humidity
- Monitor therapy by watching for adverse effects, mood and activity level changes including worsening depression and suicidal thoughts, especially at the start of therapy or following an increase or decrease in dose
- If the patient has difficulty sleeping, ensure that the last dose of bupropion is no later than 1500 h
- Ensure the patient is not currently being treated for smoking cessation with Zyban (also contains bupropion)

PATIENT INSTRUCTIONS

- Detailed instructions for patients and caregivers are provided in the Information Sheet on p. 294.

DRUG INTERACTIONS

- Clinically significant interactions are listed below

Class of Drug	Example	Interaction Effects
Amantadine		Increased side effects, including excitement, restlessness and tremor due to increased dopamine availability Case reports of neurotoxicity in elderly patients; delirium
Antiarrhythmic (Type 1c)	Propafenone, flecainidefe	Increased plasma level of antiarrhythmic due to inhibited metabolism via CYP2D6
Antibiotic	Ciprofloxacin	Seizure threshold may be reduced
	Linezolid	Due to weak MAOI activity, monitor for increased serotonergic effects
Anticholinergic	Antiparkinsonian agents, antihistamines, etc.	Increased anticholinergic effect
	Orphenadrine	Altered levels of either drug due to competition for metabolism via CYP2B6
Anticonvulsant	Carbamazepine, phenytoin, phenobarbital	Decreased plasma level of bupropion and increased level of its metabolite hydroxybupropion due to increased metabolism by the anticonvulsant
	Valproate	Increased level of hydroxybupropion due to inhibited metabolism; level of bupropion not affected
Antidepressant Cyclic (non-selective)	Imipramine, desipramine, nortriptyline	Elevated imipramine level (by 57%) and nortriptyline level (by 200%) with combination; desipramine peak plasma level and half-life increased up to 5-fold due to decreased metabolism (via CYP2D6) Seizure threshold may be reduced Additive antidepressant effect in treatment-refractory patients
Irreversible MAOI	Phenelzine	DO NOT COMBINE – dopamine metabolism inhibited
SSRI	Fluoxetine	Case of delirium, anxiety, panic and myoclonus with fluoxetine due to inhibited metabolism of bupropion and/or fluoxetine (via CYP3A2 and 2D6), competition for protein binding and additive pharmacological effects Additive antidepressant effect in treatment-refractory patients; bupropion may mitigate SSRI-induced sexual dysfunction

Class of Drug	Example	Interaction Effects
SNRI	Venlafaxine	3-fold increase in venlafaxine level due to inhibited metabolism via CYP2D6, and reduction of level of OD-metabolite Potentiation of noradrenergic effects
Antimalarial	Mefloquine, chloroquine	Seizure threshold may be reduced
Antipsychotic	Thioridazine	Increased plasma level of thioridazine due to decreased metabolism via CYP2D6; increased risk of thioridazine-related ventricular arrhythmias and sudden death. DO NOT COMBINE. Washout of 14 days recommended between drugs
	Chlorpromazine	Seizure threshold may be reduced
β-Blocker	Metoprolol	Increased plasma level of β-blocker possible due to inhibited metabolism via CYP2D6
Corticosteroid (systemic)		Seizure threshold may be reduced
Ginkgo biloba		Seizure threshold may be reduced
Hormone	Estrogen/Progesterone	Decreased metabolism (hydroxylation) of bupropion via CYP2B6
Insulin		Seizure threshold may be reduced
L-Dopa		Increased side effects, including excitement, restlessness, nausea, vomiting and tremor due to increased dopamine availability; case reports of neurotoxicity
Lithium		Additive antidepressant effect
Nicotine transdermal		Combination reported to promote higher rates of smoking cessation than either drug alone Increased risk of hypertension with combination
Nitrogen mustard analog	Cyclophosphamide, ifosfamide	Altered levels of either drug due to competition for metabolism via CYP2B6
Protease inhibitor	Ritonavir, nelfinavir, efavirenz	Increased plasma level of bupropion due to decreased metabolism via CYP2B6; risk of seizure
Stimulant	Methylphenidate, dextroamphetamine	Additive effect in ADHD
Sympathomimetic	Pseudoephedrine	Report of manic-like reaction with pseudoephedrine Seizure threshold may be reduced
Theophylline		Seizure threshold may be reduced
Tramadol		Seizure threshold may be reduced
Zolpidem		Case reports of visual hallucinations with combination

Selective Serotonin Norepinephrine Reuptake Inhibitor (SNRI)

PRODUCT AVAILABILITY

Chemical Class	Generic Name	Trade Name[A]	Dosage Forms and Strengths	Monograph Statement
Bicyclic agent (phenethylamine)	Venlafaxine	Effexor Effexor XR	Tablets: 25 mg[B], 37.5 mg, 50 mg[B], 75mg, 100 mg[B] Sustained-release tablets: 37.5 mg, 75mg, 150 mg	Not indicated for children under age 18 (see Precautions)
	Duloxetine[B]	Cymbalta	Delayed-release capsules 20mg, 30mg, 60mg	Not approved for use in children

[A] Generic preparations may be available, [B] Not marketed in Canada

INDICATIONS

Approved (for Adults)

- No approved indications for children or adolescents – Manufacturer recommends against using venlafaxine in pediatric patients due to lack of efficacy and concerns of increased hostility and suicidal ideation (rate = 2%; placebo = 1%)

- Major depressive disorder (MDD) – open-label studies suggest efficacy; two double-blind studies with patients aged 8–17 found venlafaxine and psychotherapy equal to placebo and psychotherapy
- Generalized anxiety disorder (GAD – venlafaxine) – one of two double-blind studies of venlafaxine in children aged 6–17 reported moderate efficacy; two unpublished double-blind trials found equal efficacy in placebo
- Panic disorder (venlafaxine)
- Social anxiety disorder (venlafaxine)
- Pain due to diabetic neuropathy (duloxetine)

Other Uses in Children and Adolescents

- Depressed phase of bipolar affective disorder
- Preliminary studies suggest efficacy of venlafaxine in children and adults with ADHD
- Preliminary data suggest a role in children with social anxiety disorder (venlafaxine)
- Open trial suggests benefit of venlafaxine in children and adolescents with autism spectrum disorders; improvement noted in repetitive behaviors and restricted interests, social deficits, communication and language function, inattention and hyperactivity

PHARMACOLOGY

- Potent reuptake inhibitor of serotonin and norepinephrine; inhibition of dopamine reuptake occurs at high doses
- Rapid down-regulation of β-receptors; may slow early onset of clinical activity

GENERAL COMMENTS

- Dosing is similar for MDD and GAD; some patients with GAD, however, may require a slower titration
- SNRIs should be reserved for those patients with moderate to severe mood or anxiety disorder who do not respond to or tolerate SSRIs
- Monitor all patients for worsening depression and suicidal thoughts

DOSING

Venlafaxine

- See p. 92
- In children, initiate *venlafaxine* at 12.5–25 mg with food (once daily for XR preparation and twice daily for regular preparation), and increase weekly by 12.5–25 mg increments to a maximum of 75 mg/day (in divided doses); some patients may require higher doses (in divided doses). For ADHD 0.5–3mg/kg/day

	• In adolescents (> age 12) initiate dose at 18.75–37.5 mg with food and increase weekly by 18.75–37.5 mg increments to a maximum of 225 mg/day (divided doses)

- In adolescents (> age 12) initiate dose at 18.75–37.5 mg with food and increase weekly by 18.75–37.5 mg increments to a maximum of 225 mg/day (divided doses)
- Decrease dose by 50% in hepatic disease and by 25–50% in renal disease

Duloxetine

- No dosage adjustment in mild renal impairment; avoid *duloxetine* in severe renal unsufficiency as AUC increased 100% and metabolites increased 9-fold

PHARMACOKINETICS

Venlafaxine

- Well absorbed from GI tract: food has no effect on absorption; absorption of XR formulation is slow (15 ± 6 h); XR preparation appears to be better tolerated (as to GI effects) especially at start of therapy
- Less than 35% bound to plasma protein
- Peak plasma level reached by parent drug in 1–3 h and by active metabolite (O-desmethylvenlafaxine, ODV) in 2–6 h; with XR formulation peak plasma level reached by parent drug in 6 h and metabolite in 8.8 h (mean); steady-state of parent and metabolite reached in about 3 days
- Elimination half life of oral tablet: parent = 3–7 h and metabolite = 9–13 h; XR elimination half-life is dependent on absorption half-life (15 h mean); children may metabolize venlafaxine more rapidly than adults and may require higher doses than adults on a mg/kg basis
- Parent drug metabolized by CYP2D6 and is also a weak inhibitor of this enzyme; ODV metabolite is metabolized by CYP3A3/4; major elimination is via the urine; clearance decreased by 24% in renal disease and by 50% in hepatic disease

Duloxetine

- Duloxetine: Can be given with or without meals, although food delays T_{max} by 6–10 h. There is a 3 h delay in absorption and a 30% increase in clearance with an evening dose as compared to a morning dose. Bioavailability is reduced by about 30% in smokers.
- Duloxetine is metabolized by CYP1A2 and 2D6 and is an inhibitor of CYP2D6
- In moderate liver impairment plasma clearance reduced up to 85%, AUC increased 5-fold and $T_{1/2}$ tripled
- AUC and metabolites increased in severe renal insufficiency (see Dosing, above)

ONSET AND DURATION

- Therapeutic effect seen after 14–28 days

ADVERSE EFFECTS

- Generally dose-related; see chart p. 97 for incidence of adverse effects

CNS Effects

- Both sedation and insomnia reported; disruption of sleep cycle, prolonged sleep onset latency, decreased REM sleep, increased awakenings; vivid nightmares, and reduced sleep efficiency
- Headache common
- Nervousness, agitation; may cause behavior activation and aggravate symptoms of hyperactivity; CAUTION: hostility and suicidal ideation reported in 2% of children
- Asthenia
- Risk of hypomania/mania especially where patient is experiencing the onset of bipolar disorder; increased risk in bipolar patients with comorbid substance abuse. Careful monitoring for "switch to mania" is necessary
- 10–30% of patients on venlafaxine who improve initially can have breakthrough depression after several months ("poop-out syndrome") – an increase in dosage or augmentation therapy may be of benefit
- Seizures reported rarely (< 1%) with venlafaxine
- Hyperkinesia with venlafaxine

Selective Serotonin Norepinephrine Reuptake Inhibitor (SNRI) (cont.)

Anticholinergic Effects	• May be mediated through NE-reuptake inhibition • Dry mouth common • Sweating • Constipation, urinary retention
Cardiovascular Effects	• Modest, sustained increase in blood pressure can occur, usually within two months of dose stabilization; seen in over 3% of individuals on less than 100 mg/day and about 13% of individuals on doses above 300 mg/day; may not be related to dose with duloxotine; caution in patients with history of hypertension; recommended that patients on doses above 150 mg/day have BP monitored for 2 months at each dose level • Tachycardia • Dizziness, common; hypotension occasionally reported
GI Effects	• Nausea and vomiting occurs frequently at start of therapy and tends to decrease after 1–2 weeks; less frequent with XR formulation • Anorexia, weight loss • Epistasis
Sexual Side Effects	• Sexual side effects reported in over 30% of patients including decreased libido, delayed orgasm/ejaculation, anorgasmia, no ejaculation and erectile dysfunction • Case of priapism in a child
Other	• Case of Stevens-Johnson syndrome in adult on venlafaxine • Rhinitis common (duloxetine)
DISCONTINUATION SYNDROME	• Abrupt withdrawal, even after several weeks' therapy can occur within 8–16 h of discontinuation and can last for 8 days • Symptoms include: asthenia, dizziness, headache, insomnia, tinnitus, nausea, nervousness, agitation irritability confusion, nightmares, "electric-shock" sensations, chills, cramps and diarrhea • Cases of inter-dose withdrawal reported with regular-release tablet; withdrawal reactions also reported with XR product ☞ **THEREFORE THIS MEDICATION SHOULD BE WITHDRAWN GRADUALLY AFTER PROLONGED USE**
Management	• Suggested to taper slowly over a 2–4-week period (some suggest over 6 weeks) • Substituting one dose of fluoxetine (10 or 20 mg) near the end of the taper may help in the withdrawal process
PRECAUTIONS	• Increased risk for hostility and suicidal ideation reported in children; monitor all patients for increased depression and suicidal thoughts especially at start of therapy and following any change in dose • Do not use in patients with uncontrolled hypertension, as venlafaxine can cause modest, sustained increases in blood pressure [blood pressure monitoring recommended for all patients] • May induce manic reaction in patients • AVOID duloxetine in patients with severe renal (CrCl < 30 mL/min) or chronic liver disease or substantial alcohol use

- Symptoms of toxicity include excess adrenergic stimulation, tachycardia, hypotension, arrhythmias, increase in QTc interval, bowel dysmobility, decreased level of consciousness, seizures – deaths reported following massive overdose
- Delayed onset of rhabdomyolysis or serotonin-syndrome possible

USE IN PREGNANCY

- Category C drug: Animal studies show a decrease in offspring weight, as well as stillbirths with high doses
- No teratogenic effects reported in humans, with venlafaxine to date; may be a trend toward higher rates of spontaneous abortion

Breast Milk

- The total dose of venlafaxine and its metabolite ingested by a breast-fed infant can be as high as 9% of the maternal dose

NURSING IMPLICATIONS

- A gradual titration of dosage at start of therapy will minimize nausea
- Psychotherapy and education are also important in the treatment of depression
- Monitor therapy by watching for adverse effects as well as mood and activity level changes including worsening of suicidal thoughts especially at start of therapy or following an increase or decrease in dose; keep physician informed
- Be aware that the medication may increase psychomotor activity; this may create concern about suicidal behavior
- Excessive ingestion of caffeinated foods, drugs, or beverages may increase anxiety and agitation and confuse the diagnosis
- Instruct patient not to chew or crush the sustained-release Effexor XR tablet or the delayed-release duloxetine capsules, but swallow them whole
- If a dose is missed, do not attempt to make it up; continue with regular daily schedule (divided doses)
- SNRIs should not be stopped suddenly due to risk of precipitating a withdrawal reaction

PATIENT INSTRUCTIONS

- Detailed instructions for patients and caregivers are provided in the Information Sheet on p. 297.

DRUG INTERACTIONS

- Clinically significant interactions are listed below

Class of Drug	Example	Interaction Effects
Antiarrhythmic (type 1c)	Propafenone, flecainide	Increased plasma level of venlafaxine and duloxetine due to inhibited metabolism via CYP2D6
	Quinidine	Increased plasma level of duloxetine due to inhibited metabolism
Antibiotic	Ciprofloxacin, enoxacin	Increased plasma level of duloxetine due to inhibition of metabolism via CYP1A2
	Linezolid	Due to its weak MAOI activity, monitor for increased serotonergic and noradrenergic effects
Anticholinergic	Antiparkinsonian agents, antipsychotics, etc	Increased anticholinergic effects
Antidepressant NDRI	Bupropion	3-fold increase in venlafaxine plasma level due to inhibited metabolism via CYP2D6 and reduction in level of ODV metabolite Potentiation of noradrenergic effects Bupropion may mitigate SNRI-induced sexual side effects
SSRI	Paroxetine, fluoxetine	Reports that combination with SSRIs that inhibit CYP2D6 can result in increased levels of venlafaxine and duloxetine, with possible increases in blood pressure, anticholinergic effects and serotonergic effects
	Fluvoxamine	5-fold increase in AUC and 2.5-fold increase in half-life of duloxetine due to inhibited metabolism via CYP1A2

Antidepressants

Selective Serotonin Norepinephrine Reuptake Inhibitor (SNRI) (cont.)

Class of Drug	Example	Interaction Effects
Irreversible MAOI	Phenelzine	**AVOID**; possible hypertensive crisis and serotonergic reaction
RIMA	Moclobemide	Enhanced effects of norepinephrine and serotonin; caution – no data on safety with combined use
SARI	Trazodone	Case report of serotonin syndrome with venlafaxine
Tricyclic	Imipramine	C_{max} and AUC of imipramine increased by 40% with venlafaxine
	Desipramine	Desipramine (metabolite) clearance reduced by 20% with venlafaxine; desipramine level increased 3-fold with duloxetine
		Increased levels of cyclic antidepressants metabolized by CYP2D6 possible with duloxetine
	Trimipramine	Case report of seizure in combination with venlafaxine – postulated to be a result of inhibited metabolism via CYP2D6
NaSSA	Mirtazapine	Case report of serotonin syndrome with venlafaxine
Antipsychotic	General	Increased levels of antipsychotics metabolized by CYP2D6 possible with duloxetine
	Haloperidol	Increased peak plasma level and AUC of haloperidol with venlafaxine; no change in half-life
	Thioridazine	Increased plasma level of venlafaxine and decreased concentration of ODV metabolite Possible increased plasma level of thioridazine and arrhythmias – AVOID with duloxetine
	Risperidone	Increased AUC of risperidone by 32% and decreased renal clearance by 20% with venlafaxine
β-Blocker	Propranolol	Increased plasma level of venlafaxine due to competition for metabolism via CYP2D6
H$_2$ antagonist	Cimetidine	Increased plasma level of venlafaxine due to decreased clearance by 43%; peak concentration increased by 60% Increased plasma level of duloxetine due to inhibited metabolism
Lithium		Case report of serotonin syndrome with venlafaxine
MAO-B inhibitor	Selegiline	Case reports of serotonergic reaction with venlafaxine
Metoclopramide		Case report of extrapyramidal and serotonergic effects with venlafaxine
Protease inhibitor	Ritonavir	Moderate decrease in clearance of venlafaxine with ritonavir
	Indinavir	Both increases (by 13%) and decreases (by 60%) in total concentration (AUC) of indinavir reported with venlafaxine
Stimulant	Dextroamphetamine	Case report of serotonin syndrome with venlafaxine
	Methylphenidate	Potentiated effect in the treatment of depression and ADHD
Tolterodine		C_{max} and half-life of tolterodine increased; no effect on active metabolites
Zolpidem		Case report of delirium and hallucinations with venlafaxine

Serotonin-2 Antagonists/Reuptake Inhibitors (SARI)

PRODUCT AVAILABILITY

Chemical Class	Generic Name	Trade Name[A]	Dosage Forms and Strengths	Monograph Statement
Phenylpiperidine	Nefazodone[B][D]	Serzone	Tablets: 50 mg, 100 mg, 150 mg, 200 mg, 250 mg[B]	Safety and efficacy not established in children under age 18
Triazolopyridine	Trazodone	Desyrel Desyrel Dividose	Tablets: 50 mg, 100 mg, 150 mg, 300 mg[B] Tablets: 150 mg, 300 mg	Safety and efficacy not established in children under age 18

[A] Generic preparations may be available, [B] Not marketed in Canada, [D] Withdrawn in Canada November 2003

INDICATIONS

No approved indications in children and adolescents

Approved (for Adults)

- Major depressive disorder – multicentre studies of nefazodone in children and adolescents aged 7–17 years did not demonstrate superiority over placebo
- Prophylaxis of recurrent major depression (unipolar disorder)
- Depressed phase of bipolar disorder (see Precautions)

Other Uses in Children and Adolescents

- Bulimia nervosa
- Early data report benefit in social phobia (nefazodone)
- Open trials suggest efficacy of nefazodone for sleep problems and nightmares related to posttraumatic stress disorder
- Acute and chronic insomnia and night terrors (trazodone)
- Open trials suggest benefit for premenstrual syndrome (nefazodone)
- Open trials and case reports suggest efficacy in treatment of aggression and disruptive behavior in children

PHARMACOLOGY

- Equilibrate the effects of biogenic amines through various mechanisms; cause downregulation of β-adrenergic receptors
- Nefazodone blocks 5-HT_{2A} and 5-HT_{2C} receptors, inhibits reuptake of 5-HT (at higher doses) and serves as an adrenergic antagonist

GENERAL COMMENTS

- Studies demonstrate improved outcomes in chronic depression with combination of nefazodone and psychotherapy (CBT and IPT)
- Open-label study of nefazodone in 28 children and adolescents with depression found 86% of children and 6% of adolescents were "much" or "very much" improved after 6 weeks of treatment
- Monitor all patients for worsening depression and/or suicidal thoughts

DOSING

- See p. 92
- Initiate drug at a low dose and increase every 3–5 days to a maximum tolerated dose based on side effects; there is a wide variation in dosage requirements; prophylaxis is most effective if therapeutic dose is maintained
- Trazodone should be taken on an empty stomach as food delays absorption and decreases drug effect
- Regular ingestion of grapefruit juice while on nefazodone may affect the antidepressant plasma level (see Drug Interactions p. 68)
- Once stabilized, the patient can be placed on once-daily dose of nefazodone

Antidepressants

Serotonin-2 Antagonists/Reuptake Inhibitors (SARI) (cont.)

PHARMACOKINETICS

- See p. 92
- Large percentage metabolized by first-pass effect
- Highly bound to plasma protein

Trazodone

- Completely absorbed from the gastrointestinal tract; food significantly delays and decreases peak plasma effect of trazodone
- Trazodone metabolized primarily by the liver to active metabolite m-chlorophenylpiperazine (mcPP) by CYP3A4

Nefazodone

- High ultra- and inter-individual variability seen in nefazodone plasma pharmacokinetics in children and adolescents
- Plasma levels of nefazodone and its metabolites reported to be higher in children than adolescents; half-lives of nefazodone and its metabolite are dose-dependent and appear to be shorter than in adults
- Nefazodone is a potent inhibitor of CYP3A4 and may decrease the metabolism of drugs metabolized by this isoenzyme (see Interactions p. 67–68)

ONSET AND DURATION OF ACTION

- Therapeutic effect is seen after 14–28 days
- Sedative effects are seen within a few hours of oral administration; decreased sleep disturbance reported after a few days

ADVERSE EFFECTS

- The pharmacological and side effect profile of SARI antidepressants is dependent on their affinity for and activity on neurotransmitters/receptors (see chart p. 94)
- See chart p. 96 for incidence of adverse effects at therapeutic doses; incidence of adverse effects may be greater in early days of treatment; patients adapt to many side effects over time

CNS Effects

- A result of antagonism at histamine H_1-receptors and α_1-adrenoreceptors
- Occur frequently

A. Cognitive Effects

- Drowsiness (most common adverse effect) [Management: prescribe bulk of dose at bedtime]
- Weakness, lethargy, fatigue, asthenia
- Conversely, excitement, agitation and restlessness have occurred
- Confusion, disturbed concentration, disorientation
- Nefazodone increases REM sleep and sleep quality; trazodone reported to increase stages 3/4 (slow-wave) sleep
- Improved psychomotor and complex memory performance reported with nefazodone after first dose; however, dose-related impairment noted after repeated doses
- Visual disturbances
- Precipitation of hypomania or mania, especially where patient is experiencing onset of bipolar disorder; increased risk in bipolar patients with comorbid substance abuse. Careful monitoring for "switch to mania" is necessary
- Psychosis, panic reactions, anxiety, or euphoria may occur

B. Neurological Effects

- Fine tremor
- Akathisia (rare – check serum iron for deficiency)
- Seizures can occur rarely following abrupt drug increase or after drug withdrawal; risk increases with high plasma levels

- Tinnitus
- Paresthesias reported with nefazodone
- Myoclonus; includes muscle jerks of lower extremities, jaw, and arms, and nocturnal myoclonus – may be severe
- Dysphasia, stuttering
- Headache; worsening of migraine

Anticholinergic Effects	- A result of antagonism at muscarinic receptors (ACh) - Include dry eyes, blurred vision, constipation, dry mouth [see Cyclic Antidepressants p. 75 for treatment suggestions]
Cardiovascular Effects	- A result of antagonism at α_1-adrenoreceptors, muscarinic, 5-HT$_2$ and H$_1$-receptors and inhibition of sodium fast channels - Dizziness common with nefazodone - Risk increases with high plasma levels - Bradycardia seen with nefazodone - Orthostatic hypotension
GI Effects	- A result of inhibition of 5-HT uptake and ACh antagonism - Nausea common with nefazodone - Weight gain reported with trazodone; rare with nefazodone - Peculiar taste, "black tongue," glossitis
Sexual Side Effects	- A result of altered dopamine (D$_2$) activity, 5-HT$_2$ blockade, inhibition of 5-HT reuptake, α_1-blockade, and ACh blockade - Testicular swelling, painful ejaculation, retrograde ejaculation, increased libido, inappropriate erections and priapism (with trazodone due to prominent alpha adrenergic blockade; not seen with nefazodone); spontaneous orgasm with yawning (trazodone)
Endocrine Effects	- Decreases in blood sugar levels reported (nefazodone) - Can induce SIADH with hyponatremia; risk increased with age
Allergic Reactions	- Rare - Rash, urticaria, pruritus, edema, blood dyscrasias - **HEPATOTOXICITY:** jaundice, hepatitis, hepatic necrosis and hepatic failure reported with therapeutic doses of nefazodone (laboratory evidence includes: increased levels of ALT, AST, GGT, bilirubin and increased prothrombin time); time of onset ranges from 1 to 4 months – cases of liver failure and death reported. Recommend baseline and periodic liver function tests with nefazodone. Monitor for signs of hepatotoxicity
DISCONTINUATION SYNDROME	- Likely due to serotonergic and adrenergic rebound - Abrupt withdrawal from high doses may occasionally cause a "flu-like" syndrome consisting of fever, fatigue, sweating, coryza, malaise, myalgia, headache; anxiety, dizziness, nausea, vomiting, akathisia, dyskinesia, insomnia, nightmares, and panic - Most likely to occur 24–48 h after withdrawal, or after a large dosage decrease - Rebound depression can occur (even in individuals not previously depressed – such as patients with obsessive compulsive disorders) - Paradoxical mood changes reported on abrupt withdrawal, including hypomania or mania - ☞ **THUS THESE MEDICATIONS SHOULD BE WITHDRAWN GRADUALLY AFTER PROLONGED USE**
Management	- Reinstitute the drug at a lower dose and taper gradually over several days

Serotonin-2 Antagonists/Reuptake Inhibitors (SARI) (cont.)

PRECAUTIONS

- **Monitor liver function tests periodically (3–6 times a year), and for clinical signs of liver dysfunction.** Nefazodone withdrawn from market in Canada in 2003
- Use nefazodone cautiously in patients in whom excess anticholinergic activity could be harmful (e.g., urinary retention, narrow-angle glaucoma)
- Trazodone is a substrate of CYP3A4 and its metabolism can be inhibited by CYP3A4 inhibitors; nefazodone is a potent inhibitor of CYP3A4 (see Interactions p. 67–68)
- Use caution in combination with drugs that prolong the QT interval
- Use nefazodone with caution in patients with respiratory difficulties, since antidepressants with anticholinergic properties can dry up bronchial secretions and make breathing more difficult
- May lower the seizure threshold; therefore, administer cautiously to patients with a history of convulsive disorders, organic brain disease, or a predisposition to convulsions (e.g., alcohol withdrawal)
- May impair the mental and physical ability to perform hazardous tasks (e.g., driving a car or operating machinery); will potentiate the effects of alcohol
- May induce manic reactions in patients with bipolar disorder and rarely in unipolar depression; because of risk of increased cycling, bipolar disorder is a relative contraindication
- Use caution in prescribing nefazodone for patients with a history of alcoholism or liver disorder. Monitor liver function tests at baseline and periodically during treatment, and at first symptom or clinical sign of liver dysfunction
- Combination of SARI antidepressants with SSRIs can lead to increased plasma level of the SARI antidepressant. Combination therapy has been used in the treatment of resistant patients; use caution and monitor for serotonin syndrome (see p. 46)
- Use caution when switching from a SARI antidepressant to fluoxetine and vice versa (see Drug Interactions p. 67 and Switching Antidepressants p. 98)

TOXICITY

- Acute poisoning results in drowsiness, ataxia, nausea, vomiting; deep coma as well as arrhythmias (including torsade de pointes) and AV block reported; no seizures reported

USE IN PREGNANCY

- Trazodone in high doses was found to be teratogenic and toxic to the fetus in some animal species
- Trazodone and nefazodone reported not to increase the rates of major malformations above the baseline rate of 1–3%

Breast Milk

- SARI antidepressants are excreted into breast milk
- The American Academy of Pediatrics classifies SARI antidepressants as drugs "whose effects on nursing infants are unknown but may be of concern."

NURSING IMPLICATIONS

- Psychotherapy and education are also important in the treatment of depression
- Monitor therapy by watching for adverse side effects, mood and activity level changes
- Be aware that the medication may increase psychomotor activity; this may create concern about suicidal behavior. Monitor for increased depression and suicidal thoughts especially at start of therapy and following an increase or decrease in dose
- Expect a lag time of 14–28 days before antidepressant effects will be noticed

- Reassure patient that drowsiness and dizziness usually subside after first few weeks; if dizzy, patient should get up from lying or sitting position slowly, and dangle legs over edge of bed before getting up
- Excessive use of caffeinated foods, drugs, or beverages may increase anxiety and agitation and confuse the diagnosis
- Grapefruit juice can increase the blood level of nefazodone and trazodone.
- With nefazodone, monitor for signs of hepatotoxicity including nausea, vomiting, fatigue, pruritis, dark urine, and jaundice
- These drugs should not be stopped suddenly due to risk of precipitating withdrawal reactions
- Because these drugs can cause drowsiness, caution patient that activities requiring mental alertness should not be performed until response to the drug has been determined

PATIENT INSTRUCTIONS

- Detailed instructions for patients and caregivers are provided in the Information Sheet on p. 299

DRUG INTERACTIONS

- Clinically significant interactions are listed below

Class of Drug	Example	Interaction Effects
Alcohol		Short-term or acute use reduces first-pass metabolism of antidepressant and increases its plasma level; chronic use induces metabolizing enzymes and decreases its plasma level
Antibiotic	Linezolid	Monitor for increased serotonergic effects due to weak MAOI activity of linezolid
Anticholinergic	Antiparkinsonian agents, antihistamines	Increased anticholinergic effect; may increase risk of hyperthermia, confusion, urinary retention, etc.
Anticonvulsant	Carbamazepine, phenytoin	Increased plasma level of carbamazepine or phenytoin due to inhibition of metabolism with trazodone Increased plasma level of carbamazepine with nefazodone due to inhibited metabolism via CYP3A4
	Carbamazepine, barbiturates, phenytoin	Decreased plasma level of trazodone and nefazodone due to enzyme induction via CYP3A4
Anticoagulants	Warfarin	Decreased prothrombin time with trazodone
Antidepressant Irreversible MAOI	Phenelzine, tranylcypromine	Low doses of trazodone (25–50 mg) used to treat antidepressant-induced insomnia Combined SARI and MAOI therapy has additive antidepressant effects; monitor for serotonergic effects
RIMA	Moclobemide	Additive antidepressant effect in treatment-resistant patients; monitor for serotonergic effects
SSRI	Fluoxetine, Fluvoxamine, paroxetine, sertraline	Elevated SARI plasma level (due to release from protein binding and inhibition of oxidative metabolism); monitor plasma level and for signs of toxicity Nefazodone metabolite (mCPP) level increased 4-fold with fluoxetine; case report of Serotonin syndrome with combination Additive antidepressant effect in treatment-resistant patients; nefazodone may reverse SSRI-induced sexual dysfunction and may enhance sleep
Antihistamine	Loratadine	Inhibited metabolism of antihistamine by nefazodone (via CYP3A4) leading to accumulation of parent compound and possible adverse cardiac effects (cetirizine and fexofenadine levels elevated, but considered safe)
Antihypertensive	Bethanidine, clonidine, debrisoquin, methyldopa, guanethidine, reserpine	Decreased antihypertensive effect due to inhibition of α − adrenergic receptors
	Clonidine	Additive hypotension and sedation with trazodone
	Acetazolamide, thiazide diuretics	Hypotension augmented

Serotonin-2 Antagonists/Reuptake Inhibitors (SARI) (cont.)

Class of Drug	Example	Interaction Effects
Antipsychotic	Chlorpromazine, haloperidol, perphenazine	Increased plasma level of either agent Potentiation of hypotension with trazodone
	Clozapine	Increased plasma level of clozapine and norclozapine with nefazodone due to inhibited metabolism via CYP3A4
Anxiolytic	Alprazolam, triazolam, midazolam, bromazepam, diazepam	Increased plasma level of benzodiazepines metabolized by oxidation (via CYP3A4) with nefazodone; triazolam by 500%, alprazolam by 200 ad desmethyldiazepam by 87%
Ca-channel blocker	Amlodipine	Elevated amlodipine level due to inhibited metabolism by nefazodone, via CYP3A4
CNS depressant	Hypnotics, antihistamines, benzodiazepines	Increased sedation, CNS depression
Cholestyramine		Decreased absorption of antidepressant, if given together
Digoxin		Increased digoxin plasma level, with possible toxicity, with trazodone and nefazodone
Ergot alkaloid	Ergotamine	Elevated ergotamine levels possible due to inhibited metabolism by nefazodone via CYP3A4
Ginkgo Biloba		Case report of coma with trazodone (postulated to be due to excess stimulation of GABA receptors)
Grapefruit juice		Decreased metabolism of trazodone and nefazodone via CYP3A4
Immunosuppressant	Cyclosporin, tacrolimus	Increased plasma level of cyclosporin (by approx. 70%) and tacrolimus (5-fold) with nefazodone due to inhibition of CYP3A4
Insulin		Hypoglycemia reported with nefazodone
Lithium		Additive antidepressant effect
MAO-B inhibitor	L-deprenyl (selegiline)	Reports of serotonergic reactions
Protease inhibitor	Ritonavir, indinavir	Increased plasma levels of trazodone and nefazodone due to decreased metabolism (with retonavir, trazodone clearance decreased 52%)
Sildenafil		Possible enhanced hypotension due to inhibited metabolism of sildenafil by nefazodone via CYP3A4
Statins	Simvastatin, pravastatin, atorvastatin	Inhibited metabolism of statins by nefazodone (via CYP3A4); increased plasma level and adverse effects – myositis and rhabdomyolysis reported
St. John's Wort		May augment serotonergic effects – case reports of serotonergic reactions
Sulfonylurea	Tolbutamide	Increased hypoglycemia
Thyroid drug	Triiodothyronine (T_3-liothyronine), L-thyroxine (T_4)	Additive antidepressant effect in treatment-resistant patients

Noradrenergic/Specific Serotonergic Antidepressants (NaSSA)

PRODUCT AVAILABILITY

Chemical Class	Generic Name	Trade Name[A]	Dosage Forms and Strengths	Monograph Statement
Tetracyclic agent	Mirtazapine	Remeron Remeron SolTab[B], Remeron RD[c]	Tablets: 7.5 mg[B], 15 mg[B], 30 mg, 45 mg Oral disintegrating tablets: 15 mg, 30 mg, 45 mg	Safety and efficacy has not been established in pediatric patients

[A] Generic preparations may be available, [B] Not marketed in Canada [C] Not marketed in US

INDICATIONS

Approved (for Adults)

Other Uses in Children and Adolescents

No approved indications for children and adolescents

- Major depression (with or without symptoms of anxiety) – multicentre studies in youths did not demonstrate superiority over placebo
- Preliminary reports of efficacy in panic disorder and PTSD
- Open-label study suggests improvement in aggression, self-injury, irritability, anxiety, depression and insomnia, in 35% of subjects aged 3–23 years with pervasive developmental disorder

PHARMACOLOGY

- Selective antagonist at α_2-adrenergic auto- and heteroreceptors which are involved in regulation of neuronal release of norepinephrine and serotonin (increases noradrenergic and serotonergic transmission via blockade of α-adrenoreceptors; increases the release of norepinephrine and serotonin, and blocks 5-HT_{2A+C} and 5-HT_3 receptors)

GENERAL COMMENTS

- Limited trials in pediatric patients
- Monitor all patients for worsening depression and suicidal thinking
- Reduces sleep latency and prolongs sleep duration due to H1 and 5-HT_{2A+C} blockade; may be useful when insomnia or agitation are prominent
- Has mild anxiolytic effects at lower doses

DOSING

- See p. 93
- The 15 mg and 30 mg tablets are scored for dose titration
- Initiate at 7.5–15 mg daily for 7 days; increase to 15–30 mg and maintain for at least 1–2 weeks; if ineffective, can increase to 45 mg daily

PHARMACOKINETICS

- Bioavailability is approximately 50% due to gut wall and hepatic first-pass metabolism; food slightly decreases absorption rate
- Remeron SolTabs dissolve on the tongue within 30 s; can be swallowed with or without water, chewed, or allowed to dissolve
- Peak plasma level achieved in 2 h
- Protein binding of 85%
- Females and the elderly show higher plasma concentrations than males and young adults
- Extensively metabolized via CYP1A2, 2D6, and 3A4; desmethyl metabolite has some clinical activity
- Mean half-life in adults: 20–40 h – half-life significantly longer in females (average of 37 h) than in males (average of 26 h)

Antidepressants

Noradrenergic/Specific Serotonergic Antidepressants (NaSSA) (cont.)

- Hepatic clearance decreased by 40% in patients with cirrhosis
- Clearance reduced by 30–50% in patients with renal impairment

ONSET AND DURATION OF ACTION

- Therapeutic effects seen after 14–28 days

ADVERSE EFFECTS

- See p. 97

CNS Effects

- Sedation in over 30% of patients; fatigue; less sedation at doses above 15 mg due to increased effect on α_2-receptors, an increased release of NE, as well as tolerance
- Insomnia, agitation, aggression, depersonalization, restlessness, and nervousness reported occasionally, coupled with urges of self-harm or harm to others
- Shortened sleep onset latency, decreased REM sleep and increased total sleep time; vivid (abnormal) dreams reported
- Rarely delirium, psychosis, hallucinations
- Seizures (very rare – 0.04%)
- Asthenia

Anticholinergic Effects

- Dry mouth frequent; constipation [for treatment suggestions see Cyclic Antidepressants p. 75]
- Increased sweating, blurred vision, and urinary retention reported rarely

Cardiovascular Effects

- Hypertension
- Edema
- No significant ECG changes reported

GI Effects

- Increased appetite and significant weight gain (of over 5 kg) reported (due to potent antihistaminic properties); occur primarily in the first 4 weeks of treatment and may be dose-related – may be of benefit in depressed patients with marked anorexia

Other Adverse Effects

- Sexual dysfunction reported (less than with SSRIs); risk increased with age, use of higher doses and concomitant medication
- Transient elevation of liver function tests reported
- Febrile neutropenia and agranulocytosis reported; monitor WBC if patient develops signs of infection [some recommend doing baseline and annual CBC]
- Increases in plasma cholesterol, to over 20% above the upper limit of normal reported; increases in non-fasting triglyceride levels
- Myalgia and flu-like symptoms
- Pruritus or rash
- Case of pancreatitis

DISCONTINUATION SYNDROME

- Case report of dizziness, nausea, anxiety, insomnia and paresthesia following abrupt withdrawal
- Case report of hypomania
- ☞ **THEREFORE THESE MEDICATIONS SHOULD BE WITHDRAWN GRADUALLY AFTER PROLONGED USE**

Management
- Reinstitute drug at a lower dose and taper gradually over several days

PRECAUTIONS

- Caution in patients with compromised liver function or renal impairment
- Monitor WBC if patient develops signs of infection; a low WBC requires discontinuation of therapy
- Monitor all patients for worsening depression and suicidal thoughts especially at start of therapy and following a change in dose
- May induce manic reactions in patients with BD and rarely in unipolar depression
- High potential for weight gain

TOXICITY

- Low liability for toxicity in overdose if taken alone; no changes in vital signs, with dose of 900 mg, reported
- No fatalities when drug used alone

USE IN PREGNANCY

- Early data suggests no teratogenic effects in humans

Breast Milk
- Data not available

NURSING IMPLICATIONS

- Psychotherapy and education are also important in the treatment of depression
- Monitor therapy by watching for adverse effects, mood and activity level changes including worsening of suicidal thoughts.
- Signs and symptoms of infection (e.g., sore threat, fever, mouth sores, elevated temperature) should be reported to the physician as soon as possible

PATIENT INSTRUCTIONS

- Detailed instructions for patients and caregivers are provided in the Information Sheet on p. 301

DRUG INTERACTIONS

- Clinically significant interactions are listed below

Class of Drug	Example	Interaction Effects
Anticonvulsant	Carbamazepine	Decreased plasma level of mirtazapine by 60% due to induction of metabolism via CYP3A4
Antidepressant Irreversible MAOI SSRI	Phenelzine, tranylcypromine Fluoxetine, sertraline	Possible serotonergic reaction; DO NOT COMBINE Combination reported to alleviate insomnia and augment antidepressant response; may have activating effects May mitigate SSRI-induced sexual dysfunction and "poop-out" syndrome Increased serotonergic effects possible Increased sedation and weight gain reported with combination
SNRI	Fluvoxamine Venlafaxine	Increased plasma level of mirtazapine (3- to 4-fold) due to inhibited metabolism Case report of serotonin syndrome (see p. 46)
Antiemetics ($5-HT_3$ antagonists)	Dolasetron, granisetron, ondansetron	Case reports of serotonin syndrome
CNS depressant	Alcohol, benzodiazepines	Impaired cognition and motor performance
Narcotic	Tramadol	Lethargy, hypotension and hypoxia reported
Stimulant	Phentermine, dextroamphetamine, methylphenidate	May increase agitation and risk of mania, especially in patients with bipolar disorder

Antidepressants

Nonselective Cyclic Antidepressants

PRODUCT AVAILABILITY

Chemical Class[D]	Generic Name	Trade Name[A]	Dosage Forms and Strengths	Monograph Statement
Tricyclic antidepressant (TCA)	Amitriptyline	Elavil, Endep[B]	Tablets: 10 mg, 25 mg, 50 mg, 75 mg, 100 mg, 150 mg[B] Oral suspension[C]: 10 mg/5 ml	Not recommended in children under age 12
	Clomipramine[E]	Anafranil	Tablets[C]: 10 mg, 25 mg, 50 mg Capsules[B]: 25 mg, 50 mg, 75 mg[B]	Approved for use in children > 10 years old for OCD Safety and efficacy not established for other disorders
	Desipramine	Norpramin	Tablets: 10 mg, 25 mg, 50 mg, 75 mg, 100 mg, 150 mg[B]	Safety and efficacy not established in children under age 18
	Doxepin	Sinequan, Adapin[B]	Capsules 10 mg, 25 mg, 50 mg, 75 mg, 100 mg, 150 mg Oral solution[B] 10 mg/ml	Not recommended in children under age 12
	Imipramine	Tofranil Tofranil PM[B]	Tablets: 10 mg, 25 mg, 50 mg, 75 mg[C] Capsules[B]: 75 mg, 100mg, 125 mg, 150 mg	Approved for use in children > 5 years old, for enuresis; safety and efficacy not established for other disorders
	Nortriptyline	Aventyl[C], Pamelor[B]	Capsules: 10 mg, 25 mg, 50 mg[B], 75 mg[B] Syrup[B]: 10 mg/5 ml	Safety and efficacy not established in children under age 18
	Protriptyline[B]	Vivactil	Tablets: 5 mg, 10 mg	Safety and efficacy not established in children under age 18
	Trimipramine	Surmontil	Tablets[C]: 12.5 mg, 25 mg, 50 mg, 100 mg Capsules: 25 mg[B], 50 mg[B], 75 mg[C], 100 mg[B]	Safety and efficacy not established in children under age 18

[A] Generic preparations may be available, [B] Not marketed in Canada, [C] Not marketed in USA, [D] Include: NE-reuptake inhibitors, mixed 5-HT/NE reuptake inhibitors, serotonin reuptake inhibitors, [E] Not approved for depression in USA

INDICATIONS

Approved for Children and Adolescents

- Clomipramine approved for OCD in children > 10 years of age
- Imipramine approved for enuresis in children > 5 years of age

Approved (for Adults)	• Major depressive disorder – metaanalysis of randomized controlled trials of TCAs in children aged 6–18 demonstrated a lack of efficacy; current consensus suggests that TCAs are not the medications of choice for depressed children and adolescents

• Major depressive disorder – metaanalysis of randomized controlled trials of TCAs in children aged 6–18 demonstrated a lack of efficacy; current consensus suggests that TCAs are not the medications of choice for depressed children and adolescents
• Prophylaxis of recurrent major depression (unipolar disorder)
• Treatment of secondary depression in other mental illnesses, e.g., schizophrenia, dementia
• Depressed phase of bipolar disorder (see Precautions)
• Obsessive-compulsive disorder (clomipramine)
• Treatment of enuresis (imipramine)
• Depression and/or anxiety associated with alcoholism or organic disease (doxepin – USA)
• Psychoneuroses with depression (doxepin – USA)

Other Uses in Children and Adolescents

• Bulimia/eating disorders
• School phobia, separation anxiety disorder (imipramine) – data contradictory
• Attention deficit hyperactivity disorder not responsive to other agents (amitriptyline, desipramine, imipramine, nortriptyline)
• Double-blind studies suggest efficacy for core symptoms of autism including ritualistic behavior, anger and aggression (clomipramine) or hyperactivity (desipramine, clomipramine, imipramine)
• Premenstrual dysphoric disorder (clomipramine, nortriptyline)
• Cataplexy and narcoplexy (protriptyline)
• Pain management, including migraine headache, diabetic neuropathy, postherpetic neuralgia, chronic oral-facial pain
• Tourette's syndrome (clomipramine)
• Aid in smoking cessaion (nortriptyline), alone or in combination with nicotine patch

PHARMACOLOGY

• Exact mechanism of action unknown; equilibrate the effects of biogenic amines through various mechanisms (such as reuptake blockade); cause downregulation of β-adrenergic receptors
• The action in the treatment of enuresis may involve inhibition of urination due to the anticholinergic effect and CNS stimulation, resulting in easier arousal by the stimulus of a full bladder

GENERAL COMMENTS

• In general, TCA's are less effective in children and early adolescents, for depression, than in adults; this may be due to "immature" neurophysiology of children. More than 13 controlled trials failed to show efficacy in depression, in this population (response marginally better with SSRIs)
• Monitor all patients for worsening of depression and suicidal thinking

DOSING

• Prior to treatment, a baseline ECG is recommended. When an effective daily dose is reached, a steady state serum level and ECG should be done. Do a follow-up ECG at any dose change and a plasma level every few months
• Initiate TCA at a low dose (see p. 93) and increase dose every 4–5 days to a maximum dose of 3–5 mg/kg, or based on side effects; an abrupt dose in crease can precipitate seizures

Nonselective Cyclic Antidepressants (cont.)

	• There is a wide variation in dosage requirements (partially dependent on plasma levels) (see p. 93); efficacy and toxicity appear to be dose-related • Once steady-state is reached, may give drug as a single bedtime dose; use divided doses if patient develops nightmares • Prophylaxis is most effective if therapeutic dose is maintained
PHARMACOKINETICS	• See chart p. 93 for specific agents • Completely absorbed from the gastrointestinal tract • Large percentage metabolized by first-pass effect • Peak plasma levels occur more rapidly with tertiary tricyclics, like amitriptyline (1–3 h) than with secondary tricyclics like desipramine and nortriptyline (4–8 h) • Highly lipophilic; concentrated primarily in myocardial and cerebral tissue • Highly bound to plasma protein • Metabolized primarily by the liver • Most tricyclics have linear pharmacokinetics, i.e., a change in dose leads to a proportional change in plasma concentration • Most children are able to metabolize/clear TCAs faster than adults • Elimination half-life see p. 93; steady state reached in about 5 days • Pharmacokinetics may vary between males and females; data suggest that plasma levels of tricyclic antidepressants may dip in female patients prior to menstruation
ONSET AND DURATION OF ACTION	• Tricyclics and related drugs are long-acting; they may be given in a single daily dose, usually at bedtime (except protriptyline, which is usually given in the morning) • Therapeutic effect is seen after 14–28 days • Sedative effects are seen within a few hours of oral administration, with lessened sleep disturbance after a few days • Occasionally patients may lose response to antidepressant after several months ("poop-out syndrome") [Check compliance with therapy; optimize dose (plasma level may be useful); may need to change drug]
ADVERSE EFFECTS	• The pharmacological and side effect profile of cyclic antidepressants is dependent on their affinity for and activity on neurotransmitters/ receptors (see chart p. 96) • See chart p. for incidence of adverse effects at therapeutic doses of specific agents; incidence of adverse effects may be greater in early days of treatment; patients adapt to many side effects over time
CNS Effects	• A result of antagonism at histamine H_1-receptors and $α_1$-adrenoreceptors • Occur frequently
A. Cognitive Effects	• Drowsiness (most common adverse effect) [Management: prescribe bulk of dose at bedtime] • Weakness, lethargy, fatigue

- Conversely, anxiety, excitement, agitation, restlessness, nervousness, emotional instability and insomnia have occurred; cases of worsening of depression and suicidal thinking in 2–3% of children and adolescents
- Decrease REM sleep (except for trimipramine); vivid dreaming or nightmares can occur, especially if all the medication is given at bedtime; secondary amines reduce sleep efficiency and increase wake time; tertiary amines improve sleep continuity
- Cognitive dysfunction, confusion, disturbed concentration, disorientation
- Precipitation of hypomania or mania (20–40%), especially where patient is experiencing onset of bipolar disorder – less frequent if patient receiving mood stabilizers; careful monitoring for "switch to mania" is necessary
- Psychosis, panic reactions, anxiety, or euphoria may occur

| B. Neurological Effects |

- Fine tremor
- Akathisia (rare – check serum iron for deficiency); can occur following abrupt drug withdrawal
- Seizures (more common in children with autism and patients with eating disorder) can occur following abrupt drug increase or after drug withdrawal; risk increases with high plasma levels
- Paresthesias reported
- Myoclonus – more likely with serotonergic agents; includes muscle jerks of lower extremities, jaw, and arms, and nocturnal myoclonus

| Anticholinergic Effects |

- A result of antagonism at muscarinic receptors (ACh)
- Occur frequently
- Dry mucous membranes; may predispose patient to monilial infections [Management: sugar-free gum and candy, oral lubricants (e.g., MoiStir, Ora-Care D)
- Blurred vision
- Dry eyes [Management: artificial tears, but employ caution with patients wearing contact lenses; these patients should have their dry eyes managed with their usual wetting solutions or comfort drops]
- Constipation [Management: increase bulk and fluid intake, fecal softener, bulk laxative]
- Urinary retention, delayed micturition
- Excessive sweating [Management: daily showering, talcum powder; in severe cases: Drysol solution, clonidine; drug may need to be changed]
- Confusion, disorientation, delirium, delusions, hallucinations

| Cardiovascular Effects |

- A result of antagonism at α_1-adrenoreceptors, muscarinic, 5-HT$_2$ and H$_1$-receptors and inhibition of sodium fast channels
- Risk increases with high plasma levels
- Tachycardia; may be more pronounced in younger patients
- Orthostatic hypotension
- Prolonged conduction time; contraindicated in heart block
- Arrhythmias, syncope, thrombosis, thrombophlebitis, stroke, and congestive heart failure have been reported on occasion
- Hypertension rarely reported with imipramine in patients with bulimia
- Cases of sudden unexplained deaths reported in 5 prepubescent children on desipramine (possibly due to cardiac arrhythmias)

| GI Effects |

- A result of inhibition of 5-HT uptake and ACh antagonism
- Anorexia, nausea, vomiting, diarrhea

Antidepressants

Nonselective Cyclic Antidepressants (cont.)

- Weight gain (average gain of up to 7 kg – weight gain is linear over time and is often accompanied by a craving for sweets) [Management: nutritional counseling, exercise, dose reduction, changing antidepressant]
- Constipation (see anticholinergic effects)

| Sexual Side Effects |

- A result of altered dopamine activity, 5-HT$_2$ blockade, inhibition of 5-HT reuptake, α_1-blockade, and ACh blockade
- Decreased libido, impotence
- Testicular swelling, painful ejaculation, retrograde ejaculation, increased libido and priapism; spontaneous orgasm with yawning (clomipramine)
- Breast engorgement and breast tissue enlargement in males and females
- Anorgasmia

| Endocrine Effects |

- Both increases and decreases in blood sugar levels reported
- Carbohydrate craving reported – may result in weight gain

| Allergic Reactions |

- Rare
- Jaundice, hepatitis, rash, urticaria, pruritus, edema, blood dyscrasias
- Photosensitivity, skin pigmentation (imipramine, desipramine)
- Case reports of thrombocytopenia

DISCONTINUATION SYNDROME

- Likely due to cholinergic and adrenergic rebound
- Abrupt withdrawal from high doses may cause a "flu-like" syndrome consisting of fever, fatigue, sweating, coryza, malaise, myalgia, headache; psychological symptoms: anxiety, agitation, hypomania or mania, insomnia, vivid dreams, as well as dizziness, nausea, vomiting; akathisia and dyskinesia also reported
- Most likely to occur 24–48 h after withdrawal, or after a large dosage decrease
- Rebound depression can occur (even in individuals not previously depressed – such as patients with obsessional disorders)
- Paradoxical mood changes reported on abrupt withdrawal, including hypomania or mania
- ☞ **THESE MEDICATIONS SHOULD THEREFORE BE WITHDRAWN GRADUALLY AFTER PROLONGED USE**

| Management |

- Reinstitute drug (at slightly lower dose) and gradually taper dose over several days (e.g., by 12.5–25 mg every 3–5 days)
- Alternatively, can treat specific symptoms:
    – Cholinergic rebound (e.g., nausea, vomiting, sweating) – ginger, benztropine, Atropine
    – Anxiety, agitation, insomnia – benzodiazepine (e.g., lorazepam)
    – Dizziness – dimenhydrinate
    – Neurological symptoms: akathisia – propranolol; dyskinesia – clonazepam; dystonia – benztropine

PRECAUTIONS

- The U.S. FDA defines the following ECG and examination values as unsafe in children treated with tricyclics: (a) PR interval > 200 ms, (b) QRS interval
- > 30% above a baseline (or > 120 ms), (c) BP > 140 mmHg systolic or 90 mmHg diastolic, (d) Heart rate > 130 beats/min at rest
- Sudden death (rarely) reported with desipramine, even with therapeutic plasma levels; plasma levels may be higher by 42% in children than adults, at the same dose
- Cardiac complications reported in children who smoke marihuana while on antidepressants
- Use with caution in patients with respiratory difficulties, since antidepressants with anticholinergic properties can dry up bronchial secretions and make breathing more difficult
- May lower the seizure threshold; therefore, administer cautiously to patients with a history of convulsive disorders, organic brain disease, or a predisposition to convulsions (e.g., alcohol withdrawal)
- May impair the mental and physical ability to perform hazardous tasks (e.g., driving a car or operating machinery); will potentiate the effects of alcohol
- May induce manic reactions in up to 50% of patients with bipolar disorder; because of risk of increased cycling, bipolar disorder is a relative contraindication
- Combination of cyclic antidepressants with SSRIs can lead to increased plasma level of the cyclic antidepressant. Combination therapy has been used in the treatment of resistant patients; use of serotonergic cyclic antidepressants with SSRIs can cause serotonin syndrome (see p. 46)
- Use caution when switching from a cyclic antidepressant to fluoxetine or MAOI and vice versa (see Drug Interactions p. 79 and Switching Anti-depressants p. 98)
- Concurrent ingestion of a cyclic antidepressant with high fiber foods or laxatives (e.g., bran, psyllium) can decrease absorption of the antidepressant

TOXICITY

- The therapeutic margin is low (lethal dose is about 3 times the maximum therapeutic dose); prescribe limited quantities
- Symptoms of toxicity are extensions of the common adverse effects: anti-cholinergic, CNS stimulation followed by CNS depression, myoclonus, hallucinations, respiratory depression and seizures
- Cardiac irregularities occur and are most hazardous; duration of QRS complex on the electrocardiogram (ECG) reflects the severity of the overdose; if it equals or exceeds 0.12 s, it should be considered a danger sign (normal range 0.08–0.11 s)
- High lethality in children following overdose

Management

- Activated charcoal (1–2 g/kg initially followed by 2 or 3 more doses several hours apart) decreases tricyclic antidepressant absorption and lowers its blood level
- Cathartics (sorbitol or magnesium citrate) will aid in drug evacuation. Give together with charcoal. Monitor bowel sounds to avoid impaction
- DO NOT GIVE IPECAC due to possibility of rapid neurological deterioration and high incidence of seizures
- Supportive treatment, with patient closely monitored in hospital
- Physostigmine salicylate injection (Antilirium) 1 mg IM counteracts both central and peripheral anticholinergic effects; use only in patients with coma or those with arrhythmias or convulsions resistant to standard treatment, since associated risks often outweigh the benefits
- Diazepam IV is the drug of choice for convulsions
- Forced diuresis and dialysis are of little benefit

Nonselective Cyclic Antidepressants (cont.)

USE IN PREGNANCY

- Tricyclic antidepressants have not been demonstrated to have teratogenic effects
- If possible, avoid during first trimester
- Dosage required to achieve therapeutic plasma level may increase during the third trimester of pregnancy
- Urinary retention in neonate has been associated with antidepressant use in third trimester

Breast Milk

- Tricyclic antidepressants are excreted into breast milk and it is estimated that the baby will receive up to 4% of the mother's dose; half-life of antidepressant increased in neonate 3–4-fold
- Doxepin metabolite concentration reported to reach similar plasma level in infant as in mother
- The American Academy of Pediatrics classifies antidepressants as drugs "whose effects on nursing infants are unknown but may be of concern"

MONITORING RECOMMENDATIONS

- Prior to treatment obtain baseline ECG, resting pulse and blood pressure, and weight
- Repeat pulse and blood pressure during dose titration and ECG when therapeutic dose reached, or if clinically indicated; monitor weight periodically

NURSING IMPLICATIONS

- Psychotherapy and education are also important in the treatment of depression
- Monitor therapy by watching for adverse side effects, mood and activity level changes, including worsening depression or suicidal thoughts; keep physician informed
- Be aware that the medication reduces the degree of depression and may increase psychomotor activity; this may create concern about suicidal behavior
- Expect a lag time of 7–28 days before antidepressant effects will be noticed
- Check for constipation; increase fluids and increase bulk in diet to lessen constipation
- Check for urinary retention
- Reassure patient that drowsiness and dizziness usually subside after first few weeks; if dizzy, patient should get up from lying or sitting position slowly, and dangle legs over edge of bed before getting up
- Excessive use of caffeinated foods, drugs, or beverages may increase anxiety and agitation and confuse the diagnosis
- Expect a dry mouth; suggest frequent mouth rinsing with water, and sour or sugarless hard candy or gum
- Artificial tears may be useful for patients who complain of dry eyes (or wetting solutions for those wearing contact lenses)
- Ingesting high-fiber foods or laxatives (e.g., bran) concurrently with medication may reduce the antidepressant level

PATIENT INSTRUCTIONS

- Detailed instructions for patients and caregivers are provided in the Information Sheet on p. 303

Class of Drug	Example	Interaction Effects
ACE-inhibitor	Enalapril	Increased plasma level of clomipramine due to decreased metabolism
Alcohol		Short-term or acute use reduces first-pass metabolism of antidepressant and increases its plasma level; chronic use induces metabolizing enzymes and decreases its plasma level Increased sedation, CNS depression
Anesthetic	Enflurane	Report of seizures with amitriptyline
Antiarrhythmic	Quinidine, procainamide	Prolonged cardiac conduction
	Propafenone, quinidine	Increased plasma level of desipramine (by 500%) and imipramine (by 30%)
Antibiotic	Linezolid	Monitor for increased serotonergic and noradrenergic effects due to linezolid's weak MAO inhibition
Anticholinergic	Antiparkinsonian agents, antihistamines, neuroleptics	Increased anticholinergic effect; may increase risk of hyperthermia, confusion, urinary retention, etc.
Anticoagulant	Warfarin	Increased prothrombin time with tricyclics
Anticonvulsant	Carbamazepine, barbiturates, phenytoin	Decreased plasma level of tricyclics due to enzyme induction
	Valproate, divalproex, valproic acid	Increased plasma level of tricyclic antidepressant
	Phenobarbital	Increased plasma level of phenobarbital with clomipramine
Antidepressant Irreversible MAOI	Phenelzine, tranylcypromine, isocarboxazid	If used together, do not add cyclic antidepressants to MAOI: start cyclic antidepressant first or simultaneously with MAOI; for patients already on MAOI, discontinue MAOI 10–14 days before starting combination therapy Combined cyclic and MAOI therapy has additive antidepressant effects in treatment-resistant patients
NDRI	Bupropion	Additive antidepressant effect in treatment-resistant patients Elevated imipramine level (by 57%), desipramine level (by 82%), and nortriptyline level (by 200%) with combination
SSRI	Fluoxetine, fluvoxamine, paroxetine, sertraline (less likely with citalopram or escitalopram)	Elevated tricyclic plasma level (due to release from protein binding and inhibition of oxidative metabolism); monitor plasma level and for signs of toxicity Additive antidepressant effect in treatment-resistant patients
Antifungal	Ketoconazole, fluconazole	Increased plasma level of antidepressant due to inhibited metabolism (89% with amitriptyline; 70% with nortriptyline); 20% increase with imipramine and no increase with desipramine
	Terbinafine	Prolonged increase in plasma level of amitriptyline and its metabolite nortriptyline, due to inhibited metabolism via CYP2D6
Antihistamine	Diphenhydramine	Increased plasma level of antidepressants metabolized via CYP2D6 is possible (e.g., amitriptyline, desipramine, clomipramine, imipramine) due to inhibited metabolism Additive CNS effects
Antihypertensive	Bethanidine, clonidine, debrisoquin, methyldopa, guanethidine, reserpine	Decreased antihypertensive effect due to inhibition of α-adrenergic receptors
	Acetazolamide, thiazide diuretics	Hypotension augmented
	Labetalol	Increased plasma level of imipramine (by 54%) and desipramine

Antidepressants

Nonselective Cyclic Antidepressants (cont.)

Class of Drug	Example	Interaction Effects
Antipsychotic	Chlorpromazine, haloperidol, perphenazine	Increased plasma level of either agent
	Clozapine	Possible serotonin syndrome reported in a patient taking clomipramine following the withdrawal of clozapine
Ca-channel blocker	Nifedipine Diltiazem, verapamil	May antagonize the efficacy of antidepressant drugs Increased imipramine plasma level by 30% and 15%, respectively; increased level of trimipramine
Cannabis/marihuana		Case reports of tachycardia, lightheadedness, confusion, mood lability and delirium with nortriptyline and desipramine; may evoke cardiac complications in youth
CNS depressant	Hypnotics, antihistamines, alcohol, benzodiazepines	Increased sedation, CNS depression
Cholestyramine		Decreased absorption of antidepressant, if given together
Evening primrose oil		May lower the seizure threshold
Grapefruit juice		Decreased conversion of clomipramine to metabolite due to inhibition of CYP3A4
H$_2$ antagonist	Cimetidine	Increased plasma level of antidepressant; for desipramine, inhibition of hydroxylation occurs only in rapid metabolizers
Hormone	Estrogen/progesterone oral contraceptive	Increased plasma level of antidepressant due to decreased metabolism Reduced clearance of combined oral contraceptivee possible with amitriptyline due to inhibited metabolism
Insulin		Decreased insulin sensitivity reported with amitriptyline
MAO-B inhibitor	L-deprenyl (selegiline)	Reports of serotonergic reactions
Narcotic	Methadone	Increased plasma level of desipramine (by about 108%)
	Morphine	Enhanced analgesic effect
	Codeine	Marked inhibition of conversion of codeine to morphine (active moiety) with amitriptyline, clomipramine, desipramine, imipramine and nortriptyline
Omeprazole		Increased plasma level of antidepressant due to inhibited metabolism
Oxybutynin		Increased metabolism of clomipramine (may be due to induction of CYP3A4)
Phenylbutazone		Decreased gastric emptying with desipramine leading to impaired absorption of phenylbutazone
Propoxyphene		Increased plasma level of doxepin due to decreased metabolism
Protease inhibitor	Ritonavir	Increased plasma levels of tricyclic antidepressant due to decreased metabolism (AUC of desipramine increased by 145%; peak plasma level increased 22%)

Class of Drug	Example	Interaction Effects
Rifampin		Decreased plasma level of antidepressant due to increased metabolism
Smoking – cigarettes		Increased clearance of antidepressant due to induction of CYP1A2
Stimulant	Methylphenidate	Plasma level of antidepressant may be increased Used together to augment antidepressant effect and response to symptoms of ADHD Cardiovascular effects increased with combination, in children – monitor Case reports of neurotoxic effects with imipramine, but considered rare – monitor
Sulfonylurea	Tolbutamide	Increased hypoglycemia
Sympathomimetic	Epinephrine, norepinephrine (levarterenol), phenylephrine	Enhanced pressor response from 2- to 8-fold; benefit may outweigh risks in anaphylaxis
	Isoproterenol	May increase likelihood of arrhythmias
Tamoxifen		Decreased plasma level of doxepin by 25% due to induced metabolism via CYP3A4
Triptan	Sumatriptan, zolmitriptan	Possible serotonergic reaction when combined with antidepressants with serotonergic activity (e.g., clomipramine)
Zolpidem		Case report of visual hallucinations in combination with desipramine

Antidepressants

Monoamine Oxidase Inhibitors

CLASSIFICATION

- Monoamine oxidase inhibitors can be classified as follows:

Chemical Class	Agent	Page
Reversible Inhibitor of MAO-A (RIMA)	Moclobemide	See below
Irreversible MAOIs	Isocarboxazid[A] Phenelzine Tranylcypromine[A]	See p. 86 See p. 86 See p. 86
Selective Inhibitor of MAO-B	Selegiline transdermal[A]	—

[A] Not used in children – not reviewed in this chapter

Reversible Inhibitor of MAO-A (RIMA)

PRODUCT AVAILABILITY

Chemical Class	Generic Name	Trade Name[A]	Dosage Forms and Strengths	Monograph Statement
Reversible Inhibitor of MAO-A (RIMA)	Moclobemide[C]	Manerix	Tablets: 150 mg, 300 mg	Safety and efficacy not established in children under age 18

[A] Generic preparations may be available, [C] Not marketed in USA

INDICATIONS

No approved indications in children or adolescents

Approved (for Adults)

- Major depression
- Chronic dysthymia

Other Uses in Children and Adolescents

- Open-label studies suggest improved concentration and attention in children with ADHD
- Atypical depression
- Social anxiety disorder

PHARMACOLOGY

- Benzamide derivative chemically distinct from irreversible MAOIs
- Inhibits the action of MAO-A enzyme that metabolizes the neurotransmitters Serotonin, norepinephrine, and dopamine; in chronic doses over 400 mg daily, will produce 20–30% inhibition of MAO-B in platelets
- Inhibition is reversible (within 24 h)
- Combined therapy with cyclic antidepressants or lithium may increase antidepressant effect

DOSING	• Usual dose range, 75–225 mg daily individual doses
	• Dosing is not affected by age or renal function; should be decreased in patients with liver disorder
	• Should be taken after meals to minimize tyraminerelated responses (e.g., headache)
	• Preliminary data suggest once daily dosing as effective as divided dosing

PHARMACOKINETICS

- See p. 93
- Relatively lipophilic, but at low pH is highly water-soluble
- Rapidly absorbed from gut, high first-pass effect; peak effect seen between 0.7 and 3 h
- Has low plasma-protein binding (50% – albumin)
- Plasma level increases in proportion to dose; blockade of MAO-A correlates with plasma concentration
- Metabolized by oxidation primarily via CYP2C19; elimination half-life 1–3 h; clearance decreased as dosage increased because of auto-inhibition or metabolite-induced inhibition
- Age has no effect on pharmacokinetics

ADVERSE EFFECTS

- See table p. 97

CNS Effects

- Most common: insomnia, headache and sedation
- Increased stimulation (restlessness, anxiety, agitation, and aggressivity) can occur – dose related
- Hypomania reported especially where patient is experiencing the onset of bipolar disorder; careful monitoring for "switch to mania" is necessary
- Dizziness (7%)

Anticholinergic Effects

- Dry mouth
- Blurred vision

Cardiovascular Effects

- Hypotension
- Tachycardia

GI Effects

- Nausea, abdominal pain
- Constipation
- Both weight loss and weight gain

DISCONTINUATION SYNDROME

- None known

PRECAUTIONS

- Hypertensive patients should avoid ingesting large quantities of tyraminerich foods
- Hypertensive reactions may occur in patients with thyrotoxicosis or pheochromocytoma
- Children and adolescents prescribed doses above 400 mg/day should minimize the use of tyramine-rich foods
- Use caution when combining with serotonergic drugs as "Serotonin syndrome" has been reported (see p. 46) with CNS irritability, increased muscle tone, myoclonus, diaphoresis, and elevated temperature (see Drug Interactions p. 84)
- Reduce dose by 1/2 to 2/3 in patients with severe liver impairment

Reversible Inhibitor of MAO-A (RIMA) (cont.)

TOXICITY
- Symptoms same as side effects, but intensified: drowsiness, disorientation, stupor, hypotension, tachycardia, hyperreflexia, grimacing, sweating, agitation and hallucinations; Serotonin syndrome reported
- Fatalities have occurred when combined with citalopram or clomipramine in overdose

Management
- Gastric lavage, emesis, activated charcoal may be of benefit
- Monitor vital functions, supportive treatment

USE IN PREGNANCY
- Data on safety in pregnancy is lacking
- Animal studies have not shown any particular adverse effects on reproduction

Breast Milk
- Moclobemide is secreted into breast milk at about 1% of maternal dose

NURSING IMPLICATIONS
- If patient has difficulty sleeping, ensure last dose of moclobemide is no later than 1700 h
- It is not necessary to maintain a special diet when on moclobemide; however, excessive amounts of foods with high tyramine content can lead to headache
- Administer moclobemide after meals to minimize side effects; a big meal should not be consumed after taking moclobemide
- Warn patient not to self-medicate with over-the-counter drugs or herbal preparations, but to consult the physician or pharmacist to prevent drug-drug interactions

PATIENT INSTRUCTIONS
- Detailed instructions for patients and caregivers are provided in the Information Sheet on p. 305

FOOD INTERACTIONS
- No particular precautions are required; however, excessive consumption of tyramine-containing food should be avoided to minimize hypertension risk

DRUG INTERACTIONS
- Clinically significant interactions are listed below

Class of Drug	Example	Interaction Effects
Anticholinergic	Antiparkinsonian agents drugs	Increased atropine-like effects
Antidepressant Cyclic (non-selective)	Desipramine, nortriptyline, etc.	Additive antidepressant effect in treatment-resistant patients Potentiation of weight gain, hypotension, and anticholinergic effects
	Clomipramine	Enhanced serotonergic effects – **AVOID** (see p. 46)
SNRI, SARI	Venlafaxine, nefazodone	Enhanced effects of serotonin and/or norepinephrine; no data on safety with combination
SSRI	Fluoxetine, citalopram	Use cautiously and monitor for serotonergic adverse effects, especially with citalopram and escitalopram Higher incidence of insomnia may occur; increased headache reported with fluvoxamine Fluoxetine and fluvoxamine can inhibit the metabolism of moclobemide
NDRI	Bupropion	Enhanced neurotoxic (central noradrenergic) effect

Class of Drug	Example	Interaction Effects
Anxiolytic	Buspirone	Serotonergic reaction possible (see p. 46)
Atomoxetine		Enhanced neurotoxic (central noradrenergic) effect
H₂ antagonist	Cimetidine	Decreased metabolism of moclobemide; plasma level can double
Lithium		Additive antidepressant effect in treatment-resistant patients
L-Tryptophan		"Serotonin syndrome" possible (see p. 46)
MAO-B inhibitor	L-Deprenyl (selegiline)	Caution – dietary restrictions recommended as both A + B MAO enzymes inhibited with combination
Narcotic	Meperidine, pentazocine, dextropropoxy-phene, dextromethorphan	Serotonergic reaction, increased restlessness – **AVOID**
NSAID	Ibuprofen	Enhanced effect of ibuprofen
Stimulants	Amphetamine, Methylphenidate	See Indirect acting sympathomimitic amines
Sympathomimetic amine Indirect-acting	Ephedrine, amphetamine, methylphenidate, L-dopa, etc.	Increased blood pressure and enhanced vasopressor effects if used over prolonged periods or at high doses
Direct-acting	Salbutamol, epinephrine, phenylephrine, etc.	As above
Triptan	Sumatriptan, zolmitriptan	Possibly increased serotonergic effects
	Rizatriptan	Decreased metabolism of rizatriptan; AUC and peak plasma level increased by 119% and 41%, respectively, and AUC of metabolite increased by 400%

Antidepressants

Irreversible Monoamine Oxidase Inhibitors

PRODUCT AVAILABILITY

Chemical Class	Generic Name	Trade Name[A]	Dosage Forms and Strengths	Monograph Statement
Hydrazine derivative	Phenelzine	Nardil	Tablets: 15 mg	Not recommended for children under age 16
Nonhydrazine derivative	Isocarboxazid [B][C]	Marplan	–	
	Tranylcypromine [C]	Parnate	–	

[A] Generic preparations may be available, [B] Not marketed in Canada, [C] Not used in children and not reviewed in this chapter

INDICATIONS

No approved indications in children or adolescents

Approved (for Adults)

- "Atypical" depression
- Major depression unresponsive to other antidepressants
- Phobic anxiety states or social phobia

Other Uses in Children and Adolescents

- Atypical (anergic) bipolar depression
- Panic disorder prophylaxis, agoraphobia
- ADHD not responsive to other agents
- Depression in patients with borderline personality disorder
- Chronic dysthymia
- Efficacy in posttraumatic stress disorder reported
- Separation anxiety, selective autism
- Double-blind and open trials suggest efficacy in eating disorders

PHARMACOLOGY

- Inhibit the action of MAO-A and B enzymes that metabolize the neurotransmitters responsible for stimulating physical and mental activity (Serotonin, norepinephrine, dopamine); cause down-regulation of β-adrenoceptors
- Inhibition is irreversible and lasts about 10 days
- Combined therapy with cyclic antidepressants or lithium may increase antidepressant effect
- Best response to MAOIs occurs at dosages that reduce MAO enzyme activity by at least 80%; may require up to 2 weeks to reach maximum MAO inhibition

GENERAL COMMENTS

- Rarely used in children and adolescents; use with EXTREME CAUTION for patients who have failed to respond to other classes of antidepressants
- Ability to adhere to dietary and drug restrictions should be assessed before prescribing

DOSING	• See p. 93
	• Dose should be carefully titrated and maintained between 0.3 and 1 mg/kg
	• Due to short half-life, bid dosing required; give doses in the morning and mid-day to avoid overstimulation and insomnia (occasionally cause sedation)

PHARMACOKINETICS	• See p. 93
	• Rapidly absorbed from the GI tract, metabolized by the liver and excreted almost entirely in the urine
	• With long-term use, irreversible MAOIs can impair own metabolism resulting in nonlinear pharmacokinetics and potential for drug accumulation

| **ONSET AND DURATION OF ACTION** | • May require up to 2 weeks to reach maximum MAO inhibition |
| | • Energizing effect often seen within a few days |

| **ADVERSE EFFECTS** | • See p. 97 |

CNS Effects

A. Cognitive Effects

- Drowsiness
- Stimulant effect (insomnia, restlessness, anxiety) can occur
- Increased sleep onset latency, REM sleep decreased and may be eliminated at start of therapy, reduced sleep efficiency; rebound REM on drug withdrawal
- Headache
- Hypomania and mania especially where patient is experiencing onset of bipolar disorder; careful monitoring for "switch to mania" is necessary

B. Neurological Effects

- Paresthesias or "electric shock-like" sensations; carpal tunnel syndrome (numbness) reported; may be due to vitamin B6 deficiency [Management: pyridoxine 50 mg/day]
- Myoclonic jerks, especially during sleep, tremor, muscle tension, cramps, akathisia (dose-related)

Anticholinergic Effects

- Constipation common [Management: increase bulk and fluid intake, fecal softener, bulk laxative]
- Dry mouth
- Urinary retention

Cardiovascular Effects

- Dizziness, weakness, orthostatic hypotension
- Edema in lower extremities

GI Effects

- The most common are anorexia, nausea and vomiting
- Increased appetite and weight gain

Sexual Side Effects

- Impotence, anorgasmia, decreased libido, ejaculation difficulties

Endocrine Effects

- Hyponatremia and SIADH reported

Other Adverse Effects

- Rare reports of liver toxicity

Antidepressants

Irreversible Monoamine Oxidase Inhibitors (cont.)

HYPERTENSIVE CRISIS

- Can occur with irreversible MAOIs due to ingestion of incompatible foods (containing elevated levels of tyramine) or drugs (see lists pp. 89–90)
- Not related to dose of drug

Signs and Symptoms

- Occipital headache, neck stiffness or soreness, nausea, vomiting, sweating (sometimes with fever and sometimes with cold, clammy skin), dilated pupils and photophobia, sudden nose bleed, tachycardia, bradycardia, and constricting chest pain

Management

- Withhold medication and notify physician immediately
- Monitor vital signs, ECG
- Nifedipine or captopril may decrease blood pressure (occasionally drastically – monitor)
- Phentolamine is an alternative parenteral treatment
- Patient should stand and walk, rather than lie down, during a hypertensive reaction; BP will drop somewhat

DISCONTINUATION SYNDROME

- Occur occasionally 1–4 days after abrupt withdrawal
- Reports of muscle weakness, agitation, vivid nightmares, headache, palpitations, nausea, sweating, irritability, and myoclonic jerking; acute psychosis with hallucinations reported
- REM rebound occurs
- Maintain dietary and drug restrictions for at least 10 days after stopping MAOI

PRECAUTIONS

- Should not be administered to patients with cerebrovascular disease, cardiovascular disease, or a history of hypertension
- Should not be used alone in patients with marked psychomotor agitation
- When changing from one MAOI to another, or to a tricyclic antidepressant, allow a minimum of 14 medication-free days
- Need 10–14 days to be excreted from the system before an incompatible drug or food is given, or before surgery or ECT
- Hypertensive crisis can occur if given concurrently with certain drugs or foods (see lists below)
- Use caution when combining with serotonergic drugs as "Serotonin syndrome" has been reported (see p. 46)

TOXICITY

- Symptoms same as side effects but intensified
- Severe cases progress to extreme dizziness and shock
- Overdose, whether accidental or intentional, can be fatal: patient may be symptom-free up to 6 h, then progress to restlessness-coma-death – therefore, close medical supervision is indicated for 48 h following an overdose

USE IN PREGNANCY

- Avoid; increased incidence of malformations demonstrated with use in first trimester

Breast Milk

- No data on phenelzine and isocarboxazid

NURSING IMPLICATIONS

- The incidence of orthostatic hypotension is high at the start of treatment: tell patient to get out of bed slowly
- Educate patient regarding foods and drugs to avoid; a diet sheet should be provided for each patient
- Warn patient not to self-medicate with over-the-counter drugs or herbal preparations, but to consult physician or pharmacist to prevent drug-drug interactions

- Educate patient to report headache; measure pulse and blood pressure, and report increases to physician immediately
- If patient has difficulty sleeping, ensure last dose of MAOI is no later than 1500 h

PATIENT INSTRUCTIONS

- Detailed instructions for patients and caregivers are provided in the Information Sheet on p. 307.

FOOD INTERACTIONS

There are many serious food and drug interactions that may precipitate a hypertensive crisis; maintain dietary and drug restrictions for at least 10 days after stopping MAOI

Foods to avoid:
- All matured or aged cheeses (e.g., cheddar, brick, mozzarella, parmesan, blue, gruyere, stilton, brie, Swiss, Roquefort, camembert)
- Broad bean pods (e.g., Fava) – contain dopamine
- Concentrated yeast extracts (e.g., Marmite)
- Dried salted fish, pickled herring
- Packet soup (especially miso)
- Sauerkraut
- Aged/smoked meats – sausage (especially salami, mortadella, pastrami, summer sausage); other unrefrigerated fermented meats; game meat that has been hung; liver
- Soy sauce or soybean condiments, tofu
- Tap (draft) beer, alcohol-free beer
- Improperly stored or spoiled meats, poultry, or fish

It is SAFE to use in moderate amounts (only if fresh):
- Cottage cheese, cream cheese, farmer's cheese, processed cheese, Cheez Whiz, ricotta, Havarti, Boursin, brie without rind, gorgonzola
- Liver (as long as it is fresh), fresh or processed meats, poultry or fish (e.g., hot dogs, bologna)
- Spirits (in moderation)
- Sour cream
- Soy milk
- Salad dressings
- Worcestershire sauce
- Yeast-leavened bread

Reactions have also been reported with:
- Smoked fish, caviar, snails, tinned fish, shrimp paste
- yogurt
- Meat tenderizers
- Homemade red wine, Chianti, canned/bottled beer, sherry, champagne
- Cheeses (e.g., Parmesan, muenster, Swiss, gruyere, mozzarella, feta)
- Pepperoni
- Overripe fruit, avocados, raspberries, banana (peel), plums, tomatoes, canned figs, or raisins, orange pulp
- Meat extract (e.g., Bovril, Oxo)
- Oriental foods
- Spinach, eggplant

Irreversible Monoamine Oxidase Inhibitors (cont.)

☞ **MAKE SURE ALL FOOD IS FRESH, STORED PROPERLY, AND EATEN SOON AFTER BEING PURCHASED** – products stored even under refrigeration will show an increase in tyramine content after several days
- Never touch food that is fermented or possibly "off" (spoiled)
- Avoid restaurant sauces, gravy, and soup

Over-the-counter drugs: DO NOT USE without prior consultation with doctor or pharmacist:
- Cold remedies, decongestants (including nasal sprays and drops), some antihistamines and cough medicines
- Narcotic painkillers (e.g., products containing codeine)
- All stimulants including pep-pills (Wake-ups, Nodoz)
- All appetite suppressants
- Anti-asthma drugs (Primatine P)
- Sleep aids and sedatives (Sominex, Nytol)
- Yeast, dietary supplements (e.g., Ultrafast, Optifast)

DRUG INTERACTIONS
- Clinically significant interactions are listed below

Class of Drug	Example	Interaction Effects
Anesthetic, general		May enhance CNS depression
Anorexiant	Fenfluramine, dexfenfluramine	"Serotonin syndrome" (see p. 46); **AVOID**
Anticholinergic	Antiparkinsonian agents, antipsychotics	Increased atropine-like effects
Anticonvulsant	Carbamazepine	Possible decrease in metabolism and increased plasma level of carbamazepine with phenelzine
Antidepressant Cyclic (nonselective)	Amitriptyline, desipramine	If used together, do not add cyclic antidepressants to MAOI. Start cyclic antidepressant first or simultaneously with MAOI. For patients already on MAOI, discontinue the MAOI for 10–14 days before starting combination therapy Combined cyclic and MAOI therapy has increased antidepressant effects and will potentiate weight gain, hypotension, and anticholinergic effects
	Clomipramine	"Serotonin syndrome" reported; **AVOID** (see p. 46)
SARI	Trazodone	Low doses of trazodone (25–50 mg) used to treat antidepressant-induced insomnia Combined therapy has additive antidepressant effects; monitor for serotonergic effects
SNRI	Venlafaxine	Metabolism of serotonin and norepinephrine inhibited; **AVOID**
SSRI	Fluoxetine, paroxetine, sertraline	"Serotonin syndrome" (see p. 46) and death reported with serotonergic antidepressants; **AVOID**
NDRI	Bupropion	Metabolism of dopamine inhibited; **AVOID**
NaSSA	Mirtazapine	Possible serotonergic reaction; **AVOID**
Antihypertensive	ACE inhibitors, α-blockers, β-blockers	Enhanced hypotension
	Guanethidine	Antihypertensive effects of guanethidine decreased

Class of Drug	Example	Interaction Effects
Antipsychotic	Phenothiazines, clozapine	Additive hypotension
Atropine		Prolonged action of Atropine
Anxiolytic	Buspirone	Several cases of increased blood pressure reported
Bromocriptine		Increased serotonergic effects
CNS depressant	Barbiturates, sedatives, alcohol	May enhance CNS depression
Ginseng		May cause headache, tremulousness or hypomania; case report of irritability and visual hallucinations with combination
Insulin		Enhanced hypoglycemic response through stimulation of insulin secretion and inhibition of gluconeogenesis
L-Dopa		Increased blood pressure; increased serotonergic effects Use carbidopa/L-dopa combination to inhibit peripheral decarboxylation
L-Tryptophan		Reports of "serotonin syndrome," with hyperreflexia, tremor, myoclonic jerks, and ocular oscillations (see p. 46); **AVOID**
Lithium		Increased serotonergic effects Additive antidepressant effect in treatment-resistant patients
MAO-B inhibitor	L-deprenyl (selegiline)	Increased serotonergic effects
Muscle relaxant	Succinylcholine	Phenelzine may prolong muscle relaxation by inhibiting metabolism
Narcotics and related drugs	Meperidine, dextromethorphan, diphenoxylate, tramadol	Excitation, sweating, and hypotension reported; may lead to development of encephalopathy, convulsions, coma, respiratory depression, and "serotonin syndrome" (see p. 46). If a narcotic is required, meperidine should not be used; other narcotics should be instituted cautiously
	Propoxyphene	Potentiation of catecholamine-release reported, resulting in anxiety, confusion, ataxia, hypotension
Nicotine		Low doses of tranylcypromine reported to inhibit nicotine metabolism by competitive inhibition via CYP2A6
Reserpine		Central excitatory syndrome and hypertension reported due to central and peripheral release of catecholamines
Sibutramine		Increased noradrenergic and serotonergic effects possible. DO NOT COMBINE
Stimulant	MDMA ("Ecstasy"), MDA	Case reports of "serotonin syndrome" (see p. 46)
Sulfonylurea		Enhanced hypoglycemic response
Sympathomimeticamine	*Indirect acting:* amphetamine, methylphenidate, ephedrine, pseudoephedrine, phenylpropanolamine, dopamine, tyramine	Release of large amounts of norepinephrine with hypertensive reaction; **AVOID**
	Direct acting: epinephrine, isoproterenol, norepinephrine (levarterenol), methoxamine, salbutamol	No interaction
	Phenylephrine	Increased pressor response
Tetrabenazine		Central excitatory syndrome and hypertension reported due to central and peripheral release of catecholamines
Triptan	Sumatriptan, zolmitriptan, rizatriptan	"Serotonin syndrome" (see p. 46); **AVOID;** recommend that 2 weeks elapse after discontinuing an irreversible MAOI and using sumatriptan

Antidepressants

Antidepressant Doses

Drug	Starting Dose [c]	Suggested Daily-Therapeutic Dose Range (mg)	Bioavailability	Peak Plasma Level [h]	Protein Binding (in Adults)	Elimination Halflife [h]	CYP-450 Metabolizing Enzymes[f]	CYP-450 Inhibition[g]
SSRIs								
Citalopram (Celexa)	Child: 10 mg Adolescent: 10 mg	10–40 up to 60 mg in adolescents	80%	4	80%	23–45 **(L)**	2D6[m][h], 3A4[m], 2C19[m]	2D6[w], 2C9[w], 2C19[w]
Escitalopram (Lexapro[B], Cipralex[A])	Child: 5 mg Adolescent: 5 mg	2.5–20	80%	4–5 (metab=14)	56%	27–32 **(L)(R)**	2D6[m], 3A4[m], 2C19[m]	2D6[w], 2C9[w], 2C19[w]
Fluoxetine (Prozac)	Child: 5 mg Adolescent: 5 mg	5–40[c] (up to 80 mg in autism)	72–85%	6–8 (immediate release)	94%	24–144 (parent) **(L)** 200–330 (metab)	1A2[w], 2B6[w], **2D6**[h][p], 3A4[w], **2C9**[p], **2C19**[p], 2E1	1A2[m], 2B6[w], **2D6**[w], 3A4[h][w], 2C9[w], 2C19[w]
Fluvoxamine (Luvox)	Child: 25 mg Adolescent: 25–50 mg	25–200[c] (rarely up to 300 mg)	60%	1.5–8	77–80%	9–28 **(L)**	1A, 2D6	**1A2**[w], 2B6[w], 2D6[m], 3A4[w], 2C9[m], **2C19**[p]
Paroxetine (Paxil)*** Paroxetine CR (Paxil CR)***	Child: 5 mg Adolescent: 10 mg	5–40[c] 12.5–50	>90%	5.2 (immediate release)	95%	3–65 **(L)(R)**	**2D6**[p]	1A2[w], **2B6**[p], **2D6**[p], 3A4[w], 2C9[w], 2C19[m]
Sertraline (Zoloft)	Child: 25 mg Adolescent: 50 mg	50–200[c]	70%	6	98%	22–36 (parent) **(L)(R)** 62–104 (metab)	2B6, 2D6, **3A4**[p], 2C9, 2C19[m]	1A2[w], 2B6[m], 2D6[m], 3A4[w], 2C9[w], **2C19**[p]
NDRI								
Bupropion (Wellbutrin)[B] Bupropion SR (Wellbutrin SR, Zyban)	Child: 100 mg Adolescent: 100 mg	3–6 mg/kg/day[d]	>90%	1.6 (immediate release)	80–85%	10–14 (parent) **(L)** 20–27 (metab)	1A2[w], 2A6[w], **2B6**[p], 2D6[h], 3A4[w], 2C9[w], 2E1[m]	2D6[w]
SNRI								
Venlafaxine (Effexor)*** Venlafaxine XR (Effexor XR)***	Child: 12.5 mg Adolescent: 18.75–37.5 mg	0.5–3mg/kg/day for ADHD for MDD 1–2 mg/kg/day Ages 8–12: 12.5–37.5 mg/day Ages 13–17: 25–75 mg/day; doses up to 225 mg occasionally necessary	13%	2 (immediate release) XR=5.5	27%	3–7 (parent) **(L)(R)** 9–13 (metab) 9–12 (absorption half-life)	**2D6**[p], 3A4[w], 2C9, 2C19	2D6[w], 3A4[w]
Duloxetine[A] (Cymbalta)	20 mg	20–40 up to 60 mg in adolescents	70%	6	> 95%	8–17 **(L)(R)**	1A2, 2D6	2D6 [m]
SARI								
Trazodone (Desyrel)	Child: 25 mg Adolescent: 50 mg	1–2 mg/kg/day	70–90%		93%	4–9	2D6[h], **3A4**[p]	2D6[w]

Drug	Starting Dose [c]	Suggested Daily-Therapeutic Dose Range (mg)	Bioavailability	Peak Plasma Level [h]	Protein Binding (in Adults)	Elimination Halflife [h]	CYP-450 Metabolizing Enzymes[f]	CYP-450 Inhibition[g]
Nefazodone[B]	Child: 50 mg Adolescent: 50 mg	100–300 mg to age 12 100–600 mg over age 12	15–23%	?	> 99%	2–5[e] (parent) 3–18 (metab)	2D6[h], **3A4**[p]	2B6[w], 2D6[h][w], **3A4**[p]
NaSSA Mirtazapine (Remeron)	Child: 7.5 mg Adolescent: 15 mg	15–45	50%	2	85%	20–40(L)(R)	**1A2**[p], **2D6**[h][p], **3A4**[p], 2C9	–
Tricyclic Agents Amitriptyline (Elavil)	Child: 10 mg Adolescent: 10–25 mg	45–200 Max of 1.5 mg/kg/day	43–48%	2–8	92–96%	10–46(L)	1A2[w], 2B6[w], 2D6[m], **3A4**[p], 2C9[w], **2C19**[p]	1A2[w], 2D6[m], 3A4[w], 2C9[w], 2C19[m] 2E1
Clomipramine (Anafranil)	Child: 10 mg Adolescent: 10–25 mg	3–5 mg/kg/day	48%	2–6	98%	17–37(L)	1A2[w], 2D6, 3A4[w], 2C9[w], 2C19[w]	2D6[m]
Desipramine (Norpramin)	Child: 10 mg Adolescent: 10–25 mg	2–5 mg/kg/day	50–68%	2–6	73–92%	12–76(L)	1A2, **2D6**[p]	2D6[m], 2C19[w], 2E1
Doxepin (Sinequan, Triadapin[B])	Child: 10 mg Adolescent: 10–25 mg	max. 5 mg/kg/day	25%	2–6	89%	8–36(L)	1A2[w], **2D6**[p], 3A4, 2C9[w], **2C19**[p]	–
Imipramine (Tofranil) Imipramine PM (Tofranil PM)	Child: 10 mg Adolescent: 10–25 mg	up to 250 mg max. 2.5 mg/kg/day in MDD (2–5 mg/kg/day in ADHD)	29–77%	2–6	89%	4–34(L)	1A2[w], 2B6[w], **2D6**[p], 3A4[m], 2C9[w], 2C19[m]	1A2[w], 2D6[m], 2C19[m], 2E1
Nortriptyline (Aventyl, Pamelor)	Child: 10 mg Adolescent: 10–25 mg	1–3 mg/kg/day Max of 150 mg/day in adolescents	64%	2–6	89–92%	13–88(L)	1A2, **2D6**[p], 3A4[m], 2C19	2D6, 2C19[w], 2E1
Protriptyline[B] (Vivactil)	Child: 5 mg Adolescent: 5–10 mg	up to 20 mg	75–90%	12	90–96%	54–124(L)	?	?
Trimipramine (Surmontil)	Child: 10 mg Adolescent: 10–25 mg	up to 100 mg	40%	2–6	95%	7–30(L)	2D6, 2C9, 2C19	2D6
RIMA Moclobemide[A] (Manerix)	Child: 75 mg Adolescent: 75 mg	75–450 mg	50–80%	?	50%	1–3(L)	**2C19**[p]	1A2[m], 2D6[m], 2C9, 2C19[m]
MAOI (irreversible) Phenelzine (Nardil)		0.3 to 1 mg/kg/day	?	?	?	1.5–4	2E1	

Monograph doses are just a guideline, and each patient's medication must be individualized.

*Includes sum of drug and its metabolites. ** Approximate conversion: nmol/l = 3.5 × ng/ml. *** Not recommended in children and adolescents.

(L) Increased in liver disorders – consider dose adjustment, **(R)** Increased in moderate to severe renal impairment – consider dose adjustment

[A] Not marketed in USA, [B] Not marketed in Canada, [c] SSRIs have a flat dose-response curve. For depression most patients respond to the initial (low) dose. Higher doses are used in the treatment of OCD, [d] Give in divided doses (maximum of 150 mg per dose), [e] Dose-dependent, [f] Cytochrome P450 isoenzymes involved in drug metabolism [Ref.: www. gentest.com/human_p450_database/srchh450. asp (December 2003) and www.mhc.com/Cytochromes/], [g] Cytochrome P450 isoenzymes inhibited by the drug, [h] Specific to metabolite, [m] Moderate activity, [p] Potent activity, [w] Weak activity.

Effects of Antidepressants on Neurotransmitters/Receptors*

	Amitriptyline	Clomipramine	Desipramine	Doxepin	Imipramine	Nortriptyline	Protriptyline	Trimipramine	Trazodone	Nefazodone
NE reuptake block	+++	+++	+++++	+++	+++	++++	+++++	++	+	++
5-HT reuptake block	+++	++++	++	++	+++	++	++	+	++	++
DA reuptake block	+	+	+	+	+	+	+	+	+−	+
5-HT$_1$ blockade	++	+	+	++	+	++	+	+	+++	+++
5-HT$_2$ blockade	+++	+++	++	+++	+++	+++	+++	+++	++++	+++
ACh blockade	+++	+++	++	+++	+++	++	+++	+++	−	+−
H$_1$ blockade	++++	+++	++	+++++	+++	+++	+++	+++++	++	+−
α$_1$ blockade	+++	+++	++	+++	+++	+++	++	+++	+++	+++
α$_2$ blockade	++	+	+	+	+	+	+	+	++	++
D$_2$ blockade	+	++	+	+	+	+	+	++	+	++
Selectivity	NE>5-HT	NE<5-HT	NE>5-HT	NE>5-HT	NE>5-HT	NE>5-HT	NE>5-HT	NE>5-HT	NE<5-HT	NE<5-HT

	Bupropion	Venlafaxine	Duloxetine	Citalopram	Escitalopram	Fluoxetine	Fluvoxamine	Paroxetine	Sertraline	Mirtazapine
NE reuptake	+	++	++++	+	+	++	++	+++	++	+
5-HT reuptake	+−	+++	+++++	++++	++++	++++	++++	+++++	++++	+
DA reuptake	++	+	++	+−	−	+	+−	+	++	−
5-HT$_1$ Blockade	+−	+−	−	+−	+−	+−	+−	+−	+−	−
5-HT$_2$ Blockade	+−	+−	−	+	+	++	+	+−	+	++++
ACh Blockade	+−	−	+	−		++	+−	++	++	++
H$_1$ Blockade	+	−	+	++	+	+	−	+−	+−	+++++
α$_1$ Blockade	+	−	+	+	+	+	+	+	++	++
α$_2$ Blockade	+−	+−	−	+−	?	+−	+	+	+	+++
D$_2$ Blockade	−	−		+−	+	+	++	+−	+−	+
Selectivity	NE>5-HT	NE<5-HT	NE<5-HT	NE<5-HT	NE<5-HT	NE<5-HT	NE<5-HT	NE<5-HT	NE<5-HT	NE<5-HT

* The ratio of K$_1$ values (intrinsic dissociation constant) between various neurotransmitters/receptors determines the pharmacological profile for any one drug

Key: K$_1$ (nM) > 100,000 = −; 10,000–100,000 = +−; 1000–10,000 = +; 100–1000 = ++; 10–100 = +++; 1–10 = ++++; 0.1–1 = +++++

1/K$_1^{(M)}$ < 0.001 = −; 0.001–0.01 = +−; 0.01–0.1 = +; 0.1–1 = ++; 1–10 = +++; 10–100 = ++++; 100–1000 = +++++

Adapted from Seeman, P. (1996). *Receptor Tables Vol. 2: Drug Dissociation Constants for Neuroreceptors and Transporters*. Toronto: SZ Research; Richelson, E. (1996), Synaptic effects of antidepressants. *Journal of Clinical Psychopharmacology 16(3)* (Suppl 2), 1–9, 1996

Pharmacological Effects of Antidepressants on Neurotransmitters/Receptors

NE REUPTAKE BLOCK
- Antidepressant effect
- Side effects: tremors, tachycardia, hypertension, sweating, insomnia, erectile and ejaculation problems
- Potentiation of pressor effects of NE (e.g., sympathomimetic amines)
- Interaction with guanfacine (blockade of antihypertensive effect)

5-HT REUPTAKE BLOCK
- Antidepressant, antianxiety, anti obsessional, antipanic effect
- Can increase or decrease anxiety, depending on dose
- Side effects: dyspepsia, nausea, headache, nervousness, akathisia, extrapyramidal effects, sexual side effects, anorexia
- Potentiation of drugs with serotonergic properties (e.g., L-tryptophan); caution regarding "serotonin syndrome" (p.46)

DA REUPTAKE BLOCK
- Antidepressant, antiparkinsonian effect, effect on ADHD symptoms
- Side effects: psychomotor activation, aggravation of psychosis

H_1 BLOCKADE
- Most potent action of cyclic antidepressants
- Side effects: sedation, postural hypotension, weight gain
- Potentiation of effects of other CNS drugs

ACH BLOCKADE
- Second most potent action of cyclic antidepressants
- Antidepressant effect
- Side effects: dry mouth, blurred vision, constipation, urinary retention, sinus tachycardia, QRS changes, memory disturbances, sedation, exacerbation/attack of narrow angle glaucoma
- Potentiation of effects of drugs with anticholinergic properties

A_1 BLOCKADE
- Side effects: postural hypotension, dizziness, reflex tachycardia, sedation
- Potentiation of antihypertensives acting via α_1 blockade (e.g., prazosin, doxazolin, labetalol)

A_2 BLOCKADE
- CNS arousal; possible decrease in depressive symptoms
- Side effect: sexual dysfunction, priapism
- Antagonism of antihypertensives acting as α_2 stimulants (e.g., clonidine)

$5-HT_1$ BLOCKADE
- Antidepressant, anxiolytic, and antiaggressive action

$5-HT_2$ BLOCKADE
- Anxiolytic ($5-HT_2C$), antidepressant ($5-HT_2A$), antipsychotic, antimigraine effect, improved sleep
- Side effects: hypotension, ejaculatory problems, sedation, weight gain ($5 HT_{2C}$)

D_2 BLOCKADE
- Antipsychotic effect
- Side effects: extrapyramidal (e.g., tremor, rigidity), endocrine changes, sexual dysfunction (males)

Adverse Reactions to Antidepressants at Therapeutic Doses

Reaction	TRICYCLICS								SARI		NDRI
	Amitriptyline	Clomipramine	Desipramine	Doxepin	Imipramine	Nortriptyline	Protriptyline	Trimipramine	Trazodone	Nefazodone	Bupropion
CNS Effects											
Drowsiness, sedation	> 30%	> 2%	> 2%	> 30%	> 10%	> 2%	< 2%	> 30%	30%	> 10%	> 2%
Insomnia	> 2%	> 10%	> 2%	> 2%	> 10%	< 2%	> 10%	> 2%[m]	> 2%	> 2%	> 10%
Excitement, hypomania*[b]	< 2%	< 2%	> 2%	< 2%	> 10%	> 2%	> 10%	< 2%	—[t]	> 10%	> 10%[c]
Disorientation/ confusion	> 10%	> 2%	—	< 2%	> 2%	> 10%	—	> 10%	< 2%	> 10%	> 2%
Headache	> 2%	> 2%	< 2%	< 2%	> 10%	< 2%	—	> 2%	> 2%	> 10%	> 10%
Asthenia, fatigue	> 10%	> 2%	> 2%	> 2%	> 10%	> 10%	> 10%	> 2%	> 10%	> 10%	> 2%
Anticholinergic Effects											
Dry mouth	> 30%	> 30%	> 10%	> 30%	> 30%	> 10%	> 10%	> 10%	> 10%	> 10%	> 10%
Blurred vision	> 10%	> 10%	> 2%	> 10%	> 10%	> 2%	> 10%	> 2%	> 2%[i]	> 10%	> 10%
Constipation	> 10%	> 10%	> 2%	> 10%	> 10%	> 10%	> 10%	> 10%	> 2%	> 10%	> 10%
Sweating	> 10%	> 10%	> 2%	> 2%	> 10%	< 2%	> 10%	> 2%	—	> 2%	> 10%
Delayed micturition	> 2%	> 2%	—	< 2%	> 10%	< 2%	< 2%	< 2%	< 2%	< 2%	> 2%
Extrapyramidal Effects											
Unspecified	> 2%	< 2%	< 2%	> 2%	< 2%	—	—	< 2%	> 2%	< 2%	> 2%
Tremor	> 10%	> 10%	> 2%	> 2%	> 10%	> 10%	> 2%	> 10%	> 2%	< 2%	> 10%
Cardiovascular Effects											
Orthostatic hypotension/dizziness	> 10%	> 10%	> 2%	> 10%	> 30%	> 2%	> 10%	> 10%	> 10%[n]	> 10%	> 2%[l]
Tachycardia, palpitations	> 10%	> 10%	> 10%	> 2%	> 10%	> 2%	> 2%	> 2%	< 2%[j]	< 2% [j]	> 2%
ECG changes**	> 10%[a]	> 10%[a]	> 2%[a]	> 2%[a]	> 10%[a]	> 2%[a]	> 10%[a]	> 10%[a]	> 2%	< 2%	< 2%
Cardiac arrhythmia	> 2%	> 2%	> 2%	> 2%	> 2%	> 2%	> 2%	> 2%	> 2%[g]	< 2%	< 2%
GI distress	> 2%	> 10%	> 2%	< 2%	> 10%	< 2%	—	< 2%	> 10%	> 10%	> 10%
Dermatitis, rash	> 2%	> 2%	> 2%	< 2%	> 2%	< 2%	< 2%	< 2%	< 2%	< 2%	> 10%
Weight gain (over 6 kg)	> 30%	> 10%	> 2%	> 10%	> 10%	> 2%	< 2%	> 10%	> 2%	> 2%	< 2%[k][f]
Sexual disturbances	> 2%	> 30%	> 2%	> 2%	> 30%	< 2%	< 2%	< 2%	<2%[h]	> 2%	< 2%[p]
Seizures[c]	< 2%	< 2%[d]	< 2%	< 2%	< 2%	< 2%	< 2%	< 2%	< 2%	< 2%	< 2%[o]

– None reported in literature perused, * More likely in bipolar patients, ** ECG abnormalities usually without cardiac injury

[a] Conduction delays: increased PR, QRS, or QT$_c$ interval,[b] Higher incidence in children,[c] In nonepileptic patients; risk increased with higher plasma levels, [d] Higher incidence if dose above 250 mg daily clomipramine, [f] With chronic treatment, [g] Patients with pre-existing cardiac disease have a 10% incidence of premature ventricular contractions, [h] Priapism reported, [i] Found to lower intraocular pressure, [j] Decreased heart rate reported, [k] Weight loss reported initially, [l] Hypertension reported, [m] No effect on REM sleep, [n] Less frequent if drugs given after meals, [o] Higher incidence if doses

Reaction	SNRI		SSRIs						NaSSA	MAOI	RIMA
	Venlafaxine	Duloxetine	Citalopram	Escitalopram	Fluoxetine	Fluvoxamine	Paroxetine	Sertraline	Mirtazapine	Phenelzine	Moclobemide
CNS Effects											
Drowsiness, sedation	> 10%	> 10%	> 10%	> 2%	> 10%	> 10%	> 10%	> 10%	> 30%(m)	> 10%	> 2%
Insomnia	> 10%(i)	> 10%	> 10%	> 10%	>10% (i)	> 10%	> 10%	> 10%	> 2%	> 10%(i)	> 10%(i)
Excitement, hypomania*(b)	> 10%(e)	< 2%	> 10%	< 2%	> 2%	> 10%	> 10%	> 10%	> 2%	> 10%	> 10%
Disorientation/con-fusion	> 2%	–	< 2%	< 2%	> 10%	> 2%	< 2%	< 2%	> 2%	> 2%	> 2%
Headache	> 10%	> 10%	> 10%	> 10%	> 10%	> 10%	> 10%	> 10%	> 2%	> 2%	> 10%
Asthenia, fatigue	> 10%	> 10%	> 10%	> 2%	> 10%	> 10%	> 10%	> 2%	> 10%	< 2%	< 2%
Anticholinergic Effects											
Dry mouth	> 10%	> 10%	> 10%	> 10%	> 10%	> 10%	> 10%	> 10%	> 30%	> 30%	> 10%
Blurred vision	> 2%	> 2%	> 2%	< 2%	> 2%	> 2%	> 2%	> 2%	> 10%	> 10%	> 10%
Constipation	> 10%	> 10%	> 2%	> 2%	> 2%	> 10%	> 10%	> 2%	> 10%	> 10%	> 2%
Sweating	> 10%	> 10%	> 10%	> 2%	> 2%	> 10%	> 10%	> 2%	> 2%	> 2%	> 2%
Delayed micturition	< 2%	< 2%	> 2%	–	> 2%	> 2%	> 2%	< 2%	> 2%	> 2%	< 2%
Extrapyramidal Effects											
Unspecified	> 2%	< 2%	< 2%	< 2%	> 2%	> 2%	> 2%	> 2%	< 2%	> 10%	< 2%
Tremor	> 2%	> 2%	> 2%	< 2%	> 2%	> 10%	> 10%	> 10%	> 2%	> 10%	> 2%
Cardiovascular Effects											
Orthostatic hypoten-sion/dizziness	> 10%(l)	> 10%	> 2%	> 2%	> 10%	> 2%	> 10%	> 10%	> 2%	> 10%	> 10%
Tachycardia, palpita-tions	> 2% (g)	< 2%	> 2%(j)	> 2%(j)	< 2%(j)	< 2%(j)	> 2%(j)	> 2%(a)	> 2%	> 10%(j)	> 2%
ECG changes**	< 2% (g)	–	< 2%	< 2%	< 2%	< 2%	< 2%	< 2%	< 2%	< 2%(a)	> 2%
Cardiac arrhythmia	< 2%	–	< 2%	< 2%	< 2%(d)	< 2%	< 2%	< 2%	< 2%	< 2%	> 2%
GI distress	> 30%	> 10%	> 10%	> 10%	> 10%	> 30%	> 10%	> 10%	> 2%	> 10%	> 10%
Dermatitis, rash	> 2%	> 2%	< 2%	> 2%	> 2%	> 2%	< 2%	> 2%	< 2%	< 2%	> 2%
Weight gain (over 6 kg)(f)	> 2%(k)	< 2%	> 2%	< 2%	> 2%(k)	> 2%(k)	> 10%(k)	> 2%(k)	> 30%	> 10%	< 2%
Sexual disturbances	> 30%	> 2%	> 30%	> 10%	> 30%(h)	> 30%	> 30%(h)	> 30%(h)	> 2%	> 30%	> 2%
Seizures(c)	< 2%	–	< 2%	–	< 2%	< 2%	< 2%	< 2%	< 2%	< 2%	< 2%

* More likely in bipolar patients, ** ECG abnormalities usually without cardiac injury. (a) Shortened QT_c interval, (b) Higher incidence in children, (c) In nonepileptic patients; risk increased with elevated plasma levels, (d) Slowing of sinus node and atrial dysrhythmia, (f) With chronic treatment, (g) Increased risk with higher doses, (h) Priapism reported, (i) Especially if given in the evening, (j) Decreased heart rate reported, (k) Weight loss reported initially, (l) Hypertension reported, (m) Sedation decreased at higher doses (above 15 mg), (t) Less likely to precipitate mania

Antidepressants

Switching Antidepressants

Switching from		Switching to	Wash-out Period[a]
Tricyclic (TCA)	→	TCA	No washout
	→	SSRI	5 half-lives of TCA (caution: see Drug Interactions p. 79)[b]
	→	NDRI	5 half-lives of TCA
	→	SNRI or SARI, NaSSA	No washout – taper[b]
	→	Irrev. MAOI	5 half-lives of TCA
	→	RIMA	5 half-lives of TCA
SSRI or SARI	→	TCA	5 half-lives of SSRI or SARI (caution: with fluoxetine due to long half-life of active metabolite)[b]
	→	NDRI	No washout – taper (caution: with fluoxetine)[b]
	→	SNRI	No washout – taper (caution: with fluoxetine)[b], monitor for serotonergic effects (see p. 46)
	→	Irrev. MAOI	5 half-lives of SSRI or SARI (caution: with fluoxetine) – DO NOT COMBINE
	→	RIMA	5 half-lives of SSRI or SARI (caution: with fluoxetine)
	→	SSRI or SARI, NaSSA	No washout – taper first drug over 2–5 days then start second drug (use lower doses of second drug if switching from fluoxetine; longer taper may be necessary if higher doses of fluoxetine used); monitor for serotonergic effects (see p. 46)
Irrev. MAOI	→	TCA	14 days – CAUTION
	→	SSRI or SARI	14 days – DO NOT COMBINE
	→	NDRI	14 days – DO NOT COMBINE
	→	SNRI	Minimum of 14 days – DO NOT COMBINE. Caution: case reports of Serotonin syndrome after 14 days washout
	→	NaSSA[c]	14 days – DO NOT COMBINE
	→	RIMA	Start the next day if changing from low to moderate dose; taper from a high dose. Maintain dietary restrictions for 10 days
	→	Irrev. MAOI	14 days – DO NOT COMBINE
RIMA	→	TCA	2 days – CAUTION
	→	SSRI, SARI or NaSSA	2 days – CAUTION
	→	NDRI	2 days – CAUTION
	→	SNRI	2 days – CAUTION
	→	Irrev. MAOI	Can start the following day at a low dose
NDRI	→	TCA	2 days
	→	SSRI or SARI	No washout – taper (caution with fluoxetine)[b]
	→	SNRI, NaSSA	No washout – taper[b]; monitor for noradrenergic effects[d]
	→	RIMA	5 half-lives of NDRI (3–5 days) – DO NOT COMBINE
	→	Irrev. MAOI	5 half-lives of NDRI (3–5 days) – DO NOT COMBINE
SNRI or NaSSA	→	TCA	No washout – taper[b]
	→	SSRI or SARI	No washout – taper[b]; monitor for serotonergic effects (see p. 46)
	→	NDRI	No washout – taper[b]; monitor for noradrenergic effects[d]
	→	NaSSA or SNRI	No washout – taper[b], monitor for noradrenergic and serotonergic effects
	→	Irrev. MAOI	5 half-lives of SNRI (3 days) – DO NOT COMBINE
	→	RIMA	5 half-lives of SNRI (3 days) – CAUTION

[a] Recommendations pertain to outpatients; more rapid switching may be used in inpatients (except from an irreversible MAOI or RIMA) with proper monitoring of plasma levels and synergistic effects; [b] Taper first drug over 3–7 days prior to initiating second antidepressant; consider starting second drug at a reduced dose; [c] Data on NaSSa (mirtazapine) are limited; to concur with current practice, 5 half-lives should serve as an adequate washout when switching to or from mirtazapine (except from irrev. MAOI); [d] Noradrenergic effects can include tachycardia, increased blood pressure, headache, sweating, sudden nose bleed

Antidepressant Augmentation Strategies

ANTIDEPRESSANT NONRESPONSE

- Ascertain diagnosis is correct
- Ascertain patient is compliant with therapy
- Ensure there has been an adequate trial period
- Ensure dosage prescribed is therapeutic

Factors Complicating Response

- Concurrent medical or psychiatric illness, e.g., hypothyroidism, obsessive compulsive disorder
- Concurrent prescription drugs may interfere with efficacy, e.g., calcium channel blockers
- Metabolic enhancers (e.g., carbamazepine) or inhibitors (e.g., erythromycin) will affect plasma level of antidepressant
- Drug abuse may make management difficult, e.g., cocaine, marihuana, heroin
- Psychosocial factors may affect response
- Personality disorders lead to poor outcome; however, depression may evoke personality problems which may disappear when the depression is alleviated

SWITCHING ANTIDEPRESSANTS

- Use caution when switching to or from irreversible MAOIs (see Switching Antidepressants p. 98)
- Switching from one SSRI to another can be of benefit to previously nonresponsive patients
- Switching between tricyclic agents is of questionable benefit

Advantages of Switching

- Minimizes polypharmacy
- Second agent may be better tolerated
- Less costly

Disadvantages of Switching

- Time required to taper first drug, or need for washout; risk of relapse
- Lose partial efficacy of first agent
- Delayed onset of action

AUGMENTATION STRATEGIES

Advantages of Augmentation

- May have a rapid onset
- Response > 50% with most combinations
- No need to taper first agent or have a washout

Disadvantages of Augmentation

- May have potentiation of side effects
- Increased risk of drug interactions
- Increased cost
- Potential for decreased compliance

Antidepressant Augmentation Strategies (cont.)

Antidepressant Combinations	• Combining antidepressants which affect different neurotransmitter systems may produce a better antidepressant response than either drug alone but should only be considered after several attempts at monotherapy ☞ + **DO NOT COMBINE AN IRREVERSIBLE MAOI WITH (1) SSRI, (2) SNRI, (3) NDRI, (4) SARI, (5) RIMA, or (6) NaSSA**
SSRI + Cyclic	• Open trials suggest efficacy of SSRI and clomipramine for treatment-refractory OCD; monitor for serotonergic effects • Use lower doses of TCA and monitor TCA levels to prevent toxicity including cardiovascular effects, mania and/or Serotonin syndrome; monitor ECG (see Drug Interactions p. 79) • Combination of an SSRI and a noradrenergic cyclic drug (e.g., desipramine) reported to cause greater downregulation of β-adrenergic receptors, a more rapid response, and higher remission rates
NDRI + SSRI, NDRI + SNRI	• Up to 35% of partial responders to either drug may have a mareked response to the combination' however, adverse effects (e.g., tremor, panic attacks, increased seizure risk) may limit dosage (see Drug Interactions p. 50, 56) • Bupropion may improve sleep efficacy, energy, fatigue and executive function, and mitigate SNRI- or SSRI-induced sexual disfunction
Lithium	• Up to 40% of adolescents may respond to combined treatment (with SSRIs or TCA); response may occur within 48h, but usually within 3 weeks • Unclear if there is a correlation between lithium level and clinical improvement when used as augmentation therapy; however, plasma level of 0.4–0.8mmol/l is suggested efficacy • Reponse more likely in probable bipolar patients (with a first-degree relative with bipolar disorder or with a history of hypomania)
Anticonvulsants (e.g., Carbamazepine)	• Monitor TCA levels due to increased metabolism with carbamazepine • With SSRI, monitor carbamazepine level (see Drug Interactions p. 50) • There is no significant correlation between anticonvulsant plasma level and clinical improvement
Buspirone	• Beneficial response reported in depression and in OCD; effect observed within 2–4 weeks • May help alleviate SSRI-induced sexual dysfunction • Monitor for adverse effects due to serotonergic excess • Usual dose: 15–45 mg/day
Psychostimulants	• Methylphenidate (10–30 mg) or d-amphetamine (5–30 mg) used as augmentation therapy with TCAs, SSRIs, or SNRI • Rapid symptom resolution reported in open trials; response was sustained (no tolerance observed) • May be of value in depressed pagtients with ADHD • May improve sleepiness, fatigue and executive function in patients with ADHD • Caution: observe for activation and blood pressure shanges • Irritability, anxiety and paranoia reported - use caution in patients who are anxious or agitated

Electroconvulsive Treatment	• May be used with antidepressant for acute treatment • Maintenance therapy with antidepressant or with lithium may be required
Second-Generation Antipsychotics	• 5-HT$_{2C}$ blockade suggested to increase NE, dopamine and acetylcholine levels in the prefrontal cortex; blockade of 5-HT$_{2A}$ and 5-HT$_{2C}$ receptors may improve the efficacy and side effect profile of SSRIs and enhance sleep; reported to improve cognition in MDD • Low doses of risperidone (0.5–2 mg/day), olanzapine (2.5–10 mg/day), quetiapine, ziprasidone, or aripiprazole can augment SSRIs in patients with MDD or OCD; reported to decrease anxiety, irritabilty and insomnia, improve cognition, and remission rates • Fluoxetine/olanzapine combination (Symbyax) approved in USA for treatment of bipolar depression

Antidepressants – References and Selected Readings

- Bukhari, L., Anand, A., McDougle, C.S. (200). Psychopharmacology of pediatric depression. *International Drug Therapy Newsletter 38(10)*, 73–80.
- Burry, L., Kennie, N. (2000). Withdrawal reactions. *Pharmacy Practice 16(4)*, 46–54.
- Caccia, S. (1998). Metabolism of the newer antidepressants; an overview of the pharmacological and pharmacokinetic implications. *Clinical Pharmacokinetics 34(4)*, 281–302.
- Carbone, J.R. (2000). The neuroleptic malignant and serotonin syndromes. *Emergency Medicine Clinics of North America 18(2)*, 317–325.
- Clayton, A.H., Pradko, J.F., Croft, H.A. et al. (2002). Prevalence of sexual dysfunction among newer antidepressants. *Journal of Clinical Psychiatry 63(4)*, 357–366.
- Clinical Guidelines for the Treatment of Depressive Disorders; Canadian Psychiatric Association (CANMAT) (2001). *Canadian Journal of Psychiatry 46 (Suppl.)*, 1S–47S.
- Emslie, G.J., Ryan, N.D., Wagner, K.D. (2005). Major depressive disorder in children and adolescents: Clinical trial design and antidepressant efficacy. *Journal of Clinical Psychiatry 66 (Suppl. 7)*, 14–20.
- Findling, R.L. (2001). Antidepressant pharmacology of children and adolescents with ADHD. *International Drug Therapy Newsletter 36(12)*, 89–93.
- Gerber, P.E., Lynd, L.D. (1998). Selective serotonin-reuptake inhibitor-induced movement disorders. *Annals of Pharmacotherapy 32(6)*, 692–698.
- Greenblatt, D.J., von Moltke, L.L, Harmatz, J.S. et al. (1998). Drug interactions with newer antidepressants: Role of human cytochromes P450. *Journal of Clinical Psychiatry 58 (Suppl. 15)*, 19–27.
- Hirschfeld, R.M.A., Montgomery, S., Aguglia, E. et al. (2002). Partial response or nonresponse to antidepressant therapy: Current approaches and treatment options. *Journal of Clinical Psychiatry 63(9)*, 826–837.
- Hughes, C.W., Emslie, G.H., Crismon, M.H. et al. (1999). The Texas Children's Medication Algorithm Project: Report of the Texas consensus conference panel on medication treatment of childhood major depressive disorder. *Journal of the American Academy of Child and Adolescent Psychiatry 38(11)*, 1442–1454.

Antidepressants

References and Selected Readings (cont.)

- Jellinek, M.S., Snyder, J.B. (1998). Depression and suicide in children and adolescents. *Pediatric Review 19*, 255.
- Kapczinski, F., Lima, M.S., Souza, J.S. et al. (2003). Antidepressants for generalized anxiety disorder. *Cochrane Database Syst. Rev. (2)*, CD003592.
- Klinkman, M.S. (2003). The role of algorithms in the detection and treatment of depression in primary care. *Journal of Clinical Psychiatry 64 (Suppl. 2)*, 19–23.
- Lam, R.W.,Wan, D.D.C., Cohen D.L. et al. (2002). Combining antidepressants for treatment resistant depression: A review. *Journal of Clinical Psychiatry 63(8)*, 685–693.
- Leonard, H.L., March, L., Rickler, K.C. et al. (1991). Pharmacology of the selective serotonin reuptake inhibitors in children and adolescents. *Journal of the American Academy of Child and Adolescent Psychiatry 33*, 725–736.
- Richelson, E. (2003). Interactions of antidepressants with neurotransmitter transporters and receptors and their clinical relevance. *Journal of Clinical Psychiatry 64 (Suppl. 13)*, 5–12.
- Scharko, AM (2004) Selective serotonin reuptake inhibitor-induced sexual dysfunction in adolescents: a review. *J Am Acad Child Adolesc Psychiatry 43(9)*:1071–9
- Silva, MJ. Petrycki, S. Curry, J. et al. (2004). Fluoxetine, cognitive-behavioral therapy, and their combination for adolescents with depression: Treatment for Adolescents With Depression Study (TADS) randomized controlled trial. *JAMA. 292(7)*:807–20.
- Stahl, S.M. (1998). Basic psychopharmacology of antidepressants. Part 1: Antidepressants have seven distinct mechanisms of action. *Journal of Clinical Psychiatry 59 (Suppl. 4)*, 5–14.
- Stahl, S.M. (1998). Selecting an antidepressant by using mechanism of action to enhance efficacy and avoid side effects. *Journal of Clinical Psychiatry 59 (Suppl. 18)*, 23–29.

ELECTROCONVULSIVE TREATMENT

DEFINITION

- The induction of grand mal convulsions, by means of an externally applied electric stimulus, for the treatment of certain mental disorders
- **Not** the administration of subconvulsive electric stimuli, referred to as cranial electrostimulation or electrosleep therapy; **not** the administration of aversive electric stimuli as a behavior modification protocol; and not trans-cranial magnetic stimulation (TMS; preliminary comparison of TMS with ECT indicates that TMS may be effective for major depression, but not with psychotic symptoms)
- Sometimes called electro-shock therapy and, in the animal research literature, referred to as electroconvulsive shock (ECS)

INDICATIONS

- May be necessary for childhood or early adolescent onset of severe mood disorder with suicide risk, if adequate trials of 2 or more antidepressants are ineffective; **should never be prescribed without consultation by a specialist in child and adolescent psychiatry**
- Treatment-refractory major depression; especially when associated with high suicide risk, inanition/dehydration, severe agitation, depressive stupor, catatonia, delusions, nonresponse to greater than one adequate trials of antidepressants or intolerance of therapeutic dosages
- Depressed phase of bipolar disorder
- Manic phase of bipolar disorder; adjunct to mood stabilizers and antipsychotics for severe mania (manic "delirium") and rapid-cycling illness
- Severe psychotic disorders in patients with mental retardation
- Intractable psychotic disorders; especially with concurrent catatonic and/or mood symptoms; adjunct to adequate dosage of antipsychotics for nonresponsive "positive" symptoms; after failed clozapine trial (response rate 50–60%)
- Schizoaffective disorder, first-episode psychosis; nonresponse to adequate drug trials
- Reports of efficacy in phencyclidine-induced psychosis; ECT administered only for severe/prolonged illness

GENERAL COMMENTS

- Some jurisdictions do not permit the use of ECT for youths under a specific age
- ECT should be reserved for children and adolescents with very severe illness
- Reviews suggest ECT is effective for mood disorders and generally well-tolerated in children and adolescents; rates of improvement and adverse effects similar to those in adults
- Education of patient and/or caregiver and informed consent must be obtained prior to treatment

THERAPEUTIC EFFECTS

- Vegetative symptoms of depression, such as insomnia and fatigue, and catatonic symptoms may respond initially; later improvement of affective symptoms, such as depressed mood and anhedonia; followed by improvement of cognitive symptoms, such as impaired self-esteem, helplessness, hopelessness, suicidal and delusional ideation
- Manic symptoms which respond include agitation, euphoria, motor overactivity, and thought disorder
- Some "positive" symptoms of schizophrenia and other psychoses may respond
- Most effective treatment for severe depression in that a substantial proportion of nonresponders to antidepressants do recover with ECT; "melancholic" and "psychotic" presentations respond best

Electroconvulsive
Treatment

Electroconvulsive Treatment (cont.)

MECHANISM OF ACTION

- Exact mechanism unknown
- Affects almost all neurotransmitters implicated in the pathogenesis of the mental disorders (norepinephrine, serotonin, acetylcholine, dopamine, GABA)
- Neurophysiological effects include increased permeability of the blood-brain barrier, suppression of regional cerebral blood flow and neurometabolic activity; "anticonvulsant" effects may be related to outcome (inhibitory neurotransmitters are increased by ECT)
- Affects neuroendocrine substances (CRF, ACTH, TRH, prolactin, vasopressin, metenkephalins, β-endorphins)

DOSAGE

- Brief pulse, not sine wave stimulus generators should be used for a more accurate "dosage" administration/titration method to determine seizure threshold because young people have much lower thresholds than adults
- "Dosage" may be some combination of the electrical energy/charge of the stimulus, electrode placement, seizure duration and the total number of convulsions induced; the precise duration of seizure required is unknown (perhaps must be at least 15 s) because there is no clear correlation between seizure duration and outcome; augmenting agents (e.g., caffeine) are rarely necessary
- Bilateral stimulus electrode placement (regardless of the stimulus energy/charge) has been found more effective than unilateral placement; "high-energy" bilateral may be effective for nonresponse to "threshold" bilateral treatment
- Unilateral electrode placement is effective for many patients but, when used, the stimulus energy/charge should be substantially greater than that which is just necessary to induce a convulsion (threshold stimulus); if no response after 4 to 6 treatments, recommend switch to bilateral (preliminary evidence suggests that unilateral treatment with a multiple of 5 to 6 times the threshold stimulus may be as effective as bilateral and cause fewer cognitive side effects)
- Change from bilateral to unilateral placement if the patient becomes unduly confused following bilateral treatment
- Gender, age and electrode placement affect seizure threshold: males have higher thresholds than females, thresholds increase with age and are greater with bilateral than unilateral ECT
- Total number of treatments required for a full therapeutic effect may range from approximately 6 to 20; if there is absolutely no therapeutic effect after 12 to 15 treatments, it is unlikely that further treatments will be effective

ONSET AND DURATION OF ACTION

- Therapeutic effect may be evident within three treatments but onset may require as many as 12 treatments in some cases
- Relapse rate following discontinuation is high within 1 year; prophylactic antidepressants should be administered in almost all cases; ECT for up to 6 months if antidepressant prophylaxis of rapid relapse ineffective

PROCEDURE

- Administer three times per week on alternate days; decrease frequency to twice weekly, if possible, to reduce cognitive side effects
- ECT must always be administered under general anesthesia with partial neuromuscular blockade
- Induce light "sleep" anesthesia with sodium thiopental; little clinical advantage seen with newer agents such as propofol (more expensive and almost always results in much briefer convulsions; may also raise the seizure threshold; reserve for patients with post-treatment delirium or severe nausea unresponsive to antinauseants)
- Induce neuromuscular blockade with suxamethonium or succinylcholine or a short-acting nondepolarizing agent. Post-ECT myalgia may be due to insufficient relaxation or fasciculations (attenuate the latter, if necessary, with adjunctive nondepolarizing muscle relaxant (e.g., rocuronium) which necessitates a higher dosage of succinylcholine)

- Pretreat with atropine or glycopyrrolate if excess oral secretions and/or significant bradycardia anticipated (i.e., during "threshold titration", patient on a β-blocker); post-treat with atropine if bradycardia develops
- Pretreat any concurrent physical illness which may complicate anesthesia (i.e., antihypertensives, gastric acid/motility suppressants, hypoglycemics); special circumstances require anesthesia and/or internal medicine consultation
- If possible, withhold all psychotropics with anticonvulsant properties (i.e., benzodiazepines, carbamazepine, valproate) for at least the night before and morning of each treatment
- Continue all other psychotropics, except MAOIs (see Contraindications), when clinically necessary
- Outpatient treatment can be administered if warranted by the clinical circumstances if there is no medical/anesthesia contraindication and if the patient can comply with the pre- and post-treatment procedural requirements

ADVERSE EFFECTS

- Memory loss occurs to some degree during all courses of ECT
  - Significant, patchy amnesia for the period during which ECT is administered; may persist indefinitely
  - Retrograde amnesia for some events up to a number of months pre-ECT; may be permanent; uncommonly, longer periods of retrograde amnesia
  - Patchy anterograde amnesia for 3–6 months post-ECT; no evidence of permanent anterograde amnesia
  - Cognitive impairment (concentration and attention, verbal fluency and delayed recall) reported in adolescents; recovered over several months. No evidence of long-term sequelae
  - Patients may rarely complain of permanent anterograde memory impairment; unknown if this is a residual effect of the ECT or an effect of residual symptoms of the illness for which ECT was prescribed [liothyronine may protect against memory impairment]
  - There is no evidence to suggest that ECT causes structural damage or adversely affects brain development in youths
- Mortality rate; between two and four deaths per 100,000 treatments; higher risk in those with concurrent cardiovascular disease
- Posttreatment delirium uncommon; usually of short duration
  - Reported when more than one electric stimulus is used to induce a convulsion; after prolonged seizures
  - Due to concurrent drug toxicity (e.g., lithium carbonate; clozapine – see Drug Interactions)
  - If occurs consider propofol anesthesia for subsequent treatments
- Tachycardia and hypertension may be pronounced; duration several minutes post-treatment
- Bradycardia (to the point of asystole) and hypotension may be pronounced if stimulus is subconvulsive
  - Increased risk if patient on a β-blocker
  - Attenuated by the subsequent convulsion, atropine and medication with anticholinergic effect
- Posttreatment vagal "tone" may lead to significant bradycardia in young patients
- Prolonged seizures and status epilepticus have occurred in adolescents; monitor treatment with EEG until convulsion ends; seizures should be terminated after 3 min duration (with anesthetic dosage of the induction agent, repeated if necessary, or with diazepam). Propofol may reduce risk of prolonged seizures
- Spontaneous seizures
  - Incidence of post-ECT epilepsy is approximately that found in the general population
- Headache and muscle pain common but not usually severe
  - Pretreat with rocuronium bromide (approximately 3 mg) for severe muscle pain
- Nausea common following ECT procedure [pretreat with dimenhydrinate if severe]
- Temporo-mandibular joint pain; may be reduced with bifrontal electrode placement (compared to standard bitemporal placement)

Electroconvulsive
Treatment

Electroconvulsive Treatment (cont.)

PRECAUTIONS	• Obtain pretreatment anesthesia and/or internal medicine consultation for all patients with significant pre-existing cardiovascular disease, potential gastroesophageal reflux, compromised airway, and other circumstances which may complicate the procedure (i.e., personal or family history of significant adverse effects, or delay in recovery from general anesthesia); treat as indicated • Monitor by EKG, pulse oximetry and blood pressure, before and after ECT; EEG during treatment. • Patients with insulin-dependent diabetes mellitus may have a reduced need for insulin after ECT, as ECT reduces blood glucose levels for several hours (may be related to pretreatment fasting) • 10–30% of bipolar depressed patients can switch to hypomania or mania following ECT
CONTRAINDICATION	**Note:** all contraindications should be regarded in the context of, and relative to, the risks of withholding ECT • Rheumatoid arthritis complicated by erosion of the odontoid process • Increased intracranial pressure • Extremely loose teeth which may be aspirated if dislodged • Other disorders associated with increased anesthetic risk (American Society of Anesthesiologists level 3 or 4) • Concurrent administration of an irreversible MAOI, which may interact with anesthetic agents (although most reports have implicated meperidine as the interacting drug). Severe impairment in cardiac output and hypotension during ECT may require resuscitation with a pressor agent; the choice may be limited in the presence of an irreversible MAOI. The literature therefore recommends that MAOIs be discontinued 14 days prior to elective anesthesia; if there are compelling reasons to continue the MAOI, or start ECT prior to this waiting period, obtain anesthesia consultation. The potential for a hypertensive response is much less in the presence of a selective, reversible MAOI (RIMA) such that their concurrent administration is acceptable • Concurrent drug toxicity • Clozapine (see Drug Interactions)
USE IN PREGNANCY	• Safe in all trimesters; obtain obstetrical consultation • Fetal monitoring recommended • Precaution: increased risk of gastro-esophageal reflux
PRETREATMENT WORK-UP AND DOCUMENTATION	• Assess and document patient's capacity to consent to treatment; answer patient's questions about ECT; obtain signed and witnessed consent form (valid consent requires full disclosure to the patient of the nature of the procedure, all material risks and expected benefit of ECT and those of alternative available treatments, and the prognosis if no treatment is given); if patient incapable, get written consent from eligible substitute; involve patients/guardians in consent process • Physical examination • Pregnancy test (female) • Hb, WBC and differential when clinically indicated • Assess memory if there is evidence of clinically significant cognitive impairment before treatment; reassess if treatment-emergent loss is unduly severe

- Electrolytes and creatinine for all patients on any diuretic, on lithium, or with insulin-dependent diabetes, and as clinically indicated, including patients with a history of water intoxication
- EKG for all patients being treated for hypertension, or with a history of cardiac disease and as clinically indicated
- Chest x-rays for patients with myasthenia gravis and spinal x-rays for those patients with a history of compression fracture or other injury, significant pain, and as clinically indicated; cervical spine x-rays for all patients with rheumatoid arthritis
- Sickle cell screening of all black patients; infectious hepatitis screening as clinically indicated
- Blood glucose on day of each treatment for all patients with diabetes mellitus/patients on hypoglycemic agents
- Prothrombin time (INR) and partial thromboplastin time for all patients on anticoagulants

NURSING IMPLICATIONS

- Patients must be kept NPO (especially for solid food) for approximately 8 h before treatment; continuous observation may be required. Essential medication (e.g., antihypertensives) may be administered with sip of water
- Dental appliances (excluding "fixed" braces) must be removed before treatment
- Observe and monitor vital signs until patient is recovered, oriented and alert before discharge from recovery room
- When possible avoid prn benzodiazepines the night prior to and the morning of treatment

PATIENT INSTRUCTIONS

- Detailed instructions for patients and caregivers are provided in the Information Sheet on p. 310.
- Advise patients not to operate a motor vehicle or machinery the day of each treatment; outpatients must be escorted home after treatment

DRUG INTERACTIONS

- Clinically significant interactions are listed below

Class of Drug	Example	Interaction Effects
Anesthetic	Propofol	Decreased seizure duration (may be very substantial); may increase seizure threshold
Anticonvulsant	Carbamazepine, valproate	Increased seizure threshold with potential adverse effects of subconvulsive stimuli; it is possible to over-ride the anticonvulsant effect with a modest increase in energy/charge of electric stimulus
Antidepressant Irreversible MAOI	Phenelzine	Possible need for a pressor agent for resuscitation requires that this combination be avoided
SARI, NDRI, SSRI	Trazodone, bupropion, fluoxetine	Prolonged seizures reported; clinical significance unknown. Concurrent administration not contraindicated
	Trazodone	Rare case reports of cardiovascular complications in patients with and without cardiac disease – more likely to occur at high dosages (i.e., > 300 mg/day)
Antihypertensive	β-blockers, e.g., propranolol	May potentiate bradycardia and hypotension with subconvulsive stimuli Confusion reported with combined use
Antipsychotic	Clozapine	Increased seizure duration reported in 16.6% of patients; spontaneous (tardive) seizures reported following ECT Delirium reported with concurrent, or shortly following clozapine treatment; however, there are many case reports of uncomplicated concurrent use
Benzodiazepines	Lorazepam, diazepam	Increased seizure threshold with potential adverse effects of subconvulsive stimuli or abbreviated seizure

Electroconvulsive Treatment

Electroconvulsive Treatment (cont.)

Class of Drug	Example	Interaction Effects
Caffeine		Increased seizure duration Reports of hypertension, tachycardia, and cardiac dysrhythmia
Lithium		Lithium toxicity may occur, perhaps due to an increased permeability of the blood-brain barrier; decrease or discontinue lithium and monitor patient. Concurrent administration not contraindicated if lithium level within the therapeutic range
L-Tryptophan		Increased seizure duration
Theophylline		Increased seizure duration, status epilepticus. Concurrent administration not contraindicated if serum level within the therapeutic range

Electroconvulsive Treatment – References and Selected Readings

- American Psychiatric Association (2001). *The practice of electroconvulsive therapy: Recommendations for treatment, training, and privileging.* Second edition. Washington D.C.: APA.
- Ghazuddin, N., Kutcher, S.P., Knapp, P. et al. (2004). Summary of the practice parameters for use of electroconvulsive therapy with adolescents. *Journal of the American Academy of Child and Adolescent Psychiatry 43,* December. www.aacap.org
- Patrides, G., Fink, M., Mussain, M.M. et al. (2001). ECT remission rates in psychotic versus nonpsychotic depressed patients: A report from CORE. *Journal of ECT 17,* 244–253.
- Rabheru, K. (2001). The use of electroconvulsive therapy in special patient populations. *Canadian Journal of Psychiatry 46(8),* 710–719.
- Sackeim, H.A., Pradic, J., Davanand, D.P. et al. (2000). A prospective randomized, double-blind comparison of bilateral and right unilateral electroconvulsive therapy at different stimulus intensities. *Archives of General Psychiatry 57,* 425–434.
- Walter, G., Rey, J.M., Mitchell, P.B. (1999). Practitioner Review: Electroconvulsive therapy in adolescents. *Journal of Child Psychology and Psychiatry 40(3),* 325–334.

CLASSIFICATION

- Antipsychotics can be classified as follows:

Chemical Class	Agent	Page
"Second-Generation" Antipsychotics[A] (SGA)		
Benzisoxazole	Risperidone	See p. 115
Dibenzodiazepine	Clozapine	See p. 115
Dibenzothiazepine	Quetiapine	See p. 115
Thienobenzodiazepine	Olanzapine	See p. 115
Benzothiazolylpiperazine	Ziprasidone[D]	See p. 115
"Third-Generation" Antipsychotic (TGA)		
Dihydrocarbostyril	Aripiprazole [D]	See p. 127
"First-Generation" Antipsychotics[B] (FGA)		
Butyrophenone	Haloperidol, Droperidol[C][E]	See p. 130
Dibenzoxazepine	Loxapine	See p. 130
Dihydroindolone	Molindone[D][E]	–
Diphenylbutylpiperidine	Pimozide	See p. 130
Phenothiazines:		
– aliphatic	Example: chlorpromazine	See p. 130
– piperazine	Example: trifluoperazine	See p. 130
– piperidine	Example: thioridazine[D][F]	See p. 131
Thioxanthenes	Example: thiothixene	See p. 131

[A] Formerly called "atypical". "Atypical" antipsychotics (1) may have low affinity for D_2 receptors and are readily displaced by endogenous dopamine in striatum (e.g., clozapine, molindone, quetiapine); (2) may have high D_2 blockade and high muscarinic blockade-anticholinergic activity; (3) may block both D_2 and $5-HT_2$ receptors (e.g., risperidone, clozapine, olanzapine, quetiapine); (4) may have high D_4 blockade (e.g., clozapine, olanzapine, loxapine); (5) may lack a sustained increase prolactin response (e.g. clozapine, quetiapine, olanzapine); (6) show mesolimbic selectivity (e.g., olanzapine, clozapine, quetiapine).
[B] Formerly called "typical or conventional antipsychotics." [C] Injectable drug used primarily in the emergency setting (see below). [D] Not marketed in Canada. [E] Not generally used in children – not reviewed in this chapter. [F] Thioridazine restricted to treatment of refractory schizophrenia in adults; not recommended in children and adolescents

GENERAL COMMENTS

- Significant pharmacological characteristics of antipsychotics:
  - Antipsychotic activity
  - Absence of deep coma or anesthesia with administration of large (not toxic) doses
  - Absence of physical or psychic dependence
- Generally sedating; different antipsychotics are associated with different efficacy and safety profiles – therapy needs to be individually optimized
- Second-generation antipsychotics are used as first-line therapy in most clinical situations in children and adolescents because of their decreased risk for extrapyramidal side effects, dysphoric effects, and tardive dyskinesia; most conventional antipsychotics are primarily used on a "PRN" or short-term basis, or in persons who do not respond or cannot tolerate novel agents
- All classes prescribed to treat positive symptoms of psychosis, including hallucinations and delusions. No particular antipsychotics have proven efficacy for primary negative symptoms of psychosis (i.e., affective flattening, alogia, amotivation, social withdrawal). SGAs or

Antipsychotics (Neuroleptics) (cont.)

TGAs may be preferred but their advantage over FGAs may be due to an improvement in secondary negative symptoms (e.g., depression, parkinsonism), to an improved side effect profile, or because they don't worsen primary negative symptoms.
- May improve cognition: e.g., attention/information processing, reaction time and verbal fluency (clozapine); attention, executive functioning, and working memory (risperidone, quetiapine); verbal learning and memory, verbal fluency and executive functioning (olanzapine); episodic memory, attention/vigilance, executive function and visuomotor speed (ziprasidone)
- Accumulating evidence for SGAs reducing affective symptomatology in schizophrenia, bipolar disorder and treatment-resistant depression; some evidence suggests SGAs may reduce cognitive symptoms in schizophrenia
- SGAs often prescribed to children and adolescents to decrease symptoms of severe aggression, agitation, or hyperactivity
- May be helpful in tic disorders and children with autism
- In autism, antipsychotics are frequently used to reduce target symptoms such as stereotypies, temper tantrums, aggression, self-injurious behavior, and hyperactivity
- In mania, reduce euphoria, excitement, irritability, expansiveness, energy, thought disorder, and pressure of ideas
- Risperidone found to be superior to haloperidol in preventing relapse in first episode psychosis (relapse rate 42% with risperidone and 55% with haloperidol)
- Accumulating evidence from studies suggests a correlation between earlier treatment of psychotic disorders with antipsychotics and better prognosis. Novel antipsychotics shown (in in-vivo studies) to alter brain-derived neurotropic factor levels in the hippocampus and may provide neuroprotection
- Non-compliance with antipsychotic therapy estimated to be up to 75% in outpatients on oral medication – results in high incidence of relapse (adult population)

PHARMACOLOGY
- See pp.146–147
- Exact mechanism of action unknown – primary action has been attributed to D2 blockade, although "second- and third-generation" compounds have suggested a role for other dopamine receptors (e.g., D3 and D4) and other neurotransmitters (e.g., serotonin,)
- In contrast to FGAs, most SGA and TGA drugs appear to activate dopamine neurons in the prefrontal cortex and limbic regions (e.g., nucleus accumbens) with less effect in the striatum; this may explain the low incidence of EPS and the greater effect on negative symptoms with these drugs. Fast dissociation from the D_2 receptor, allowing it to periodically accomodate endogenous dopamine has also been postulated as an explanation of their action
- Receptor specificity varies with different antipsychotics: e.g., clozapine, olanzapine, quetiapine, risperidone and ziprasidone have greater $5\text{-}HT_2$ blockade than D2 blockade (see p. 146). The relative lower affinity for the D2 receptor by second-generation antipsychotics appears to be determined by their faster rate of disassociation (i.e., unbinding) from the D2 receptor
- Novel antipsychotics selectively block mesolimbic (A10) dopamine neurons; other antipsychotics block both A10 and A9 (nigrostriatal neurons)

DOSING
- See pp. 141–145
- With the exception of chlorpromazine and haloperidol, most monographs for antipsychotic drugs state that safety and efficacy have not been established in younger children

- Start doses low and increase slowly; limit dose and duration of therapy; assess dosage requirements and continued need for drug and monitor for early signs of tardive dyskinesia; higher incidence of tardive dyskinesia with conventional antipsychotics – see p. 153 for risk factors
- Acute patients may require slightly higher doses than chronic patients; manic patients may need even higher doses; maintenance doses for bipolar patients tend to be about half those used in schizophrenia
- Behavioral toxicity can occur when high doses used; this includes: worsening of symptoms, impairment of learning, apathy, irritability, tics, or hallucinations
- Lower doses and slower titration are recommended in children, and in patients with compromised liver or renal function
- Schizophrenia: in newly diagnosed children and adolescents who have been symptom-free for 6–12 months, consider gradual drug withdrawal and monitor for relapse

BLOOD LEVELS

- The usefulness of serum levels have not been demonstrated in children and adolescents
- Threshold plasma level suggested for response to clozapine: 350 ng/ml (or 1050 nmol/l) suggested by some; 250 ng/ml (or 750 nmol/l) by others

PHARMACOKINETICS

- Vary with individual agents – see pp. 141–145

Oral

- In general, younger individuals have lower plasma levels of antipsychotics than adults, at equivalent mg/kg doses; this may be due to increased clearance of the drug
- Peak plasma levels of oral doses reached 1–4 h after administration
- Highly bound to plasma proteins
- Metabolized extensively in the liver; specific agents inhibit cytochrome P-450 metabolizing enzymes (see pp. 141–145)
- Once-daily dosing is appropriate for many antipsychotics (but not all) because of long elimination half-life
- Increased excretion reported in smokers with many antipsychotics (see Drug Interactions pp. 126, 140)

Short-Acting Injection

- Generally peak plasma level reached sooner than with oral preparation
- Bioavailability usually greater than with oral drug; dosage should be adjusted accordingly (loxapine excepted)

Depot Injection

- See pp. 117 and 150–151
- Long-acting antipsychotic formulations have been proven to improve compliance and reduce consequences of missed doses, which include relapse, progression of illness, and personality deterioration
- Depot antipsychotics provide improved bioavailability and more consistent blood levels without the peaks and troughs observed with short-acting oral therapy
- Depot antipsychotics have not been adequately studied in children and adolescents. They should be reserved only for youths with documented chronic psychotic symptoms and a history of poor compliance. Not recommended in very early onset of schizophrenia

ADVERSE EFFECTS

- See SGAs (pp. 118–122), TGAs (p. 128), FGAs (pp. 133–136), and charts (pp. 149)
- Differential percentages of blockage of different receptors, as well as the rate of dissociation from the receptors account for observed side effects, e.g., the faster an antipsychotic dissociates from the D2 receptor, the lower the rate of EPS, prolactin elevation, and possibly the risk of TD
- When determining the need for intervention, consideration should be given to: (1) how bothersome the side effect is, (2) duration of the side effect, (3) the expected duration of treatment with the antipsychotic, (4) the benefit of treatment vs risk of relapse that might occur with dosage reduction or drug switch, (5) advantages or disadvantages of adding another agent to treat the adverse effect (e.g., adverse effects, drug interactions, cost, etc.)

Antipsychotics (Neuroleptics)

Antipsychotics (Neuroleptics) (cont.)

MONITORING RECOMMENDATIONS	• *Baseline:* prior to initiating antipsychotics in children and adolescents, a thorough medical, substance use, family history, and psychiatric evaluation should be done, including the following baseline tests: liver and renal function, CBC, electrocardiogram, BP, pulse, height, weight, waist circumference and BMI, fasting blood glucose (including HbAlc) and lipids
	• Continued monitoring is recommended as follows:

- Body mass index, height, and weight monthly for first 3 months, then after every 3 months while on a stable antipsychotic dose
- Fasting blood glucose, triglyceride and cholesterol levels, whenever the antipsychotic is changed, and annually thereafter (recommended every 3 months in patients with obesity or a family history of diabetes, or in patients who gain > 5% of their body weight while on medication or experience a rapid increase in weight measurement)
- Blood pressure and pulse during dosage titration with clozapine, risperidone, quetiapine, chlorpromazine, thioridazine
- ECG: prior to prescribing thioridazine, pimozide and ziprasidone, and periodically during course of therapy; DO NOT PRESCRIBE these drugs if patient's QT_c > 450 ms and use caution with other antipsychotics
- EEG: if seizures or myoclonus occurs.
- Slit lamp ophthalmic examinations recommended with quetiapine, at baseline and at 6-month intervals, as per product monograph risk is low; no documented cases of ophthalmological problems seen in humans
- Thyroid function tests (T_4, TSH) with quetiapine, especially in patients at risk for hypothyroidism
- Symptoms related to prolactin elevation (e.g., menstrual disturbances, galactorrhea, amenorrhea or sexual dysfunction) monthly for 3 months, then yearly; order prolactin level if symptomatic

☞ **Clozapine monitoring: WBC (= white blood count) and granulocyte counts must be done weekly (after 6 months (Canada) and 12 months (USA) can be done monthly if patient had no abnormalities). "Green": WBC = 3.5×10^9/l or ANC (= absolute neutrophil count) = 2.0×10^9/l; "Yellow": WBC $2–3.5 \times 10^9$/l or ANC $1.5–2 \times 10^9$/l – do blood work twice weekly till normal; "Red": WBC < 2×10^9/l or ANC < 1.5×10^9/l – STOP clozapine and monitor bloodwork and clinical symptoms for 4 weeks. DO NOT rechallenge**

- Laboratory tests are also indicated in the following situations:
  - With fever, rigidity and diaphoresis – monitor white blood cell count and CPK (rule out neuroleptic malignant syndrome)
  - With pruritus or signs of jaundice – monitor liver function tests; some clinicians suggest annual liver tests (e.g., risperidone has caused hepatotoxicity)
  - With seizures, polydipsia – monitor electrolytes
  - Monitor serum potassium and magnesium prior to prescribing thioridazine, and ziprasidone, and periodically during course of therapy

MEDICOLEGAL ISSUES

- Antipsychotic therapy has been a source of litigation
- Be frank with patients and caregivers; antipsychotics are not innocuous; however, continuing psychosis is very destructive
- Provide educational material, drug education groups, answer questions of family and patients
- Keep educating and re-educating patients and caregivers about the illness and medications as levels of retention of material are low; a policy of ongoing education is better than written consent, though in some jurisdictions written consent is necessary
- No antipsychotic is perfectly safe; for tardive dyskinesia some may be safer than others: SGAs and TGA have a lower risk of TD than FGAs (0.6% vs 4.6%) and may also have antidyskinetic effects; document a baseline assessment for movement disorders, and monitor regularly (e.g., every 3–12 months) – more frequently if patient at high risk for developing TD

- Careful observation, data collection, and documentation of patient behavior patterns prior to drug administration, as well as during therapy, are essential nursing measures
- Care is essential in minimizing side effects; patients should be educated and reassured about side effects to promote positive attitudes toward taking medication; allow patient to discuss fears about medication. Unrecognized and untreated side effects (e.g., akathisia, sexual dysfunction) may play a major role in nonadherence to treatment
- Prn antiparkinsonian agents may be required during first few weeks of treatment; patient should take antiparkinsonian agents (e.g., benztropine, procyclidine) only for the extrapyramidal side effects (EPS) of antipsychotics; excess use of these agents may precipitate an anticholinergic delirium. Prophylactic antiparkinsonian agents may be required on a temporary basis, by adolescent males, or by individuals with a history of EPS on low doses of antipsychotics, when given FGAs or risperidone
- Blurred vision is usually transient; near vision only is affected; if severe, pilocarpine eye drops or neostigmine tablets may be prescribed
- Weight gain may occur in some patients receiving antipsychotics (especially some SGAs); proper diet, exercise and avoidance of calorie-laden beverages is important; monitor height, weight, waist circumference, and body mass index during course of treatment
- Monitor patient's intake and output; urinary retention can occur, especially in the elderly; bethanechol (Urecholine) can reverse this
- Anticholinergics reduce peristalsis and decrease intestinal secretions leading to constipation; increasing fluids and bulk (e.g., bran, salads), as well as fruit in the diet is beneficial; if necessary, bulk laxatives (e.g., Metamucil, Prodiem) or a stool softener (e.g., docusate) can be used; lactulose is effective in chronic constipation
- Avoid photosensitivity reactions by providing sunscreen agents with UVA protection and suggest that protective clothing be worn until response to sun has been determined; patients should wear UVA-protective sunglasses in bright sunlight
- Be aware that akathisia can be misdiagnosed as anxiety or psychotic agitation and the incorrect treatment prescribed [propranolol may decrease akathisia]
- Hold dose and notify physician if patient develops acute dystonia, severe persistent extrapyramidal reactions (longer than a few hours), or has symptoms of jaundice or blood dyscrasias (fever, sore throat, infection, weakness)
- Check patients on depot injections for indurations; "Z"-track technique is recommended for most depot injections
- "Older" multi-punctured vials of **fluphenazine decanoate** may contain hydrolyzed ("free") fluphenazine, which can result in higher peak plasma levels within 24 h of injection – monitor for EPS
- Recommend patient visit general practitioner yearly for a physical examination, including neurological and ophthamological examination
- Sublingual preparations of **risperidone** or **olanzapine** can be administered with a noncarbonated beverage (e.g., water, milk, juice)
- If half tablets of **olanzapine** are required, break tablet carefully and wash your hands after this procedure. Avoid exposure to powder as dermatitis, eye irritation and allergic reactions reported. Store broken tablet in tight, light-resistant container (tablet discolors), and use within 7 days
- **Olanzapine** powder for solution for injection should be reconstituted using 2.1 ml of sterile water for injection; must be used within 1 h of mixing (see directions in package); recommend vital signs be evaluated prior to IM administration - monitor for oversedation and cardio-respiratory depression (see Interactions p. 125)
- Store **risperidone depot** dose pack in the refrigerator; the powder and solvent should be allowed to come to room temperature prior to reconstitution; it should then be used as soon as possible (see directions in package). Do not combine/mix two different dose strengths of Risperdal Consta. To minimize pain on injection use alternate buttocks as injection sites. Use only supplied teflon-coated needles – use of smaller gauge may impede passage of microspheres
- Patients should avoid exposure to extreme heat and humidity as antipsychotics affect the body's ability to regulate temperature

Antipsychotics (Neuroleptics) (cont.)

- Because antipsychotics can cause sedation, caution patient not to perform activities requiring alertness until response to the drug has been determined
- Monitor patients for symptoms that may be associated with QT prolongation (e.g., dizziness, fainting spells, palpitation, nausea and vomiting)
- Excessive use of caffeine (colas, coffee, tea, chocolate) may worsen anxiety and agitation and counteract the beneficial effects of antipsychotics
- **Ziprasidone** should be taken with meals. Avoid grapefruit juice with antipsychotics as it may interfere with drug effects. **Risperidone** solution should not be taken with tea or colas. Pectinate in apple juice reported to have a physical incompatibility with **perphenazine** and **fluphenazine** – unknown if this interaction occurs with other antipsychotics

PATIENT INSTRUCTIONS

- Detailed instructions for patients and caregivers are provided in the Information Sheets on pp. 312 and 315

PRODUCT AVAILABILITY

Chemical Class	Generic Name	Trade Name[(A)]	Dosage Forms and Strengths	Monograph Statement
Benzisoxazole	Risperidone	Risperdal Risperdal M-Tab Risperdal Consta	Tablets: 0.25 mg, 0.5 mg, 1 mg, 2 mg, 3 mg, 4 mg, 5 mg[(C)] Oral solution: 1 mg/ml Oral disintegrating tablets: 0.5 mg, 1 mg, 2 mg, 3 mg, 4 mg Long-acting injection: 25 mg/vial, 37.5 mg/vial, 50 mg/vial	Safety and efficacy not established in children
Dibenzodiazepine	Clozapine	Clozaril Fazaclo ODT[(B)]	Tablets: 12.5 mg[(B)], 25 mg, 50 mg[(B)], 100 mg, 200 mg[(B)] Oral disintegrating tablet[(B)]: 25 mg, 100 mg	Safety and efficacy not established in children
Thienobenzodiazepine	Olanzapine	Zyprexa Zyprexa Zydis Zyprexa Intramuscular	Tablets: 2.5 mg, 5 mg, 7.5 mg, 10 mg, 15 mg[(B)], 20 mg[(B)] Injection: 10 mg/vial Oral dissolving tablets: 5 mg, 10 mg, 15 mg[(B)], 20 mg[(B)] Powder for solution for injection: 10 mg/vial	Safety and efficacy not established in children Contraindicated in children
Dibenzothiazepine	Quetiapine	Seroquel	Tablets: 25 mg, 50 mg[(B)], 100 mg, 200 mg, 300 mg, 400 mg[(B)]	Safety and efficacy not established in children
Benzothiazolylpiperazine	Ziprasidone[(B)]	Geodon	Capsules: 20 mg, 40 mg, 60 mg, 80 mg Injection: 20 mg/ml	Safety and efficacy not established in children

[(A)] Generic preparations may be available, [(B)] Not marketed in Canada, [(C)] Not marketed in USA

INDICATIONS

No approved indications in children and adolescents

Approved (for Adults)

- Treat symptoms of acute and chronic psychoses (i.e., schizophrenia, manic phase of bipolar disorder, delusional disorder, schizoaffective disorder)
- Maintenance in schizophrenia
- Treatment-resistant schizophrenia (clozapine); benefit reported in treatment resistant childhood schizophrenia
- Maintenance of treatment response in schizophrenia (olanzapine, risperidone)
- Delaying relapse in long-term treatment of schizophrenia (risperidone – USA)
- Prophylaxis of bipolar disorder
- Maintenance treatment of bipolar disorder (olanzapine, quetiapine – USA)
- Acute mania, bipolar mania; acute treatment of manic or mixed episodes in BD (olanzapine, risperidone, quetiapine, ziprasidone) small-scale studies and case reports report positive results in children and adolescents with all SGAs; efficacy reported wih risperidone in pediatric mania; good response seen when quetiapine used to augment valproate in adolescents with mania or mixed states; ziprasidone reported effective in children with treatment-refractory BD
- Agitation associated with schizophrenia (ziprasidone IM) and bipolar mania (olanzapine IM and ziprasidone IM)
- Quetiapine: monotherapy or adjunct therapy for short-term treatment of acute manic episodes of Bipolar I disorder
- Clozapine – reduces risk of recurrent suicidal behavior in patients with schizophrenia or schizoaffective disorder (USA); also reported with olanzapine
- Bipolar depression (olanzapine/fluoxetine combination)

Second-Generation Antipsychotics (Neuroleptics) (cont.)

Other Uses in Children and Adolescents	• Early onset psychosis/schizophrenia (risperidone, quetiapine, olanzapine) • Clozapine found effective in treatment-resistant childhood schizophrenia • Behavioral disturbance and psychotic symptoms associated with a wide range of childhood psychiatric disorders; efficacy reported in the management of irritability, aggression, stereotypies and explosive behavior in pervasive developmental disorders, mental retardation, oppositional defiant disorder, and conduct disorder • Used in managing aggression, temper tantrums, psychomotor excitement, stereotypies, and hyperactivity unresponsive to other therapy • Delusional major depression • Augmentation in refractory obsessive-compulsive disorder and related disorders (risperidone, olanzapine, clozapine) – but occasional reports of worsening of OCD symptoms • Double-blind and open trials report efficacy in tic disorders (risperidone and ziprasidone), and Tourette's Syndrome (risperidone, olanzapine, ziprasidone). • Good response noted when quetiapine used to augment valproate in adolescents with manic or mixed episodes • Risperidone reported to prevent relapse of disruptive behavior of autism after 6 months of therapy (12.5% relapse with risperidone vs 62.5% with placebo) • Psychosis associated with psychostimulant use (risperidone) • Self-mutilation and aggressive behavior in different populations (risperidone, clozapine) • Personality disorders (e.g., borderline patients) – marginal efficacy • Reactive attachment disorders • Reported to decrease motor symptoms in a number of movement disorders (e.g., tremor, dyskinesia and bradykinesia, essential tremor, akinetic disorders, blepharospasm, Meige syndrome, etc.) • Studies suggest clozapine and olanzapine decrease suicidality in patients with schizophrenia • Open-label studies suggest benefit in anorexia nervosa (olanzapine, risperidone) • Pediatric insomnia (risperidone)
PHARMACOLOGY	• See p. 146–147 • Second-generation antipsychotics are distinguished as a class by (a) greater 5-HT$_2$ versus D$_2$ blockade, (b) fast dissociation from the D$_2$ receptor, and (c) limbic selectivity • Ziprasidone is a 5-HT$_{1A}$ agonist (increases DA release in the prefrontal cortex which has been implicated in improving cognition and mood), a 5-HT$_{1D}$ antagonist (causing increased serotonin release), and a moderate inhibitor of 5-HT, DA, and NE transporters (i.e., reuptake)
DOSING	• There are few clinical trials which have evaluated dosing in children and adolescents • See pp. 141–142 • In patients with mental retardation doses should be lower and titration rate slower than in individuals with normal intelligence • Slower dose titration will minimize side efferts, especially sedation and orthostatic hypotension

- Dosage requirements of olanzapine may be higher in young males who smoke
- Recommended that doses of clozapine above 300 mg be divided due to seizure risk; prescribing restrictions apply (see p. 112)
- It is recommended that quetiapine and ziprasidone be given twice daily (due to short half-life)
- Risperidone may need to be given bid in children and some adolescents to sustain effect throughout the day

ADMINISTRATION

Oral Medication

- Medication may be given with meals or at bedtime followed by a glass of water, milk or orange juice; avoid apple or grapefruit juice as they may interfere with drug effect. Do not give liquid risperidone with tea or colas
- Food increases the bioavailability of ziprasidone; fatty foods increase the absorption of ziprasidone
- Do not give oral medication within 2 h of an antacid or antidiarrheal drug, as absorption of the antipsychotic may be decreased
- Use liquid (risperidone) or quick-dissolving tablets (olanzapine, risperidone) if patient has difficulty swallowing or is suspected of being noncompliant. Olanzapine Zydis can be administered in a noncarbonated liquid (e.g. water, milk, juice)

Short-Acting Injection

- Ziprasidone: IM injection used for rapid control of acute agitation in schizophrenia. May be used concomitantly with benztropine – no data in children
- Olanzapine (powder for solution): IM injection – no data in children. Should not be combined with a benzodiazepine (see Interactions)

Depot Injection

- See p. 111 and chart pp. 150–151
- Risperidone depot is provided as a powder and solvent that must be reconstituted prior to use; recommended that dose pack be allowed to come to room temperature before reconstitution and injection. Should be used as soon as possible - shelf life is 6 h (nursing administration instructions are provided with the drug); some clinicians recommend a test oral dose of 1–2 mg/day for 2 days if the patient has never taken risperidone. Only use needles supplied with the kit as use of lower gauge may impede the passage of microspheres. If clogging occurs, change needle to same or larger gauge.
- Shake the preparation within 2 min before administering; give deep IM into gluteal muscle; rotate sites and specify in charting
- DO NOT massage injection site

PHARMACOKINETICS

Oral

- See pp. 111 and 141–142

- Differences in plasma concentration between males and females demonstrated with clozapine (40–50% increase in females) and with olanzapine (30% increase in females)
- Free clozapine + active metabolite norclozapine contribute to both efficacy and adverse effects in youth. There is no difference in dose-normalized plasma concentrations between children and adults.
- Olanzapine pharmacokinetics reported to be similar in children (age 10–18) as in nonsmoking adults
- Quetiapine pharmacokinetics appear to be similar in children and adults
- Risperidone, and metabolite, elimination is decreased by 60% in patients with moderate to severe renal disease
- On discontinuation, clozapine and quetiapine are rapidly eliminated from the plasma and brain – may result in rapid re-emergence of symptoms

Dissolving Tablets

- Supralingual preparations of olanzapine (Zydis) and risperidone (M-Tabs) dissolve in saliva within 30 s (can be swallowed with or without liquid) – bioequivalent to oral tablet
- Useful in children and adolescents who have difficulty swallowing tablets
- Help to ensure the patient is receiving the medication

Antipsychotics (Neuroleptics)

Second-Generation Antipsychotics (Neuroleptics) (cont.)

Short-Acting Injection	• Ziprasidone peak plama level is reached within 30 min and is dose-related • Bioavailability of IM olanzapine is approximately 5 times greater than with oral drug and C_{max} occurs in 15–45 min rather than 5–8 h; half-life is < 3 h)
Depot Injection	• See p. 111 and chart on pp. 150–151 • Depot antipsychotics provide improved bioavailability and more consistent blood levels without the peaks and troughs observed with short-acting oral therapy • Risperidone: about 1% of risperidone is released from the depot formulation immediately; erosion of microspheres and absorption of risperidone occurs 3–6 days after injection. The main release begins 3 weeks after injection and peak plasma levels are seen in 4–6 weeks - oral supplementation is recommended in the first 3 weeks following start of depot (given q 2 weeks); steady state is reached after four injections (6–8 weeks), and plasma concentrations are maintained for 4–6 weeks after the last injection - complete elimination in about 7–8 weeks
ADVERSE EFFECTS	• See chart on p. 149 for incidence of adverse effects • Children and adolescents may be more sensitive to adverse effects • Many adverse effects are transient; persistent ones often have remedies, but are often best dealt with by changing the dosing schedule or dose, or by a change in medication
CNS Effects	• A result of antagonism at H_1, ACh and α_1-receptors and dopamine
Cognitive Effects	• Sedation and fatigue common (up to 20% incidence), especially during the first 2 weeks of therapy (primarily with clozapine, and quetiapine; moderate with olanzapine) [Management: prescribe bulk of dose at bedtime] • Insomnia (up to 20% incidence – risperidone, olanzapine, ziprasidone); vivid dreams, nightmares (risperidone, clozapine) • Confusion, disturbed concentration, disorientation (more common with high doses • Dysphoria, asthenia (of more concern in children with mental retardation) • May cause exacerbation of obsessive-compulsive symptoms • Increased agitation and anxiety reported with olanzapine and quetiapine – up to 25% incidence; case reports of mania in adolescents receiving olanzapine and ziprasidone
Neurological Effects	• A result of antagonism at dopamine D_2 receptors (extrapyramidal reactions correlated with D_2 binding above 80%). D_2 receptor densities are higher in children and adolescents than in adults, therefore the risk of EPS is increased • Headache • Lowered seizure threshold; caution in patients with a history of seizures. Risk of seizures with clozapine 1% (doses below 300 mg), 2.7% (300–600 mg) and 4.4% (above 600 mg); may be preceded by myoclonus; 4% risk of seizures and up to 82% risk of EEG abnormalities in children with clozapine [Management: Valproate or Topiramate in therapeutic doses]; nonspecific EEG abnormalities reported with olanzapine, including cases of seizures; seizures rare with quetiapine (0.8%) and risperidone (0.3%) • Myoclonic jerks, tics or cataplexy reported with clozapine; may be precursor of generalized seizure [decrease dose or add anticonvulsant] • Extrapyramidal reactions less common with "second-generation" antipsychotics than conventional antipsychotics and are dose-dependent with olanzapine (> 20 mg/day), risperidone (> 4 mg/day), and ziprasidone (see p. 149). Children and adolescents with developmental

disabilities are at higher risk for EPS, including dystonias and dyskinesias (reported incidence of 17.5% with risperidone and 21% with olanzapine) – young girls are at highest risk. Clozapine and quetiapine have the lowest risk of EPS and may ameliorate existing symptoms
- Akathisia (rare) can be misdiagnosed in children as worsening of psychosis, as they may not be able to verbalize their symptoms; low iron may predispose to akathisia
- Loss of gag reflex (especially in males)
- Dysphagia (difficulty swallowing); of greater concern in males; sialorrhea (especially with clozapine) – see GI Effects
- Urinary incontinence (overflow incontinence); enuresis reported with clozapine; case reports with olanzapine and risperidone [may respond to desmopressin or DDAVP nasal spray or tablets, oxybutynin]
- Withdrawal dyskinesias common in children (see p. 122)
- Tardive dyskinesia (TD) (see p. 154). Risk lower with SGAs (0.6% with risperidone and olanzapine) and TGA, and these drugs may reduce TD symptoms. Clozapine has the lowest TD risk, based on current data and has demonstrated a significant reduction in existing TD (especially tardive dystonia)

| Anticholinergic Effects |

- A result of antagonism at muscarinic receptors (ACh)
- Common; effects are additive if given concurrently with other anticholinergic agents
- Dry mucous membranes [Management: sugar-free gum and candy, oral lubricants (e.g., MoiStir, OraCare D)]; may predispose patient to monilial infection
- Blurred vision, dry eyes [Management: artificial tears, wetting solutions; pilocarpine 0.5% eye drops]
- Constipation (up to 14% incidence) [Management: increase bulk and fluid intake, fecal softener (e.g., docusate), bulk laxative (e.g., Prodiem, Metamucil)]
- Urinary retention [Management: bethanechol]
- Use of high doses or in combination with other anticholinergic drugs may result in anticholinergic toxicity with both central and peripheral effects including disorientation, confusion, memory loss, fever, tachycardia, etc.

| Cardiovascular Effects |

- A result of antagonism at α_1-adrenergic and muscarinic receptors
- Hypotension (up to 7% incidence). **DO NOT USE EPINEPHRINE**, as it may further lower the blood pressure; phenylephrine may be used. Risperidone, quetiapine or clozapine dose increases should be gradual to minimize hypotension as well as sinus and reflex tachycardia (3–7% incidence) [Treatment options include dividing the daily dose, increasing fluid and salt intake]
- Transient increases in blood pressure and tachycardia reported with clozapine (usually during treatment initiation); rare cardiac deaths
- Dizziness (up to 20% incidence)
- ECG changes (T-wave inversion, ST segment depression, QT_c lengthening – may increase risk of arrhythmias) reported with ziprasidone and clozapine at higher doses and rarely with risperidone, olanzapine, and quetiapine.
- Risk factor for QT_c prolongation include female gender, electrolyte imbalance, long QT syndrome, history of cardiac disease and concomitant drugs that prolong the QT interval (see Drug Interactions pp. 124–126)
- Rare reports of arrhythmias, myocardial infarction with olanzapine in adults

| GI Effects |

- Weight gain (a result of multiple systems including dopamine, $5-HT_{1B}$, $5-HT_{2C}$, α_1, and H_1 blockade, prolactinemia, gonadal and adrenal steroid imbalance and increase in circulating leptin); may be related to insulin resistance (increased blood glucose); may also be due to carbohydrate craving and excessive intake of high-calorie beverages to alleviate drug-induced thirst and dry mouth);
  - Common with most "second-generation" antipsychotics; not seen with ziprasidone, moderate risk with quetiapine and risperidone, and frequent with clozapine and olanzapine

Second-Generation Antipsychotics (Neuroleptics) (cont.)

- Children and adolescents are more susceptible to weight gain than adults – a major factor in drug compliance; more common in children with tic disorders, PDD and mental retardation
- Over 50% of children and adolescents given clozapine or olanzapine gain at least 10% of their body weight. Patients with low BMI tend to gain more weight than patients with higher BMI at baseline. Maximal increase occurs in first 8 weeks of treatment (except with clozapine). May be dose-related (controversial); caution in women with polycystic ovaries. Weight gain may not plateau with time
- Weight gain may predispose to coronary artery disease, hyperglycemia (for each kg increase in weight, risk for in diabeties increases 4–9%; see Endocrine Effects) and obstructive sleep apnea; may be of concern in individuals with juvenile onset diabetes mellitus, Prader-Willi syndrome, Turner's syndrome or Trisomy-21 [Management: consultation with a dietitian, exercise; the following drugs have been tried with varying degrees of success: topiramate, metformin, orlistat, nizatidine (300–600 mg/day); consider switching antipsychotic if patient gains > 5% of his/her body weight]
- Monitor weight, BMI, waist circumference, fasting blood sugar and lipid levels (300–600 mg/day)
- Anorexia, dyspepsia, dysphagia, occasionally diarrhea
- Reflux esophagitis (approx. 11% incidence reported with clozapine)
- Sialorrhea, difficulty swallowing, gagging (with clozapine up to 90%; case reports with olanzapine and risperidone); suggested to be more frequent in children than adults. May be due to stimulation of M_4 muscarinic or α_2 receptors in salivary glands [reduce dose, chew sugarless gum; preliminary evidence suggests amitriptyline (25–100 mg), benztropine (1–4 mg), atropine "eye" drops (1 drop sublingually, 1–2 times per day) or clonidine (0.05–0.4 mg/day) may be effective in treatment]
- Severe constipation with clozapine has resulted in cases of gastrointestinal complications including fecal impaction, mucosal necrosis

Sexual Side Effects

- A result of altered serotonin, dopamine (D_2) activity, ACh, α_1, H_1, and 5-HT_2 blockade
- Decreased libido
- Erectile difficulties, impotence
- Inhibition of ejaculation, abnormal ejaculation, retrograde ejaculation (risperidone), anorgasmia
- [Treatment options may include: dosage reduction, waiting 1–3 months to see if tolerance occurs, switching antipsychotic or adding a second drug to treat the problem]

Endocrine Effects

- Elevated prolactin level (related to 50–75% D_2 occupancy) – increases occur several hours after dosing and normalize by 12–24 h with clozapine, olanzapine, ziprasidone and quetiapine; with risperidone levels rise and peak within 1–2 months (incidence 8–15%); adolescents and children appear to be at higher risk; elevated prolactin levels may be associated with arrested growth and delayed puberty
- In females: breast engorgement and lactation, amenorrhea (with risk of infertility), menstrual irregularities, changes in libido, hirsutism (due to increased testosterone) osteoporosis and osteopenia (due to decreased estrogen) [Management: reduce dose, change antipsychotic; bromocriptine (low doses) or amantadine if prolactin level elevated]
- In males: gynecomastia, rarely galactorrhea, decreased libido and erectile or ejaculatory dysfunction [Management: reduce dose, change antipsychotic, bromocriptine if prolactin level elevated]
- Metabolic syndrome (also called syndome x or insulin resistance syndrome) describes a constellation of disorders. It is diagnosed in adults, if 3 or more of the following occur:

- obesity: waist circumference > 88 cm (34.6") in adult females and > 102 cm (40.2") in adult males
- disturbed glucose metabolism and /or disturbed insulin metabolism (insulin resistence, hyperinsulinemia or type 2 diabetes): fasting glucose > 6.2–7.0
- dysregulation of plasma lipids; HDL < 1 mol/L (females) and < 1.3 mol/L (males); triglycerides > 1.7 mol/L
- hypertension: BP > 130/85

• Hyperglycemia, glycosuria, and high or prolonged glucose tolerance tests (risk highest and greatest increases seen with clozapine and olanzapine, intermediate with risperidone and quetiapine, and lowest with ziprasidone); tend to occur within 6 months of starting medication and are often associated with substantial weight gain and seems not to be dose-dependent. Cases of exacerbation of "type 2" diabetes as well as de novo onset, and diabetic ketoacidosis in nondiabetic patients, reported with clozapine, risperidone, quetiapine, and olanzapine (induce dose-dependent insulin resistance). Risk factors include obesity or a family history of diabetes mellitus [screen for hyperglycemia periodically-see p. 112, obtain consultation for severe or symptomatic hyperglycemia and monitor for presence of diabetic ketoacidosis]

• Dyslipidemia reported: including increased cholesterol and triglyceride concentrations; greatest increases seen with clozapine and olanzapine, moderate with risperidone and quetiapine, while ziprasidone reported to lower levels of cholesterol and triglycerides independent of changes in body mass index. Have been correlated with blood glucose and insulin levels and body weight; a positive correlation reported between insulin and leptin (see weight gain p. 149); [screen for hyperlipidemia periodically –see p. 112]

• Disturbances in antidiuretic hormone function – hyponatremia with polydipsia and polyuria; increased risk in smokers and alcoholics; risk may be decreased with clozapine. Monitor Sodium levels to decrease risk of seizures in chronically treated patients (especially with clozapine) [Management: fluid restriction, demeclocycline up to 900 mg/day; replace electrolytes]

• Dose-dependent decrease in total T_4 and free T_4 concentrations reported with quetiapine – clinical significance unknown

Ocular Effects

• Lens changes can occur after chronic use of quetiapine (reported incidence of 0.005%) – slit lamp examinations recommended, in monograph, at start of therapy and at 6-month intervals (controversial)

• Case report of esotropia (form of strabismus) with olanzapine

Hematological Effects

• Children are at increased risk of hematological side effects from clozapine. Neutropenia reported in 13% of 172 children and agranulocytosis in 1 child (0.6%) over an 8 month period

• Eosinophilia reported with clozapine frequently between weeks 3 and 5 of treatment; higher incidence in females. Neutropenia can occur concurrently. Transient eosinophilia also reported with olanzapine

• Agranulocytosis
  - Occurs in less than 0.1% of patients within first 12 weeks of treatment
  - Occurs in about 1–2% of patients on clozapine (0.38% risk with monitoring), may be due to metabolite formed via CYP3A4 pathway; monitor WBC and differential; more frequent in children and adolescents, females, and certain ethnic groups (i.e., Ashkenazi Jews)
  - Mortality high if drug not stopped and treatment initiated
  - Signs include sore throat, fever, weakness, mouth sores
  - Recurrence of previous clozapine-induced neutropenia reported after olanzapine started

• Case reports of leukopenia with olanzapine and risperidone

• Transient leukocytosis

Hypersensitivity Reactions

• Usually appear within the first few months of therapy (but may occur after the drug is discontinued)

• Photosensitivity and photoallergy reactions including sunburn-like erythematous eruptions which may be accompanied by blistering

• Skin reactions, rashes (up to 5% incidence), rarely abnormal skin pigmentation (risperidone)

Second-Generation Antipsychotics (Neuroleptics) (cont.)

- Cholestatic jaundice (reversible if drug stopped)
  - Occurs in less than 0.1% of patients on antipsychotics within first 4 weeks of treatment
  - Signs include yellow skin, dark urine, pruritus
- Transient asymptomatic transaminase elevations (ALT/SGPT 2–3 times the upper limit of normal) reported with olanzapine (dose-related), clozapine, quetiapine, and ziprasidone; case reports of liver enzyme abnormalities and fatty liver with risperidone
- Reports of pancreatitis with olanzapine, risperidone, quetiapine, and clozapine (possibly secondary to hypertriglyceridemia or hyperglycemia) generally occurs within first 6 months of therapy
- Case report of myalgia, progressing to rhabdomyolysis in adolescent (on Lithium) following the addition of olanzapine
- Rarely, asthma can be exacerbated
- Neuroleptic malignant syndrome (NMS) – rare disorder characterized by muscular rigidity, tachycardia, hyperthermia, altered consciousness, autonomic dysfunction, and increase in CPK; dystonia more common in children
  - Can occur with any class of antipsychotic agent, at any dose, and at any time (increased risk in hot weather and tends to follow an increase in antipsychotic dose); other risk factors include polypharmacy, mood disorders, dehydration, exhaustion, agitation, low serum Sodium. Case reports in pediatric patients taking olanzapine, risperidone, ziprasidone or clozapine
  - NMS with clozapine, and other novel agents, may present with fewer extrapyramidal symptoms, a lower rise in CPK and increased autonomic effects; reported incidence with clozapine is 0.2%
  - Potentially fatal unless recognized early and medication is stopped; supportive therapy must be instituted as soon as possible, especially fever reduction, fluids, and correction of electrolytes (mortality rate up to 10%)
  - Dantrolene, amantadine and bromocriptine may be helpful (controversial); ECT has also been used successfully

Temperature Regulation

- Altered ability of body to regulate response to changes in temperature and humidity; may become hyperthermic or hypothermic; more likely in temperature extremes due to inhibition of the hypothalamic control area
- Transient temperature elevation can occur with clozapine in up to 50% of patients, usually within the first three weeks of treatment; may be accompanied by an elevation in WBC

Other Adverse Effects

- Mild elevations in uric acid (olanzapine)
- Rhinitis – higher incidence with risperidone; nosebleeds (risperidone)

DISCONTINUATION SYNDROME

- Most likely to occur 24–48 h after abrupt drug withdrawal, or after a large dosage decrease and may last up to 14 days
- Abrupt cessation of high doses may rarely cause gastritis, nausea, vomiting, dizziness, tremors, feelings of warmth or cold, sweating, tachycardia, headache, and insomnia in some patients; [if severe, reinstitute drug and taper slowly]
- Agitation, aggression, delirium, worsening of psychosis, diaphoresis and abnormal movements associated with rapid clozapine withdrawal (suggested taper of 25–50 mg/week)
- Rebound neurological symptoms may occur including akathisia, dystonia and parkinsonism (within the first few days), withdrawal dyskinesia reported within 1–4 weeks
- Tardive neurological symptoms may emerge

- Supersensitivity psychosis (acute relapse) has been described after acute withdrawal, in some patients – more common with clozapine and quetiapine
- ☞ **THEREFORE THESE MEDICATIONS SHOULD BE WITHDRAWN GRADUALLY OVER WEEKS OR MONTHS AFTER PROLONGED USE**

PRECAUTIONS

- Use with caution in the presence of cardiovascular disease, chronic respiratory disorder, and convulsive disorders
- Caution in prescribing to patients with known or suspected hepatic disorder; monitor clinically and measure transaminase level (ALT/AST), periodically
- Monitor if QT interval exceeds 420 ms and discontinue drug if patient symptomatic or if QT interval exceeds 500 ms. DO NOT USE ziprasidone in patients with a history of QT_c prolongation or in combination with drugs known to prolong the QT_c interval. Patients with hypokalemia or hypomagnesemia may also be at risk
- Do not use clozapine in patients with severe cardiac disease. In patients with a family history of heart failure, perform a thorough cardiac evaluation prior to starting therapy
- Cigarette smoking is reported to induce the metabolism and decrease the plasma level of most antipsychotics

TOXICITY

- Symptoms of toxicity are extensions of common adverse effects: anticholinergic, cardiovascular (tachycardia hypotension, dysrhythmia), CNS stimulation followed by CNS depression; EPS is less common than with conventional agents and may be delayed up to 12–24 h.
- Postural hypotension may be complicated by shock, coma, cardiovascular insufficiency, myocardial infarction, and arrhythmias
- Convulsions appear late, except with clozapine; symptoms may persist as drug elimination may be prolonged following intoxication
- Toxic doses in children < age 6 reported as: olanzapine 0.5 mg/kg; clozapine 2.5 mg/kg

Management

- Supportive treatment should be given
- Monitor vital signs and ECG for at least 6 h and admit the patient for at least 24 h if significant intoxication apparent
- Overdose with ziprasidone or clozapine should include continuous ECG monitoring; avoid drugs that produce additive QT prolongation (e.g., disopyramide, procainamide, and quinidine)

USE IN PREGNANCY

- Most antipsychotics have not been demonstrated to have an increased risk of teratogenic effects in humans (risk category C)
- Greatest risk of fetal malformations associated with use during the first trimester. Consider the potential effects on delivery and for withdrawal effects in newborn when used in third trimester
- Risk category B for clozapine – concentration of clozapine in plasma of fetus exceeds that in the mother; floppy infant syndrome and neonatal seizures reported. Rare cases of congenital malformations and perinatal syndromes reported in infants. Suggested to monitor WBC of newborn infants if mother on clozapine
- There may be increased weight gain and risk of hyperglycemia in pregnant women taking clozapine, olanzapine during gestation

Breast Milk

- Antipsychotics have been detected in breast milk, clinical significance in the newborn is unclear
- The American Academy of Pediatrics (2001) classifies antipsychotics as drugs "whose effect in the nursing infant is unknown but may be of concern"
- Suggested that patients taking clozapine not breast feed as concentration of drug in breast milk exceeds that in mother's plasma and can cause sedation, decreased suckling, restlessness or irritability, cardiovascular instability and seizures; if mother does breastfeed, recommend WBC of infant be monitored regularly
- Mothers should avoid breastfeeding within 6 h of taking a dose of an antipsychotic (during peak plasma and breast milk levels) to minimize infant exposure to the drug

Antipsychotics (Neuroleptics)

Second-Generation Antipsychotics (Neuroleptics) (cont.)

LABORATORY TESTS/ MONITORING
- See p. 112
- Specific guidelines apply to clozapine (p. 112)

DRUG INTERACTIONS
- Clinically significant interactions are listed below

Class of Drug	Example	Interaction Effects
Adsorbent	Antacids, activated charcoal, cholestyramine, attapulgite (kaolinpectin)	Oral absorption decreased significantly when used simultaneously; give at least 1 h before or 2 h after the antipsychotics
Antiarrhythmic	Amiodarone	Increased plasma level of risperidone due to inhibited metabolism via CYP2D6
	Quinidine	Increased plasma level of clozapine and risperidone due to inhibited metabolism via CYP2D6 Possible synergism or prolongation of QT interval with ziprasidone. Concurrent use with antiarrhythmics contraindicated
Antibiotic	Ciprofloxacin	Increased clozapine (by up to 80%) and olanzapine level due to inhibited metabolism via CYP1A2 Possible synergism or prolongation of QT interval with ziprasidone. DO NOT COMBINE
	Erythromycin, clarithromycin	Increased plasma level and decreased clearance of clozapine (by 33–54% with erythromycin) and of quetiapine due to inhibition of metabolism via CYP3A4
Anticholinergic	Antiparkinsonian agents drugs, antidepressants, antihistamines	Potentiate atropine-like effects causing dry mouth, blurred vision, constipation, etc.; may produce inhibition of sweating, and may lead to paralytic ileus; high doses can bring on a toxic psychosis Variable effects seen on metabolism, plasma level, and efficacy of antipsychotic
Anticoagulants	Warfarin	Decreased PT ratio or INR response with quetiapine
Anticonvulsant	Carbamazepine	Increased clearance and decreased antipsychotic plasma level (by 63% with clozapine, 44% with olanzapine, 4-fold with quetiapine; also with risperidone) (ziprasidone AUC decreased by 35%) Avoid clozapine due to risk of agranulocytosis with either agent
	Lamotrigine	Combination with antipsychotic found beneficial in treatment-refractory schizophrenia (see p. 157); case report of increased plasma level of clozapine. Monitor blood work as both drugs can depress bone marrow function
	Phenytoin, Phenobarbital	Decreased antipsychotic plasma level due to induction of metabolism; up to 24-fold decrease reported with quetiapine and phenytoin With phenobarbital, plasma level of clozapine decreased by 35% and ratio of metabolite to parent drug increased
	Valproate (divalproex, valproic acid)	Both increased and decreased clozapine levels reported; changes in clozapine/norclozapine ratio. Case report of hepatic encephalopathy Elevated valproate level reported with risperidone (possibly due to displacement from protein binding) Combination of valproate with olanzapine or risperidone associated with a high rate of weight gain Combination of valproate with olanzapine or risperidone associated with greater elevations of hepatic enzymes than with either agent alone

Class of Drug	Example	Interaction Effects
Antidepressant Cyclic, SARI	Amitriptyline, clomipramine, trimipramine, trazodone	Additive sedation, hypotension, and anticholinergic effects Increased plasma level of either agent Possible case of serotonin syndrome after withdrawal of clozapine in a patient taking clomipramine
SSRI	Fluoxetine, paroxetine, fluvoxamine, sertraline, citalopram	Increased plasma level of antipsychotic (76% increase of **clozapine** with fluoxetine and 40–45% increase with paroxetine or sertraline, increased AUC by 119% and decreased clearance by 50% of **olanzapine** with fluvoxamine (**risperidone** level increased with paroxetine and sertaline, and up to 2.8-fold with fluoxetine) – case report of serotonin syndrome with paroxetine; **quetiapine** level may be increased with fluvoxamine due to inhibited metabolism via CYP3A4 Fluvoxamine increases steady-state plasma **clozapine** level 5–10-fold, decreases the norclozapine/clozapine ratio and inhibits its metabolism (via multiple CYP isoenzymes); this results in a reduction of metabolic side effects (attributed to norclozapine) and a need to use a lower dose of clozapine to achieve therapeutic effects. Potentially significant increase in **clozapine** level with citalopram Case reports of dose-related mania when **risperidone** or **ziprasidone** added to SSRI Case reports of possible serotonin syndrome in combination with olanzapine (see p. 46)
SARI	Nefazodone	Increased plasma level of quetiapine and clozapine due to inhibited metabolism via CYP3A4
Irrev. MAOI, RIMA	Tranylcypromine, moclobemide	Additive hypotension
Antifungal	Ketoconazole, fluconazole, itraconazole	Increased levels of clozapine, olanzapine, quetiapine and ziprasidone (AUC increased by 35–40%) due to inhibition of metabolism via CYP3A4; monitor for effects on cardiac conduction with clozapine and ziprasidone
Antihypertensive	Methyldopa, enalapril, clonidine, guanethidine	Additive hypotensive effect possible
Antipsychotic combination	General	Increased risk of EPS and elevated prolactin level when combining a FGA with a SGA, or when combining 2 SGAs
	Clozapine + risperidone	Competitive inhibition of clozapine with risperidone for CYP2D6 metabolism resulting in elevated total clozapine level; risperidone level may also be increased; case report of NMS with combination
	Thioridazine + quetiapine	Increased clearance of quetiapine by 65%
	Olanzapine or clozapine + pimozide	Potential for cardiac side effects with combination of novel drug with pimozide, due to competition for metabolism via CYP1A2 and risk of elevated plasma level
	Quetiapine and ziprasidone	Case report of increased QT_c prolongation possibly due to increased plasma level of either drug due to competitive inhibition via CYP3A4
	Phenothiazine or pimozide + ziprasidone	Possible synergism or increased QT interval prolongation
Antitubercular drug	Rifampin	Decreased clozapine level (by 600%) and decreased haloperidol plasma level due to induction of metabolism
Anxiolytic Benzodiazepines	Diazepam, clonazepam, lorazepam	Increased incidence of dizziness (collapse) and sedation when combined with clozapine; cases of ECG changes, delirium and respiratory arrest reported – more likely to occur early in treatment when clozapine added to benzodiazepine regimen (estimated risk 0.36 to 7.7%) Synergistic effect with antipsychotics; used to calm agitated patients
	Lorazepam	Synergistic increase in somnolence with IM olanzapine. DO NOT administer together; recommend Lorazepam be given at least 1 h after IM olanzapine

Second-Generation Antipsychotics (Neuroleptics) (cont.)

Class of Drug	Example	Interaction Effects
Ca-channel blocker	Diltiazem, verapamil	Increased plasma level of quetiapine due to inhibited metabolism via CYP3A4
Caffeine	Coffee, tea, cola	Increased akathisia/agitation Increased plasma levels of clozapine due to competition for metabolism via CYP1A2
CNS depressants	Antidepressants, hypnotics, antihistamines Alcohol	Increased CNS effects Alcohol may worsen EPS Olanzapine absorption increased Additive CNS effects and orthostatic hypotension with olanzapine and quetiapine
Disulfiram		Decreased metabolism and increased plasma level of clozapine
Donepezil		Exacerbation of EPS possible with combination
Grapefruit juice		Increased plasma level of quetiapine due to inhibition of metabolism via CYP3A4; AVOID (data contradictory with clozapine)
H$_2$ antagonist	Cimetidine	Inhibited metabolism of clozapine, olanzapine, risperidone and quetiapine, with resultant increase in plasma level and adverse effects
	Nizatidine	Higher doses of nizatidine reported to increase plasma level of quetiapine (used in combination with paroxcitne), due to inhibited metabolism via CYP3A4, resulting in akathisia, bradykinesia, mild rigidity and bilateral tremor in upper extremities
Lithium		Possibly increased risk of agranulocytosis and seizures with clozapine
Metoclopramide		Increased risk of EPS
Modafinil		Case of clozapine toxicity – increased plasma level of clozapine due to inhibited metabolism via CYP2C19
Oral contraceptive		Estrogen potentiates hyperprolactinemic effect of antipsychotics
Protease inhibitors	Ritonavir, indinavir	Decreased metabolism and increased plasma level of clozapine due to inhibited metabolism via CYP3A4; AVOID due to effects on cardiac conduction Increased plasma level and moderate increase in AUC of risperidone reported Decreased olanzapine level; increased AUC (by 53%) and clearance (by 116%) with ritonavir due to enzyme induction via CYP1A2
Smoking – cigarettes		Decreased plasma level of clozapine and olanzapine by 20–100% due to induction of metabolism; caution when patient stops smoking as level of antipsychotic will increase – case report of clozapine toxicity following smoking cessation
Statin	Lovastatin	Case report of prolonged QT$_c$ interval with quetiapine, possibly due to competitive inhibition of CYP3A4
Stimulant	Amphetamines	Antipsychotics can counteract many signs of stimulant toxicity
	Methylphenidate	Case reports of worsening of tardive movement disorder and prolongation or exacerbation of withdrawal dyskinesia following antipsychotic discontinuation
Sympathomimetic	Epinephrine, norepinephrine	May result in paradoxical fall in blood pressure (due to α-adrenergic block produced by antipsychotics); benefits may outweigh risk in anaphylaxis; phenylephrine is a safe substitute for hypotension

Third-Generation Antipsychotics (Neuroleptics)

Chemical Class	Generic Name	Trade Name	Dosage Forms and Strengths	Monograph Statement
Dihydrocarbostyril	Aripiprazole[B]	Abilify	Tablets: 2 mg, 5 mg, 10 mg, 15 mg, 20 mg, 30 mg Oral solution: 1 mg/ml	Not approved for use in children

[B] Not marketed in Canada; available only through Special Access Program.

INDICATIONS

No approved indications in children and adolescents

Approved for Adults

- Schizophrenia; 89% of children aged 10–17 ($n = 19$) with schizophrenia, schizophreniform disorder or BD were improved "or very much improved" in an open trial of 20–30 mg/day
- Bipolar mania including manic and mixed episodes; 71% of pediatric patients ($n = 41$) with BD taking 16 mg (+/-8 mg) for 5 months were very much or much improved
- Maintenance treatment of bipolar disorder

Other Uses in Children and Adolescents

- Schizoaffective disorder
- Aggressive behavior in conduct disorders and oppositional defiant disorders was reduced in an open trial in children and adolescents

PHARMACOLOGY

- See p. 146–147
- Aripiprazole demonstrates high affinity, partial agonism at dopamine D_2 receptors (both pre and post-synaptic) and serotonin $5HT_{1A}$ receptors, and antagonism at serotonin $5HT_{2A}$ receptors
- Called a dopamine system stabilizer (DSS), the net effect of dopamine partial agonism depends on whether there is a hypo or hyperdopaminergic state. In areas of hypodopaminergic activity, partial D_2 agonism results in an increase in dopaminergic function (postulated as an explanation for benefit in negative symptoms and affective symptoms and less EPS). In areas of hyperdopaminergic activity, partial D_2 agonism results in a net decrease in dopaminergic function (postulated as explanation for improvement of positive symptoms).
- Aripiprazole demonstrates moderate affinity for histamine H_1 receptors and adrenergic α_1 receptors. It has no appreciable affinity for cholinergic M_1 receptors.

GENERAL COMMENTS

- Decreases both positive and negative symptoms of schizophrenia without producing motor side effects or elevating the prolactin level
- Improves depressive symptoms

DOSING

- See p. 142
- Begin at 1–10 mg once daily (if < 25 kg, start with 1mg; 25–50 kg, give 2 mg; 50–70 kg give 5 mg; and > 70 kg, give 10 mg); can increase gradually after 2 weeks, up to a maximum of 30 mg/day (dosing not affected by food); effective dose range: 10–30 mg/day
- Dose adjustment not required in renal or hepatic impairment, nor in smokers

Third-Generation Antipsychotics (Neuroleptics) (cont.)

PHARMACOKINETICS	<list><li>See p. 142</li><li>Pharmacokinetics in children is similar to that of adults</li><li>Can be taken with or without food; peak plasma concentration in 3–5 h</li><li>Metabolite dehydroaripiprazole is active, represents 40% of parent drug exposure in plasma, and has similar affinity for D_2 receptors</li><li>Because of long half-life, steady-state occurs in about 14 days</li><li>Metabolized primarily by CYP3A4 and 2D6; poor metabolizers of 2D6 have a 60% higher exposure to active drug, and half-life increases to 146 h</li></list>
ADVERSE EFFECTS	<list><li>See p. 150</li><li>Dose-related</li></list>
CNS Effects	<list><li>Most common: headache, agitation, insomnia, anxiety, nervousness, sedation, asthma</li><li>Dizziness, lightheadedness</li><li>Akathisia reported</li><li>Low risk of extrapyramidal side effects; cases of tremor dystonia, parkinsonian gait and weakness reported</li><li>Case reports of seizures</li></list>
Cardiovascular Effects	<list><li>Orthostatic hypotension reported</li><li>Minimal change in QT_c interval; in some patients QT_c interval was shortened</li><li>Edema, chest pain</li></list>
GI Effects	<list><li>Nausea and vomiting commonly seen at start of therapy; higher with increased doses</li><li>Low incidence of weight gain; weight loss reported</li><li>Constipation</li></list>
Endocrine Effects	<list><li>Minimal effect on prolactin</li><li>Effect on glucose is unclear; case reports of hyperglycemia and one report of diabetic ketoacidosis in adults</li><li>Does not appear to affect lipid profiles, nor increase total cholesterol or low-density lipid cholesterol (may improve HDL), and it does not have a deleterious effect on triglyceride levels</li></list>
Other Adverse Effects	<list><li>Rash</li><li>Cases of neuroleptic malignant syndrome including report in an adolescent</li></list>
DISCONTINUATION SYNDROME	<list><li>Withdrawal symptoms reported, similar to those seen with other classes of antipsychotics</li></list>

- Caution in patients with known cardiovascular disease, cerebrovascular disease, or conditions that predispose patients to hypotension

TOXICITY

- GI (vomiting) and CNS (drowsiness) symptoms reported following overdose; significant cardiovascular effects not seen
- Vomiting and lethargy reported lasting 30 h in 2 yr old boy following ingestion of 40 mg; a six yr old boy experienced lethargy, drooling and flaccid facial muscles after 2 doses of aripiprazole
- Toxic dose in children < 6 years of age reported as 3 mg/kg

Management

- Supportive treatment. Early intervention may include administration of charcoal to lesson GI absorption

USE IN PREGNANCY

- Teratogenic effects seen in animal studies; effects in humans unknown. One case of healthy child following 85 days of maternal exposure in late pregnancy

Breast Milk

- Unknown if drug or metabolites excreted into human milk

DRUG INTERACTIONS

- Clinically significant interactions are listed below

Class of Drug	Example	Interaction Effects
Antiarrhythmic	Quinidine	Increased AUC of aripiprazole by 112% due to decreased metabolism via CYP2D6; AUC of metabolite increased by 52% – dosage adjustment may be required
	Amiodarone	Increased plasma level of aripiprazole possible due to inhibited metabolism via CYP2D6
Antibiotic	Erythromycin, clarithromycin	Increased plasma level of aripiprazole due to inhibited metabolism
Anticonvulsant	Carbamazepine, oxcarbazepine	Decreased plasma level of aripiprazole due to increased metabolism via CYP3A4; C_{max} and AUC of drug and metabolite decreased by about 70% – dosage adjustment may be required
	Valproate	C_{max} and AUC of aripiprazole decreased by 25%; of low clinical significance
Antidepressant – SSRI	Fluoxetine, paroxetine, fluvoxamine	Increased plasma level of aripiprazole due to inhibited metabolism; case reports of EPS symptoms Case of CNS toxicity including delusions and hallucinations in 13 yr old on high doses of aripiprazole and fluoxetine
Antifungal	Ketoconazole, itraconazole	Increased plasma levels of aripiprazole due to decreased metabolism via CYP3A4; AUC of aripiprazole and metabolite increased by 63% and 77%, respectively – dosage adjustment may be required
CNS depressant	e.g., hypnotics, narcotics	Potentiation of CNS effects (e.g. sedation, fatigue)
H_2 antagonist	Famotidine	Decreased rate (C_{max}) and extent (AUC) of absorption of aripiprazole and its active metabolite; of low clinical significance
	Cimetidine	Increased plasma level of aripiprazole due to inhibited metabolism

First-Generation Antipsychotics (FGAs) (Neuroleptics)

PRODUCT AVAILABILITY

Chemical Class	Generic Name	Trade Name[A]	Dosage Forms and Strengths	Monograph Statement
Butyrophenone	Haloperidol	Haldol Haldol Decanoate	Tablets: 0.5 mg, 1 mg, 2 mg, 5 mg, 10 mg, 20 mg Oral solution: 2 mg/ml, 1 mg/ml[B] Injection: 5 mg/ml Injection (depot): 50 mg/ml, 100 mg/ml	Not recommended in children under age 3
Dibenzoxazepine	Loxapine	Loxapac[C] Loxitane[B]	Tablets[C]: 2.5 mg, 5 mg, 10 mg, 25 mg, 50 mg Extended-release capsules[B]: 5 mg, 10 mg, 25 mg, 50 mg Oral solution: 25 mg/ml Injection: 50 mg/ml	Safety and efficacy not established in children
Dihydroindolone	Molindone[B][D]	Moban	–	–
Diphenylbutylpi-peridine	Pimozide	Orap	Tablets: 2 mg, 4 mg	Limited data on use and efficacy in children under age 12
Aliphatic Pheno-thiazine	Chlorpromazine	Largactil[C], Thorazine[B]	Tablets: 10 mg[B], 25 mg, 50 mg, 100 mg, 200 mg[B] Oral solution: 30 mg/ml[B], 40 mg/ml[C], 44.5 mg/ml[C], 100 mg/ml[B] Oral syrup: 10 mg/5 ml[B] Injection: 25 mg/ml	Not recommended in children under 6 months
	Methotrimeprazine[C]	Nozinan	Tablets: 2 mg, 5 mg, 25 mg, 50 mg Injection: 25 mg/ml	Children under age 12 should not exceed 40 mg/day
Piperazine pheno-thiazine	Fluphenazine	Moditen[C], Prolixin[B] Modecate[C], Prolixin decanoate[B]	Tablets: 1 mg, 2 mg[C], 2.5 mg, 5 mg, 10 mg[B] Oral solution: 2.5 mg/5 ml, 5 mg/ml[B] Injection: 2.5 mg/ml[B] Injection (depot): 25 mg/ml, 100mg/ml[C]	Safety and efficacy not established in children under age 12
	Perphenazine	Trilafon	Tablets: 2 mg, 4 mg, 8mg, 16 mg Oral solution: 16 mg/5ml Injection: 5 mg/ml	Dosage recommendations available for children over age 12
	Thioproperazine[D][C]	Majeptil	–	–
	Trifluoperazine	Stelazine	Tablets: 1 mg, 2 mg, 5 mg, 10 mg, 20 mg[C] Oral solution: 1 mg/ml[C], 10 mg/ml	Dosage recommendations available for children age 6–12

Chemical Class	Generic Name	Trade Name[A]	Dosage Forms and Strengths	Monograph Statement
Piperidine pheno-thiazine	Pericyazine[C]	Neuleptil	Capsules: 5 mg, 10 mg, 20 mg Oral solution: 10 mg/ml	Dosage recommendations provided for children
	Pipotiazine[C][D]	Piportil L4	–	–
	Thioridazine[B][E]	Mellaril	Tablets: 10 mg, 15 mg, 25 mg, 50 mg, 100 mg, 150 mg, 200 mg Oral solution: 30 mg/ml, 100 mg/ml	Dosage recommendations provided for children over 2 yrs of age
Thioxanthene	Flupenthixol	Fluanxol Fluanxol Depot[C]	Tablets: 0.5 mg, 3 mg Injection (depot): 20 mg/ml, 100 mg/ml	Safety and efficacy not established in children
	Thiothixene	Navane	Capsules: 1 mg[B], 2 mg, 5 mg, 10 mg, 20 mg[B] Oral solution[B]: 5 mg/ml Powder for injection[B]: 5 mg/ml	Safety and efficacy not established in children under age 12
	Zuclopenthixol[C]	Clopixol Clopixol Acuphase Clopixol Depot	Tablets: 10 mg, 25 mg Injection: 50 mg/ml Injection (depot): 200 mg/ml	Safety and efficacy not established in children under age 18

[A] Generic preparations may be available, [B] Not marketed in Canada, [C] Not marketed in USA, [D] Not generally used in children – not reviewed in this chapter [E] restricted use in treatment-refractory schizophrenia in adults – not recommended in children

INDICATIONS

Approved in Children and Adolescents	• Management of aggressive and agitated behavior in patients with chronic brain syndrome and mental retardation, or children with severe behavior problems (e.g., hyperexcitability, explosiveness, impulsivity, aggression – haloperidol, chlorpromazine) • Symptomatic control of Tourette syndrome (haloperidol)

Approved (for Adults)	• Treatment of acute and chronic psychosis (i.e., schizophrenia, manic phase of bipolar disorder, delusional disorder, toxic psychosis) • Prophylaxis of schizophrenia • Acute mania, mixed states, and prophylaxis of bipolar affective disorder • Agitated aggressive and self-injurious behavior of dementia and mental retardation • Control of impulsivity and aggression in psychosis (pericyazine, haloperidol) • Tourette's syndrome (haloperidol, pimozide) • Anti-emetic (chlorpromazine, trifluoperazine, perphenazine, methotrimeprazine) • Nausea, vomiting, anxiety associated with acute intermittent porphyria (chlorpromazine) • An adjunct to anesthesia, analgesia, refractory hiccups and in the treatment of tetanus (chlorpromazine, methotrimeprazine) • Sedation (methotrimeprazine, chlorpromazine)

Antipsychotics (Neuroleptics)

First-Generation Antipsychotics (FGAs) (Neuroleptics) (cont.)

Other Uses in Children and Adolescents	• Conduct disorder accompanied by severe aggressiveness and explosiveness (haloperidol, pimozide) • Augmentation for refractory obsessive-compulsive disorder and related disorders (e.g., pimozide); data suggest efficacy of haloperidol in trichotillo-mania • Autism Spectrum Disorders: double-blind studies show efficacy in treatment of aggression, hyperactivity, stereotypies, and social withdrawal of children with autism (haloperidol, thiothixene, pimozide)
PHARMACOLOGY	• See pp. 146–147 • All FGAs are distinguished as a class by binding to D_2 receptors throughout the brain as powerful long-acting antagonists
DOSING	• See pp. 143–145 • Current opinion suggests use of lower doses (i.e., haloperidol 1–6 mg daily, or equivalent); clinical efficacy correlated with D_2 binding above 60% (see p. 146); outcome studies show patient response at low doses similar to high doses, with decreased adverse effects • Slower titration will minimize side effects such as sedatian and orthostatic hypotension
ADMINISTRATION	
Oral Medication	• Medication may be given with meals or at bedtime followed by a glass of water, milk or orange juice. Avoid apple or grapefruit juice as they may interfere with drug effect • Protect liquids from light • Discard markedly discolored solutions; however, a slight yellowing does not affect potency • Dilute liquids with milk, orange juice, or semisolid food just before administration as some drugs may be bitter in taste • Some liquids such as chlorpromazine and methotrimeprazine have local anesthetic effects and should be well diluted to prevent choking • Do not give oral medication within 2 h of an antacid or antidiarrheal drug, as absorption of the antipsychotic will be decreased • If patient is suspected of not swallowing tablet medication, liquid medication can be given
Short-Acting Injection	• Watch for orthostatic hypotension, especially with parenteral administration of chlorpromazine or methotrimeprazine; keep patient supine or seated for 30 minutes afterwards; monitor BP before and after each injection • Give IM into upper outer quadrant of buttocks or the deltoid (deltoid offers faster absorption due to better blood perfusion); alternate sites, charting (L) or (R); massage slowly after, to prevent sterile abscess formations, and tell patient the injection may sting • Do not let drug stay in syringe for longer than 15 min as plastic may adsorb drug
Depot Injection	• Use a needle of at least 21 gauge; give deep IM into large muscle (using Z-track method); rotate sites and specify in charting • SC administration can be used for fluphenazine

- Do not let drug stand in syringe for longer than 15 min as plastic may adsorb drug
- DO NOT massage injection site

PHARMACOKINETICS

- See pp. 111, 143–145

Oral Medication

- Most phenothiazines and thioxanthenes have active metabolites

Short-Acting Injection

- See p. 111

Depot Injection

- See p. 111 and chart on p. 150
- Presence of "free" fluphenazine in multi-dose vials of fluphenazine decanoate is responsible for high peak plasma level seen within 24 h of injection – monitor for EPS
- Injections can be painful; greatest pain reported 5 min after administration and tends to decrease gradually over 2–10 days

Zuclopenthixol Acuphase

- Short-acting depot injection
- Peak plasma level: 24–36 h; elimination half-life = 36 h (mean); long-acting depot formulation also available

ADVERSE EFFECTS

- See chart on p. 148 for incidence of adverse effects; the incidence of adverse effects may differ between different dosage forms of the same drug (e.g., oral vs depot vs acuphase)
- Children and adolescents may be more sensitive to adverse effects
- Many adverse effects are transient; persistent effects often have remedies, but are often best dealt with by changing the dosing schedule, the dose, or the medication

CNS Effects

- A result of antagonism at H1, ACh, and α_1-receptors and dopamine

A. Cognitive Effects

- Sedation common, especially during the first 2 weeks of therapy (incidence up to 81%, depending on drug) [Management: prescribe bulk of dose at bedtime]
- Confusion, disturbed concentration, disorientation (more common with high doses)
- May improve attention/information processing; antipsychotics do not seem to affect memory or psychomotor performance unless anticholinergic effects prominent (e.g., chlorpromazine) or excessive dysphoric effects present

B. Neurological Effects

- A result of antagonism at dopamine D_2 receptors (extrapyramidal reactions correlated with D2 binding above 75–80%). D_2 receptor densities are higher in children and adolescents than in adults therfore the probability of EPS is increased
- Lowered seizure threshold; caution in patients with a history of seizures. May occur if dose increased rapidly or may be secondary to hyponatremia in SIADH
- Extrapyramidal reactions (see pp. 152–154) seen primarily with the high potency antipsychotics are dose and drug-related, (incidence 12–73%) and include: dystonias, dyskinesias, and pseudoparkinsonism; akathisia and akinesia occur less frequently in children (low cal-

First-Generation Antipsychotics (FGAs) (Neuroleptics) (cont.)

cium levels may predispose to extrapyramidal reactions and low iron to akathisia). Rare cases of "Pisa Syndrome." Suggested that patients who lack CYP2D6 isoenzyme may be at higher risk for chronic movement disorder from drugs metabolized primarily by this isoenzyme. Increased sensitivity to EPS may be related to increased amount of D_2 receptors in the striatum in children and adolescents

- Loss of gag reflex (especially in males)
- Dysphagia (difficulty swallowing); of greater concern in males; sialorrhea – see GI Effects
- Urinary incontinence (overflow incontinence) [can be managed with desmopressin or DDAVP nasal spray or tablets, oxybutynin]
- Withdrawal dyskinesias common in children (see p. 122)
- Tardive dyskinesia (see p. 154). TD and withdrawal dyskinesias are the most common (12–34%) long-term untoward side effect of FGAs and their greatest limitation. Risk in adolescents estimated to be 17.6%; risk in children with heterogeneous disorders is less than in adults (estimated at 5.9%); children with autism are at high risk (25% by 11 months, 40% by 2.5 years, and 75% by 3.5 years) – difficult to distinguish between emerging dyskinesias and breakthrough autistic symptomatology. Persistent or tardive dyskinesias appear late in therapy, rarely sooner than 3–6 months, and often persist after termination of therapy; symptoms often appear when the antipsychotic is discontinued or the dosage lowered; symptoms are not alleviated by antiparkinsonian medication and may be made worse by it; symptoms disappear during sleep and can be suppressed by voluntary effort and concentration; they are exacerbated by stress. Risk factors include: mood disorders, lower IQ, presence of obstetrical complications at birth, and cumulative antipsychotic exposure

| Anticholinergic Effects |

- A result of antagonism at muscarinic receptors (ACh)
- Common; effects are additive if given concurrently with other anticholinergic agents
- Dry mucous membranes [Management: sugar-free gum and candy, oral lubricants (e.g., MoiStir, OraCare D)]; may predispose patient to monilial infection
- Blurred vision, dry eyes [Management: artificial tears, wetting solutions; pilocarpine 0.5% eye drops]
- Constipation [Management: increase bulk and fluid intake, fecal softener (e.g., docusate), bulk laxative (e.g., Prodiem, Metamucil), osmotic laxative (e.g., lactulose)]
- Urinary retention [Management: bethanechol]
- Use of high doses or in combination with other anticholinergic drugs may result in anticholinergic toxicity with both central and peripheral effects including disorientation, confusion, memory loss, fever, tachycardia, etc.

| Cardiovascular Effects |

- A result of antagonism at α_1-adrenergic and muscarinic receptors
- Hypotension, most frequent with parenteral use. **DO NOT USE EPINEPHRINE**, as it may further lower the blood pressure [treatment options may include dividing the daily dose, increasing fluid and/or salt intake, or phenylephrine may be used]
- Dizziness, fainting [change antipsychotic; if not possible: sodium chloride tablets, caffeine, increase fluids]
- Tachycardia, nonspecific ECG changes (including ST segment depression, flattened T waves and increased U wave amplitude), QT_c lengthening – in rare cases "torsades de pointes" arrhythmia has occurred (especially with droperidol, thioridazine, and pimozide); electrolyte abnormalities including hypokalemia, hypomagnesemia and hypocalcemia can contribute to the development of torsades de pointes
- Sudden death of patients on antipsychotics is probably due to arrhythmias (rare)

GI Effects	

- Weight gain (a result of multiple systems including dopamine, 5-HT$_{1B}$, 5-HT$_{2C}$, α_1, H$_1$ blockade, hyperprolactinemia, gonadal and adrenal steroid imbalance, and an increase in circulating leptin; may be related to insulin resistance (increased blood glucose); may also be due to carbohydrate craving and excessive intake of high calorie beverages to alleviate drug-induced thirst and dry mouth): more likely to occur early in treatment; more common with low-potency agents (e.g., chlorpromazine – mean gain 3–5 kg) and depot preparations, and may be dose-dependent; women reported to be at higher risk; weight loss also reported (loxapine)
- Anorexia, dyspepsia, constipation, occasionally diarrhea
- Vomiting common after prolonged treatment, especially in smokers
- Sialorrhea, difficulty swallowing, gagging

Sexual Side Effects	

- A result of altered dopamine (D$_2$) activity, ACh blockade, α_1 blockade, sedative effects
- Reported incidence in males is 16–60% and females 7–33%
- Decreased libido
- Erectile difficulties, impotence
- Inhibition of ejaculation, retrograde ejaculation or absence of ejaculation (especially thioridazine), pain at orgasm (males and females) and anorgasmia
- Priapism (especially with thioridazine, chlorpromazine)
- [Treatment options may include: dosage reduction, waiting 1–3 months to see if tolerance occurs, switching antipsychotics, or adding a second drug to treat the problem]

Endocrine Effects	

- Prolactin level may be elevated depending on drug and dose (related to 50–75% D2 occupancy) –develops over the first week of treatment and remains elevated throughout use of drug (some suggest levels can decline with chronic use); returns to normal within 3 weeks when drug stopped; may take up to 6 months with depots. Children and adolescents appear to be at higher risk. High prolactin levels may be associated with sexual side effects, menstrual disturbances, infertility, reduced bone density as well as polydipsia
- In females: breast engorgement, lactation, amenorrhea, menstrual irregularities, changes in libido, hirsutism and possibly osteoporosis (due to decreased estrogen) [Management: re-evaluate dose, change antipsychotic; bromocriptine (low doses) or amantadine if prolactin level elevated]
- False positive pregnancy test
- In males: gynecomastia, rarely galactorrhea, decreased libido and erectile or ejaculatory dysfunction [Management: reduce dose, switch to another agent, bromocriptine if prolactin level elevated or change to alternate medication with lower risk of elevating prolactin (e.g., quetiapine)]
- Increased appetite, weight gain (see GI Effects p. 134)
- Hyperglycemia, glycosuria, and high or prolonged glucose tolerance tests (in patients on oral and depot antipsychotics)
- Hypoglycemia
- Hyperlipidemia reported: increases in cholesterol and triglyceride levels
- Disturbance in antidiuretic hormone function – hyponatremia with polydipsia and polyuria; reported to occur in 6–20% of chronic patients; risk increased in smokers and alcoholics; suggestion that risk may be increased with depot haloperidol; monitor sodium levels to decrease risk of seizures in chronically treated patients [Management: fluid restriction, demeclocycline; replace electrolytes]

Ocular Effects	

- Lenticular pigmentation
  - Related to long-term use of antipsychotics (primarily chlorpromazine)
  - Presents as glare, halos around lights or hazy vision
  - Granular deposits in eye

First-Generation Antipsychotics (FGAs) (Neuroleptics) (cont.)

- – Vision usually is not impaired; may be reversible if drug stopped
- – Often present in patients with antipsychotic-induced skin pigmentation or photosensitivity reactions
- Pigmentary retinopathy (retinitis pigmentosa)
  - – Primarily associated with chronic use of thioridazine or chlorpromazine [annual ophthalmological examination recommended]
  - – Reduced visual acuity (may occasionally reverse if drug stopped)
  - – Blindness can occur
- With chronic use, chlorpromazine can cause pigmentation of the endothelium and Descemet's membrane of the cornea; it can color the conjunctiva, sclera and eyelids a slate-blue color – may not be reversible when drug stopped
- Association reported between phenothiazine use and cataract formation

Hypersensitivity Reactions

- Usually appear within the first few months of therapy (but may occur after the drug is discontinued)
- Photosensitivity and photoallergy reactions including sunburn-like erythematous eruptions which may be accompanied by blistering
- Skin reactions, rashes, abnormal skin pigmentation
- Cholestatic jaundice (reversible if drug stopped)
  - – Occurs in less than 0.1% of patients within first 4 weeks of treatment, with most antipsychotics
  - – Occurs in less than 1% of patients on chlorpromazine
  - – Signs include yellow skin, dark urine, pruritus
- Low potency agents may be a risk factor for venous thrombosis in predisposed individuals – case reports of deep vein thrombosis in adult patients on chlorpromazine – usually occurs in first 3 months of therapy
- Transient asymptomatic transaminase elevations (ALT/SGPT 2–3 times the upper limit of normal) reported with haloperidol (up to 16% of patients)
- Agranulocytosis
  - – Occurs in less than 0.1% of patients within first 12 weeks of treatment with most antipsychotics
  - – Mortality high if drug not stopped and treatment initiated
  - – Signs include sore throat, fever, weakness, mouth sores
- Rarely, asthma, laryngeal, angioneurotic or peripheral edema, and anaphylactic reactions occur
- Neuroleptic malignant syndrome (NMS) – rare disorder characterized by muscular rigidity, tachycardia, hyperthermia, altered consciousness, autonomic dysfunction, and increase in CPK
  - – Can occur with any class of antipsychotic agent, at any dose, and at any time (more common in the summer); other risk factors include young age, mood disorders, dehydration, exhaustion, agitation, low serum Sodium, or rapid or parenteral administration of antipsychotic. Children receiving low-potency antipsychotics reported to have poorer outcomes
  - – Potentially fatal unless recognized early and medication is stopped; supportive therapy must be instituted as soon as possible, especially fluid and electrolytes (mortality rate 4%)
  - – Dantrolene, amantadine and bromocriptine may be helpful (controversial)
- Cases of systemic lupus erythematosus reported with chlorpromazine in adults

| Temperature Regulation | • Altered ability of body to regulate response to changes in temperature and humidity; may become hyperthermic or hypothermic in temperature extremes due to inhibition of the hypothalamic control area |

DISCONTINUATION SYNDROME

- Most likely to occur 24–48 h after withdrawal, or after a large dosage decrease
- Abrupt cessation of high doses may rarely cause gastritis, nausea, vomiting, dizziness, tremors, feelings of warmth or cold, sweating, tachycardia, headache, and insomnia in some patients; symptoms begin 2–3 days after abrupt discontinuation of treatment and may last up to 14 days
- Rebound neurological symptoms may occur including akathisia, dystonia and parkinsonism (within the first few days), withdrawal dyskinesia reported (in up to 51% of individuals) within 1–4 weeks; more common in children and adolescents with autism
- Tardive neurological symptoms may emerge
- Supersensitivity psychosis (acute relapse) has been described after acute withdrawal in some patients
- ☞ **THEREFORE THESE MEDICATIONS SHOULD BE WITHDRAWN GRADUALLY OVER WEEKS TO MONTHS AFTER PROLONGED USE**

Management

- Maintain antiparkinsonian drug for a few days after stopping the antipsychotic to minimize EPS reactions
- If symptoms are moderate to severe, reinstitute previous dose and withdraw more slowly

PRECAUTIONS

- Hypotension occurs most frequently with parenteral use, especially with high doses; the patient should be in supine position during short-acting IM administration and remain supine or seated for at least 30 minutes; measure the BP before and following each IM dose
- IM injections should be very slow; the deltoid offers faster absorption as it has better blood perfusion. Need to ensure child has adequate muscle mass in deltoid; gluteal or thigh may be alternatives
- Use with caution in the presence of cardiovascular disease, chronic respiratory disorder, and convulsive disorders
- Caution in prescribing to patients with known or suspected hepatic disorder; monitor clinically and measure transaminase level (ALT/AST), periodically
- Prior to prescribing thioridazine or pimozide, baseline ECG, and serum potassium should be done, and monitored periodically during the course of therapy. DO NOT USE thioridazine in patients with QT_c interval over 450 ms
- Monitor if QT interval exceeds 420 ms and discontinue drug if exceeds 500 ms; do not exceed 325 mg thioridazine or 10 mg pimozide daily
- Cigarette smoking is reported to induce the metabolism and decrease the plasma level of most antipsychotics

TOXICITY

- Symptoms of toxicity are extensions of common adverse effects: anticholinergic, cardiovascular, and CNS stimulation followed by CNS depression; extrapyramidal effects (e.g., dystonias) may be delayed up to 24 h
- Postural hypotension may be complicated by shock, coma, cardiovascular insufficiency, myocardial infarction, and arrhythmias
- Convulsions appear late
- Overdose with thioridazine, droperidol, and pimozide should include continuous ECG monitoring; avoid drugs that produce additive QT prolongation (e.g., disopyramide, procainamide, and quinidine)
- Toxic doses in children < 6 years of age reported as: chlorpromazine 15 mg/kg, thioridazine 1.4 mg/kg, haloperidol 0.15 mg/kg

Management

- Supportive treatment should be given

First-Generation Antipsychotics (FGAs) (Neuroleptics) (cont.)

USE IN PREGNANCY

- Antipsychotics have been clearly demonstrated to have teratogenic effects
- If possible, avoid during first trimester; suggested that high-potency agents offer less risk
- Use of moderate to high doses of FGAs in the last trimester may produce extrapyramidal reactions in newborn and impair temperature regulation after birth

Breast Milk

- Antipsychotics have been detected in breast milk in concentrations of 0.2–11%; clinical significance in the newborn is unclear
- The American Academy of Pediatrics classifies antipsychotics as drugs "whose effect in the nursing infants is unknown but may be of concern"

DRUG INTERACTIONS

- Clinically significant interactions are listed below

Class of Drug	Example	Interaction Effects
Adsorbent	Antacids, activated charcoal, cholestyramine, attapulgite (kaolin-pectin)	Oral absorption decreased significantly when used simultaneously; give at least 1 h before or 2 h after the antipsychotic
Anesthetic	Enflurane	Additive hypotension with chlorpromazine
Antiarrhythmic	Quinidine	Increased plasma level of haloperidol due to inhibited metabolism via CYP2D6
	Quinidine, procainamide, amiodarone, disopyramide, bretylium	Additive cardiac depression and impaired conduction with thioridazine, chlorpromazine, pimozide – DO NOT COMBINE
Antibiotic	Clarithromycin, erythromycin	Decreased clearance of pimozide by 80%; DO NOT COMBINE due to effects on cardiac conduction – deaths reported
Anticholinergic	Antiparkinsonian agents drugs, antidepressants, antihistamines	Potentiate atropine-like effects causing dry mouth, blurred vision, constipation, etc.; may produce inhibition of sweating, and may lead to paralytic ileus; high doses can bring on a toxic psychosis Variable effects seen on metabolism, plasma level, and effcacy of antipsychotic
Anticoagulant	Warfarin	Decreased PT ratio or INR response with haloperidol
Anticonvulsant	Carbamazepine	Increased level of carbamazepine and metabolite with loxapine and haloperidol Increased clearance and decreased antipsychotic plasma level (up to 100% with haloperidol), also reported with zuclopenthixol and flupenthixol
	Phenytoin, phenobarbital	Decreased antipsychotic plasma level due to induction of metabolism; reported with haloperidol and phenothiazines
	Valproate (divalproex, valproic acid)	Increased neurotoxicity, sedation, and other side effects due to decreased clearance of valproic acid with chlorpromazine Increased plasma level of haloperidol by an average of 32%

Class of Drug	Example	Interaction Effects
Antidepressant Cyclic, SARI	Amitriptyline, trimipramine, trazodone	Additive sedation, hypotension, and anticholinergic effects Increased plasma level of either agent
SSRI	Fluoxetine, paroxetine, fluvoxamine, sertraline	Increased plasma level of antipsychotic (up to 100% increase in **haloperidol** level with fluoxetine or fluvoxamine, and 4-fold increase with paroxetine); (3-fold increase in plasma level of **thioridazine** with fluvoxamine); (up to 21-fold increase in peak plasma level of **perphenazine** with paroxetine) (40% increase in AUC and C_{max} of **pimozide** with sertraline and increase in AUC and C_{max} with paroxetine by 151% and 62%, respectively) DO NOT COMBINE **thioridazine** with fluoxetine, fluvoxamine or paroxetine, or **pimozide** with sertraline, due to risk of cardiac conduction slowing Increased EPS and akathisia
Irrev. MAOI, RIMA	Tranylcypromine, moclobemide	Additive hypotension
Antifungal	Ketoconazole, itraconazole, voriconazole	Increased pimozide level due to inhibition of metabolism via CYP3A4; monitor for effects on cardiac conduction
	Fluconazole	Fluconazole does not inhibit CYP3A4, but potential for additive QT prolongation exists
Antihypertensive	Methyldopa, enalapril, clonidine	Additive hypotensive effect
	Guanethidine	Reversal of antihypertensive effect with chlorpromazine, haloperidol, and thiothixene (not reported with molindone) due to blockade of guanethidine uptake into postsynaptic neurons
Antipsychotic combination	General	Increased risk of EPS and prolactin elevation when combining a FGA with a SGA, or when combining two FGAs
	Thioridazine, quetiapine	Increased clearance of quetiapine by 65%
	Thioridazine, fluphenazine, haloperidol	Increase in plasma of free (unbound) fluphenazine or haloperidol (by 30% and 50%, respectively) when combined with thioridazine
	Olanzapine, clozapine, pimozide	Potential for cardiac side effects with combination of novel drug with pimozide, due to competition for metabolism via CYP1A2 and risk of elevated plasma level
Antitubercular drug	Isoniazid	Increased plasma level of haloperidol due to inhibited metabolism
	Rifampin	Decreased haloperidol plasma level due to induction of metabolism
Anxiolytic Benzodiazepines	Alprazolam	Increased plasma level of haloperidol (by 19%)
	Clonazepam, lorazepam	Synergistic effect with antipsychotics; used to calm agitated patients
Buspirone		May increase extrapyramidal reactions Increased haloperidol and metabolite plasma level (by 26% and 83%, respectively)

First-Generation Antipsychotics (FGAs) (Neuroleptics) (cont.)

Class of Drug	Example	Interaction Effects
β-Blocker	Propranolol	Increased plasma level of both chlorpromazine and propranolol reported Thioridazine level increased 3–5-fold – DO NOT COMBINE
	Pindolol	Increased plasma level of both thioridazine and pindolol reported – DO NOT COMBINE
Ca-channel blocker	Diltiazem, verapamil	Additive Ca-channel blocking effects with thioridazine and pimozide – caution, as may lead to conduction abnormalities
Caffeine	Coffee, tea, cola	Increased akathisia/agitation
CNS depressant	Alcohol, hypnotics, antihistamines	Increased CNS effects (e.g. sedation, fatigue)
Disulfiram		Decreased plasma level of perphenazine and an increase in its metabolite
Donepezil		Exacerbation of EPS possible with combination
Grapefruit juice		Increased plasma level of pimozide due to inhibition of metabolism via CYP3A4; AVOID
H₂ antagonist	Cimetidine	Inhibited metabolism of thiothixene, with resultant increase in plasma level and adverse effects
Hormone	Oral contraceptive	Estrogen potentiates hyperprolactinemic effect of antipsychotic
Lithium		Increased neurotoxicity at therapeutic doses; may increase EPS; increased plasma level of molindone and haloperidol
Narcotic	Codeine	Marked inhibition of conversion of codeine to active metabolite, morphine, with chlorpromazine, methotrimeprazine, haloperidol and thioridazine
Protease inhibitor	Ritonavir	Decreased metabolism and increased plasma level of pimozide due to inhibited metabolism via CYP3A4; AVOID due to effects on cardiac conduction Moderate increase in AUC of chlorpromazine, haloperidol, perphenazine and thioridazine
Smoking – cigarettes		Decreased plasma level of antipsychotic (chlorpromazine, haloperidol, fluphenazine, thiothixene) by 20–100% due to induction of metabolism
Stimulant	Amphetamine	Antipsychotics can counteract many signs of stimulant toxicity
	Methylphenidate	Case reports of worsening of tardive movement disorder and prolongation or exacerbation of withdrawal dyskinesia following antipsychotic discontinuation
Sympathomimetic	Epinephrine, norepinephrine	May result in paradoxical fall in blood pressure (due to α-adrenergic block produced by antipsychotics); benefits may outweigh risk in anaphylaxis; phenylephrine is a safe substitute for hypotension

Antipsychotic Doses

Drug	Compara-ble Daily Dose (mg)*	Suggested Doses for Psychosis in Children and Adolescents	Bio-avail-ability	Peak Plasma level (h) T_{max}	Protein Bind-ing	Elimina-tion Half-life (h)	CYP-450 Metabolizing Enzymes[i]	CYP-450 Inhibitor[j]	D_2 Receptor Occupancy[a] (dose & plasma Level)[b]	5-HT$_{2A}$ Occu-pancy (dose)	5-HT$_{2A}$: D2 Affinity Ratio
SECOND-GENERATION AGENTS (SGAs)											
Benzisoxazole											
Risperidone (Risperdal)	2–2.5	0.25 mg bid to start and in-crease gradually Suggested daily dose ranges:[n] Children 1–2 mg Adolescents: 2.5–4 mg Doses above 10 mg/day do not usually produce further Improvement	60–80%	1–1.5 (parent) 3 (metab)	88–90% (parent) 77% (metabo-lite)	**3–15** (par-ent) 20–24 (active metab) Increased in hepatic or renal disease p. 150	**2D6**[p], 3A4 P-gp	2D6, 3A4[w]	60–75% (2–4 mg) 63–85% (2–6 mg; 36–252 nmol/l)	60–90% (1–4 mg)	8:1
Risperidone Consta	1.8–25 mg q 2 weeks	12.5–25 mg q 2 weeks	–	–	as above		**2D6**[p], 3A4 P-gp	2D6, 3A4[w]	59–83% (50–75 mg q 2 weeks)	?	
Dibenzodiazepine											
Clozapine (Clozaril)[g]	200–250	6.25–12.5 mg on day 1, 25–50 mg on day 2, then increase gradually by 6.25–2.5 mg weekly to the suggested dose range (in divided doses) Suggested daily dose ranges:[n] Children: 100–350 mg Adolescents: 225–450 mg Prescribing restrictions: – Canada: max of 7-day prescription for 6 months, then, if approved, can prescribe every 2 weeks – USA: max of 7-day prescrip-tion (other countries may have less stringent regulations)	40–60%	1–6	95%–97% (to 1-acid glyco-protein)	6–33 (11–105 metab)	**1A2**[p], 2D6[w], **3A4**[p], 2C9[w], 2C19[w], 2E1[w], FMO, UGT, P-gp[w]	1A2[w], 2D6[w], 3A4[w], 2C9, 2C19	38–68%[e] (300–900 mg; 600–2500 nmol/l)	85–94% (>125 mg)	30:1
Quetiapine (Seroquel)	300–400	12.5 mg bid to start; increase by 12.5–25 mg per day, as tolerated, to the suggested dose range (given bid) Suggested daily dose ranges:[n] Children: 150–400 mg Adolescents: 250–550 mg Doses above 800 mg/day not recommended	Absolute bioavail-ability unknown	.5–3	83%	5.3 Clearance reduced in hepatic impairment	2D6[w], **3A4**[p]	1A2[w], 2D6[w], 3A4[w], 2C9[w], 2C19[w]	20–44%[e] (300–700 mg) 13% (150mg)	21–80%[h] (150–600 mg) 38% (150mg)	1:1

Antipsychotic Doses (cont.)

Drug	Compara-ble Daily Dose (mg)*	Suggested Doses for Psychosis in Children and Adolescents	Bio-avail-ability	Peak Plasma level (h) T_{max}	Protein Bind-ing	Elimina-tion Half-life (h)	CYP-450 Metabolizing Enzymes[i]	CYP-450 Inhibitor[j]	D$_2$ Receptor Occupancy[a] (dose & plasma Level)[b]	5-HT$_{2A}$ Occu-pancy (dose)	5-HT$_{2A}$: D2 Affinity Ratio
Thienobenzodiaz-epine											
Olanzapine (Zyprexa)	7.5–10	2.5–5 mg daily to start; increase by 2.5–5 mg weekly Suggested daily dose ranges:[n] Children: 5–10 mg Adolescents: 10–15 mg Doses above 20 mg/day not recommended	57–80%	4–6 (oral) 75–45 min (IM)	93% (to albu-min and l-acid glyco-protein)	20–70 reduced in smokers	1A2, 2D6[w] FMO U6T	1A2, 2D6[w], 3A4[w], 2C9[w], 2C19[w]	55–80%(5–20 mg; 59–187 nmol/l) 83–88% (30–40 mg)	90–98% (5–20 mg)	50:1
Benzothiazolylpi-perazine											
Ziprasidone (Geodon)[c]	40–80	5 mg daily to start and increase gradually to the suggested dose range Suggested daily dose ranges:[n] Children: 40–100 mg Adolescents: 80–140 mg	30% (60% with food) AUC incr 40–67% in renal impair-ment and 26% in cirrhosis	3–6 (C_{max} incr. by 32–72% in mild renal impair-ment)	99%	4–10 (dose-dependent)	**3A4**[p], 1A2[w], 2D6, 2C18, 2C19	2D6[w], 3A4[w]	45–75% (40–80 mg)	80–90% (40–80 mg)	11:1
THIRD-GENERATION AGENT (TGA)											
Aripiprazole (Abilify)	5–10	Initial dosing: (if < 25 kg, start with 1 mg; 25–50 kg, give 2 mg; 50–70 kg give 6 mg; and > 70 kg, give 10 mg) Suggested daily dose ranges:[n] Children: 5–15 mg Adolescents: 10–20 mg	87%	3–5	99%	47–75 (metab - 94) no change in renal or hepatic impairment	2D6, 3A4	–	40–95% (0.5–30 mg)	?	?

Drug	Comparable Daily Dose (mg)*	Suggested Doses for Psychosis in Children and Adolescents	Bioavail-ability	Peak Plasma level (h) T_{max}	Protein Binding	Elimination Half-life (h)	CYP-450 Metabolizing Enzymes[i]	CYP-450 Inhibitor[j]	D_2 Receptor Occupancy[a] (dose & plasma Level)[b]
FIRST–GENERATION AGENTS (FGAs)									
Butyrophenone									
Haloperidol (Haldol)	2	Age 3–12 (15–40 kg wt): 0.5 mg to start; can increase by 0.5 mg q 5–7 days (given bid or tid) Psychotic Disorders: 0.05–0.15 mg/kg/day Suggested daily dose ranges:[n] Children: 1–4 mg Adolescents: 2–10 mg Nonpsychotic Disorders: 0.05–0.075 mg/kg/day Doses above 10 mg/day not recommended	40–80%	0.5–3	92% (to 1-acid gly-coprotein)	12–36	1A2[w], 2D6[w], **3A4[p]**	2D6[p], 3A4 P-gp	75–89% (4–6 mg; 6–13 nmol/l)
Haloperidol decanoate (Haldol LA)	0.7 (20 mg q 4 weeks)	Suggested daily dose ranges:[n] Children: 15–50 mg q 4 weeks Adolescents: 50–150 mg q 4 weeks	–	p. 150	92% (to 1-acid gly-coprotein)	p. 150	as above	as above	60–85% (30–70 mg q 4 weeks; 9 nmol/l)
Dibenzoxazepine									
Loxapine (Loxa-pac, Loxitane)	15	Initial dose: 5–10 mg/day and increase gradually by 10 mg/day Usual dose: 50–100 mg daily	33%	?	?	8–30 (multiple active metab with long $T_{1/2}$	1A2, 2D6, 3A4 UGT	—	60–80% (15–30 mg)
Diphenylbutyl-piperidine									
Pimozide (Orap)	2	Initial dose: 0.05 mg/kg at bedtime; may increase every 3 days to a maximum of 0.2 mg/kg (10 mg/day) Usual dose: 1–5 mg/day	15–50%	8	97%	29–55[f]	1A2, **3A4[p]**	**2D6[p]**, 3A4[w], 2C19[w], 2E1, P-gp	77–79% (4–8 mg)
Phenothiazines – Aliphatic									
Chlorpromazine (Largactil, Thorazine)	100	6–12 years old: Oral 0.5 mg/kg q 4–6 h, Rectal: 1 mg/kg q 6–8 h IM: 0.5 mg/kg q 6–8 h Psychosis: Suggested daily dose ranges:[n] Children: 150–200 mg Adolescents: 225–375 mg	25–65%	0.5–1	95–99% (to 1-acid glycopro-tein)	16–30	1A2[w], **2D6[p]**, 3A4, UGT, P-gp	1A2, **2D6[p]**, 3A4[w], 2C9[w], 2C19, 2E1, P-gp	78–80% (100–200 mg; 10 nmol/l)

Antipsychotic Doses (cont.)

Drug	Comparable Daily Dose (mg)*	Suggested Doses for Psychosis in Children and Adolescents	Bioavail-ability	Peak Plasma level (h) T_{max}	Protein Binding	Elimination Half-life (h)	CYP-450 Metabolizing Enzymes[i]	CYP-450 Inhibitor[j]	D_2 Receptor Occupancy[a] (dose & plasma Level)[b]
Methotrime-prazine[d] (Nozinan)	70	Initial dose: 0.25 mg/kg/day in 2 to 3 divided doses; increase gradually to ef-fective dose. Maximum of 40 mg/day in children under age 12	?	1–3	?	16–78	1A2, 2D6	**2D6**[p]	?
Phenothiazines – Piperazine									
Fluphenazine HCl (Moditen, Pro-lixin)	2	Suggested daily dose ranges:[n] Children: 1.5–5 mg Adolescents: 2.5–10 mg; 0.04 mg/kg/day or 0.5–10 mg/day	1–50%	1.5–2	90–99%	13–58	1A2, 2D6, P-gp	1A2, **2D6**[p], 3A4[w], 2E1, 2C8/9, P-gp	?
Fluphenazine decanoate (Modecate, Pro-lixin decanoate)	0.46 (13 mg q 4 weeks)	Suggested daily dose ranges:[n] Children: 6.25–12.5 mg q 2–3 weeks Adolescents: 12.5–25 mg q 2–3 weeks	–	p. 150	90–99%	p. 128	2D6	1A2, **2D6**[p], 3A4, 2E1	?
Perphenazine (Trilafon)	10	Suggested daily dose ranges:[n] Children: 6–12 mg Adolescents: 12–22 mg	25%	1–4	91–92%	9–21	1A2, **2D6**[p], 3A4, 2C9, 2C19	1A2[w], **2D6**[p], 3A4, 2C9, 2C19, P-gp	79% (4–8 mg)
Trifluoperazine (Stelazine)	5	Age 6–12: start at 1 mg od or bid and increase gradually to a maximum of 10 mg/day Usual daily dose range [n] Children: 2–10 mg Adolescents: 6–15 mg/day IM: for severe symptoms 1 mg od-bid	?	?	95–99%	13	1A2 P-gp	P-gp	75–80% (5–10 mg)
Phenothiazines – Piperidine									
Pericyazine[d] (Neuleptil)	15	Over age 5: 2.5–10 mg am and 5–30 mg hs (approx. 1–3 mg per year of age per day)	?	?	?	?	2D6	?	?
Thioridazine (Mellaril)[c][k]	100	Age 1–5: 1 mg/kg/day Over age 5: 75–150 mg/day; Usual daily dose range:[n] Children: 100–250 mg Adolescents: 225–325 mg	10–60%	1–4	97–99%	9–30	1A2[w], 2D6, 2C19[w]	1A2, **2D6**[p], 2C8/9, 2E1, P-gp, Inducer of 3A4	74–81% (100–400 mg; 620– 900 nmol/l)

Drug	Comparable Daily Dose (mg)*	Suggested Doses for Psychosis in Children and Adolescents	Bioavail-ability	Peak Plasma level (h) T_{max}	Protein Binding	Elimination Half-life (h)	CYP-450 Metabolizing Enzymes[i]	CYP-450 Inhibitor[j]	D$_2$ Receptor Occupancy[a] (dose & plasma Level)[b]
Thioxanthenes									
Flupenthixol (Fluanxol)	5	Children: 0.4–2 mg daily Adolescents: up to 3 mg daily as maintenance dose; up to 12 mg daily used in some patients	30–70%	3–8	99%	26–36	?	2D6[w]	70–74% (6 mg; 2–5 nmol/l)
Flupenthixol decanoate (Fluanxol inj.)[d]	1.8 (50 mg q 4 weeks)	20–40 mg q 2–3 weeks; up to 60 mg/injection	–	p. 150	99%	p. 128	?	2D6[w]	81% (40 mg q 7 days; 19 nmol/l)
Thiothixene (Navane)	5	0.26 mg/kg/day Suggested daily dose ranges:[n] Children: 4–7 mg, Adolescents: 4–20 mg	50%	1–3	90–99%	34	**1A2**[p]	2D6[w]	?
Zuclopenthixol (Clopixol)[d]	12	10–25 mg to start; increase by 10–20 mg every 2 to 3 days Usual daily dose: 20–60 mg; doses above 100 mg daily not recommended	44%	2–4	98%	12–28	**2D6**[p]	2D6	?
Zuclopenthixol acetate (Clopixol acuphase)[d]	30 mg q 2–3 days	Usual dose: 25–100 mg IM and repeat every 2–3 days as needed to a maximum of 4 injections (a second injection may need to be given 1–2 days after the first, in some patients)	–	24–48	98%	36	as above	as above	?
Zuclopenthixol decanoate (Clopixol depot)[d]	4.3 (60 mg q 2 weeks)	Usual maintenance dose: 100–250 mg q 2 to 4 weeks	–	p. 150	98%	p. 128	as above	as above	81% (200 mg q 14 d; 50 nmol/l)

NOTE: Comparable doses are only approximations. Generally doses used are higher in adolescents than in children and in the acute stage of the illness than in maintenance. Monograph doses are just a guideline, and each patient's medication must be individualized. Plasma levels are available for some antipsychotics but their clinical usefulness is limited. The use of conversion ratios from an oral to a depot preparation is appropriate as a starting point, but wide intra- and interindividual variations in pharmacokinetic parameters require careful clinical monitoring of the patient. It is recommended that the initially effective dose be reduced, or the injection interval increased, after 4–6 weeks to prevent possible accumulation of the drug as plasma concentrations approach steady-state.

*Based on clinical studies, on D$_2$ affinity, and/or on pharmacokinetics.

[a] D$_2$ receptor occupancy correlates better with plasma level than with dose, and appears to correlate with clinical efficacy in controlling positive symptoms of schizophrenia, [b] Approximate conversion: nmol/l = 3 × ng/ml, [c] Not marketed in Canada, [d] Not marketed in USA, [e] Occupancy higher 2 h vs 12 h post dose, [f] Half-life longer (mean 66–111 h) in children and adults with Tourette's syndrome, [g] Prescribing/monitoring restrictions in Canada and the USA, [i] Cytochrome P-450 isoenzymes involved in drug metabolism [Ref. www.gen-test.com/human_P450_database/srchh450.asp (December 2003) and www.mhc.com/Cytochromes], [j] Cytochrome P-450 isoenzymes inhibited by drug, [k] Not recommended in children or adolescents; indicated only for adults with schizophrenia who cannot tolerate other antipsychotic drugs or who fail to respond to them, [l] Specific to metabolite, [m] Moderate activity, [n] Based on Expert Consensus Guideline. *Journal of Clinical Psychiatry* 64 (Suppl 12) 2003; doses outside these ranges may be necessary for some individuals, [p] Potent activity, [w] Weak activity

P-gp = P-glycoprotein, a transporter of hydrophobic substances in or out of specific body organs (e.g., block absorption in the gut)

UGT = uridine diphosphate glucurnosy transferase – involved in Phase 2 reactions (conjugation)

FMO = flavin moxooxygenase enzyme involved in N-oxidation reactions.

Antipsychotics (Neuroleptics)

Effects of Antipsychotics on Neurotransmitters/Receptors*

	Chlorproma-zine	Methotrime-prazine	Pericyazine	Thioridazine	Fluphenazine	Perphenazine	Trifluoperazine	Haloperidol	Loxapine
Blockade D_1	+++	?	?	+++	+++	+++	+++	+++	+++
Blockade D_2	+++	+++	++++	+++++	+++++	++++	+++++	+++++	++++
Blockade D_3	++++	?	?	++++	+++++	?	?	++++	?
Blockade D_4	++++	?	?	++++	++++	?	+++	+++++	++++
Blockade H_1	+++	+++++	?	+++	+++	++++	++	+	+++
Blockade M_1	+++	++++	?	+++	+	+	+	+	++
Blockade α_1	++++	?	?	++++	+++	+++	+++	+++	+++
Blockade α_2	++	?	+	+	+	++	+	+	+
Blockade $5\text{-}HT_{1A}$	+	+++	?	+	+	+	+	+	+
Blockade $5\text{-}HT_{2A}$	++++	++++	?	++++	++++	++++	++++	+++	++++
DA reuptake	+	?	?	+	+	+	?	+	?

	Pimozide	Flupenthixol	Thiothixene	Zuclopen-thixol	Clozapine	Risperidone	Olanzapine	Quetiapine	Ziprasidone	Aripiprazole
Blockade D_1	++	++++	++	+++++	+++	+++	+++	+	+++	?
Blockade D_2	++++	++++	++++	+++++	++	+++++	+++	++	++++	+++++[A]
Blockade D_3	++++	++++	?	?	++	++	++++	++	++++	+++++
Blockade D_4	+++	?	?	++++	++++	+++++	++++	−	+++	+++
Blockade H_1	+	+++	+++	+++	++++	+++	++++	++++	+++	+++
Blockade M_1	+	+++	+	++	+++	+−	++++	+	−	−
Blockade α_1	+++	+++	++	++++	+++	++++	+++	++++	+++	+++
Blockade α_2	++	++	++	++	+++	++++	++	+++	+−	?
Blockade $5\text{-}HT_{1A}$	+−	+	+	+	++	++	+	++	++++	++++
Blockade $5\text{-}HT_{2A}$	+++	++++	+++	++++	++++	+++++	++++	+++	+++++	++++
DA reuptake	++	++	?	++	+−	+	?	?	?	?

*The ratio of K_i values between various neurotransmitters/receptors determines the pharmacological profile for any one drug.

Key: K_i (nM) > 100,000 = −; 10,000–100,000 = +−; 1000–10,000 = +; 100–1000 = ++; 10–100 = +++; 1–10 = ++++; 0.1–1 = +++++

$1/K_i$ < 0.001 = − 0.001–.01 = +−; .01–.1 = +; .1–1 = ++; 1–10 = +++; 10–100 = ++++; 100–1000 = +++++

See p. 125 for Pharmacological Effects on Neurotransmitters.

Adapted from: Seeman, P. (1993). *Receptor Tables Vol. 2: Drug Dissociation Constants for Neuroreceptors and Transporters.* Toronto: SZ Research; Leysen, J.E. et al. (1993). *Psychopharmacol. 112,* S40–S54; Seeman, P. et al. (1996). *Jpn. J. of Pharmacol. 77,* 187–204; Richelson, E. (1996). *J. Clin. Psychiatry 57 (Suppl 11)* 4–11; Seeman, P. (2002). *Can. J. Psychiatry 47,* 27–38.

[A] Partial agonist

Pharmacological Effects of Antipsychotics on Neurotransmitters/Receptors

DOPAMINE BLOCKADE

- Additive or synergistic interactions occur between various dopamine receptor subtypes

D_1 Blockade

- May mediate antipsychotic effect

D_2 Blockade

- In mesolimbic area – antipsychotic effect: correlates with clinical efficacy in controlling positive symptoms of schizophrenia; an inverse relationship exists between D_2 blockade and therapeutic antipsychotic dosage (i.e., potent blockade = low mg dose)
- In nigrostriatal tract – side effect: extrapyramidal (e.g., tremor, rigidity, etc.)
- In tuberinfundibular area – side effect: prolactin elevation (e.g., galactorrhea, etc.)

D_3 Blockade

- May mediate antipsychotic effect on positive and negative symptoms of schizophrenia

D_4 Blockade

- Effect unclear

DA REUPTAKE BLOCK

- Antidepressant, antiparkinsonian
- Side effects: psychomotor activation, aggravation of psychosis

H_1 BLOCKADE

- Anti-emetic effect
- Side effects: sedation, drowsiness, postural hypotension, weight gain
- Potentiation of effects of other CNS drugs

(ACH) M_1 BLOCKADE

- Mitigation of extrapyramidal side effects
- Side effects: dry mouth, blurred vision, constipation, urinary retention and incontinence, sinus tachycardia, QRS changes, memory disturbances, sedation
- Potentiation of effects of drugs with anticholinergic properties

α_1 BLOCKADE

- Side effects: postural hypotension, dizziness, reflex tachycardia, sedation, hypersalivation, urinary incontinence
- Potentiation of antihypertensives acting via α_1 blockade (e.g., prazosin)

α_2 BLOCKADE

- May lead to increased release of acetylcholine and increased cholinergic activity
- Side effect: sexual dysfunction
- Antagonism of antihypertensives acting as α_2 stimulants (e.g., clonidine)
- Antidepressant, anxiolytic, and antiaggressive action

5-HT$_{1A}$ BLOCKADE

- Antidepressant, anxiolytic, and antiaggressive action.

5-HT$_{2A}$ BLOCKADE

- May correlate with clinical efficacy in decreasing negative symptoms of schizophrenia (data speculative); may modulate (decrease) extrapyramidal effects caused by D_2 blockade
- Anxiolytic (5-HT$_{2C}$), antiaggressive (5-HT$_{2A}$), and antipsychotic effect
- Side effects: hypotension, sedation, weight gain (5-HT$_{2C}$)

Antipsychotics (Neuroleptics)

Frequency (%) of Adverse Reactions to Antipsychotics at Therapeutic Doses

	FIRST-GENERATION AGENTS (FGAs)								
	Phenothiazines – Aliphatic		Phenothiazines – Piperidine		Phenothiazines – Piperazine				
Reaction	Chlorpromazine	Methotrimeprazine	Pericyazine	Thioridazine	Fluphenazine	Perphenazine	Trifluoperazine	Haloperidol	Loxapine
Drowsiness, sedation Insomnia, agitation	> 30 < 2	> 30 < 2	> 30 < 2	> 30 < 2	> 2 > 2	> 10 > 10	> 2 > 2	> 30[h] > 10	> 30 < 2
Extrapyramidal Effects[i] Parkinsonism Akathisia Dystonic reactions	> 10 > 2 > 2	> 10 > 2 < 2	> 2 > 30 < 2	> 2 > 2 < 2	> 30 > 10 > 10	> 10 > 10 > 10	> 30[j] > 10 > 10	>30[j] > 30 > 30[j]	> 30 > 30 > 10
Cardiovascular Effects Orthostatic hypotension Tachycardia ECG abnormalities* QTc prolongation (> 450 ms)	> 30[b] > 10 > 30[h] > 2[h]	> 30[b] > 10 > 10 > 2	> 10 > 2 > 2 > 2	> 30 > 10 > 30[h] > 10[h]	> 2 > 10 > 2 < 2[h]	>10 > 10 > 2 < 2	> 10 > 2 > 2 < 2	> 2 < 2 > 2 < 2[h]	> 10 > 10 < 2 –
Anticholinergic Effects	> 30	> 30	> 30	> 30	> 2	> 10	> 10	> 2	> 10
Endocrine Effects Sexual dysfunction[e] Galactorrhea Weight gain Hyperglycemia Hyperlipidemia	> 30[f] > 30 > 10 >30 >30	> 2[f] > 30 > 10 ? ?	> 10[f] > 10 > 10 ? ?	> 30[f] > 30 > 30 ? >30	>30[f] > 10 > 30 >10 ?	> 10[f] > 10 > 10 >10 >2[s]	> 30[f] > 10 > 10 >2 ?	> 30[f] < 2 > 2 >10 >2	> 2 < 2 < 2[d] >2[s] >10
Skin Reactions Photosensitivity Rashes Pigmentation[a]	> 10 > 10 > 30[h]	> 10 > 2 < 2	> 2 > 2 –	> 10[h] > 10 > 2	< 2 <2 –	< 2 < 2 –	> 2 < 2 –	< 2 < 2 < 2	< 2 > 2 –
Ocular Effects[a] Lenticular pigmentation Pigmentary retinopathy	> 2 > 2[a]	> 2 > 2[a]	> 2 –	> 2 > 10[a]	< 2 –	< 2 < 2	< 2 < 2	< 2 –	< 2 < 2
Blood dyscrasias Hepatic disorder Seizures[g]	< 2 < 2 < 2[b]	< 2 < 2 < 2	< 2 < 2 < 2	< 2 < 2 < 2	< 2 < 2 < 2	< 2 < 2 < 2	< 2 < 2 < 2	< 2 < 2 < 2	< 2 < 2 < 2

	FIRST-GENERATION AGENTS (FGAs)				SECOND-GENERATION AGENTS (SGAs)					TGA
		Thioxanthenes								
Reaction	**Pimozide**	**Flupenthixol**	**Thiothixene**	**Zuclopenthixol**	**Clozapine**	**Risperidone**	**Olanzapine**	**Quetiapine**	**Ziprasidone**	**Aripiprazole**
Drowsiness, sedation	> 10[c]	> 2	> 30	> 30	> 30	> 10[b] [p]	> 30 [p]	> 30 [p]	> 10	> 10[h]
Insomnia, agitation	> 2	< 2	> 10	> 10	> 2	> 10	> 2	> 10	> 30	> 10
Extrapyramidal Effects[i]										
Parkinsonism	> 30	> 30	> 30	> 30	> 2	> 10[h]	> 2	> 2	> 2	> 2
Akathisia	> 10	> 30	> 30	> 10	> 10	> 10[h]	> 10	> 2	> 2	> 10
Dystonic reactions	> 2	> 10	> 30	> 10[j]	< 2	< 2[h]	< 2	< 2	> 2	< 2
Cardiovascular Effects										
Orthostatic hypotension	> 2	> 2	> 2	> 2	> 30	> 30[b]	> 2	>10	> 2	> 2
Tachycardia	> 2	> 2	> 2	> 2	> 30	> 10	> 2[o]	> 2	> 2	> 2
ECG abnormalities*	> 2[c]	> 2	< 2	≳ 2	> 30[h]	< 2	< 2	< 2	> 2[h]	< 2
QTc prolongation (>450 ms)	> 2[c]	< 2	< 2	< 2	< 2[h]	< 2	< 2	< 2	< 2[h]	–
Anticholinergic Effects	> 2	> 10	> 2	> 10[k]	> 30[k]	> 10	> 10	> 10	> 10	> 2
Endocrine Effects										
Sexual dysfunction[e]	> 30	> 30[f]	> 2[f]	> 30[f]	< 2[f]	> 30[f]	> 30[f]	> 30[f]	< 2[f]	< 2
Galactorrhea	< 2	–	< 2	–	< 2	> 10	< 2	–	> 2	< 2
Weight gain	> 2[d]	> 10	> 10	> 10	> 30[p]	> 30[p]	> 30[p]	> 10	> 2	> 2
Hyperglycemia	> 2	> 10	> 2[s]	?	> 30	> 10	> 30	> 30	> 30	< 2
Hyperlipidemia	?	?	?	?	> 30	> 10	> 30	> 10	< 2	< 2
Skin Reactions										
Photosensitivity	–	< 2	< 2	< 2	> 2	> 2	–	–	–	< 2
Rashes	> 2	> 2	< 2	< 2	> 2	< 2	< 2	< 2	> 2	> 2
Pigmentation[a]	–	–	< 2	< 2	–	< 2	–	–	–	–
Ocular Effects[a]										
Lenticular pigmentation	< 2	< 2	< 2	< 2	–	–	–	< 2	–	–
Pigmentary retinopathy	–	< 2	< 2	–	–	–	–	–	–	–
Blood dyscrasias	< 2	< 2	< 2	< 2	< 2[l]	< 2	< 2	–	< 2	< 2
Hepatic disorder	< 2	< 2	< 2	< 2	> 2	< 2	< 2	> 2	–	< 2
Seizures[g]	< 2	< 2	< 2	> 2	< 2[m]	< 2	< 2	< 2	–	< 2

Comparisons of adverse effects are based on currently used/approved doses, usually dose related. Data are pooled from separate studies and are not necessarily comparable
– None reported in literature perused, * ECG abnormalities usually without cardiac injury including ST segment depression, flattened T waves, and increased U wave amplitude
[a] Usually seen after prolonged use, [b] May be higher at start of therapy or with rapid dose increase, [c] Pimozide above 20 mg daily poses greater risk, [d] Weight loss reported, [e] Includes impotence, inhibition of ejaculation, anorgasmia, [f] Priapism reported in adults, [g] In nonepileptic patients, [h] Higher doses pose greater risk, [i] More frequent in autism, [j] Lower incidence with depot preparation, [k] Sialorrhea reported, [l] Risk < 2% with strict monitoring (legal requirement in North America), [m] Risk lower with doses below 300 mg, and increased at higher doses or single doses above 300 mg, [o] Bradycardia frequent with IM olanzapine, often accompanied by hypotension, [p] More frequent in children with PDD or mental retardation, [s] reported, but exact incidence unknown.

Antipsychotics
(Neuroleptics)

Comparison of Depot Antipsychotics

	Flupenthixol decanoate (Fluanxol)	Fluphenazine decanoate (Modecate; Prolixin)	Haloperidol decanoate (Haldol LA)	Zuclopenthixol decanoate (Clopixol Depot)	Risperidone (Risperdal Consta)
Chemical class	Thioxanthene	Piperazine phenothiazine	Butyrophenone	Thioxanthene	Benzisoxazole
Form	Esterified with decanoic acid (a 10-carbon chain fatty acid) and dissolved in vegetable oil; must be hydrolyzed to free flupenthixol; metabolites inactive	Esterified with decanoic acid and dissolved in sesame oil; must be hydrolyzed to free fluphenazine	Esterified with decanoic acid and dissolved in sesame oil; must be hydrolyzed to free haloperidol	Esterified with decanoic acid in coconut oil; must be hydrolyzed to free zuclopenthixol	Encapsulated in a polymer as microspheres in an aqueous base
Strength supplied	(2%)–20 mg/ml (10%)–100 mg/ml	25 mg/ml 100 mg/ml	50 mg/ml 100 mg/ml	200 mg/ml	25 mg/vial, 37.5 mg and 50 mg/vial
Usual dose range	20–40 mg	20–40 mg	50–200 mg	100–250 mg	20–50 mg
Usual duration of action	2–3 weeks	2–4 weeks	4 weeks	2–4 weeks	2 weeks
Pharmacokinetics					
Peak plasma level*	4–7 days	First peak within 24 h (due to presence of hydrolyzed "free" fluphenazine); level drops, then peaks again in 8–12 days	3–9 days	3–7 days	See Depot Injection p. 118
Elimination half-life**	8 days (after single injection), 17 days (multiple dosing)	Over 14 days (single injection), up to 102 days (multiple dosing)	18–21 days	19 days	See Depot Injection p. 118
Adverse Effects*	Similar to oral flupenthixol	Similar to oral fluphenazine	Similar to oral haloperidol	Similar to oral zuclopenthixol	Similar to oral risperidone
CNS	Both sedating and alerting effect reported; can cause excitation (may have more activating effects at low doses)	Both drowsiness and insomnia reported	Both drowsiness and insomnia reported	Both drowsiness and insomnia reported (less frequent than with oral Zuclopenthixol)	Drowsiness, insomnia, headache and anxiety
Extrapyramidal	Frequent	Less frequent than with oral preparation Note: increased frequency of dystonia noted with use of "older" multipunctured multi-dose vials due to presence of "free" fluphenazine	Frequent, however, reported less often than with oral haloperidol	Reported in 5–15% of patients	Akathisia and parkinsonism in 7% Hyperkinesia in 12%
Skin and local reactions	Indurations rarely seen (at high doses) Photosensitivity and hyperpigmentation very rare; dermatological reactions seen	Dermatological reactions have been reported	Inflammation and nodules at injection site (may be more common with 100 mg/ml preparation) Less common if deltoid used	No indurations but local dermatological reactions reported	Pain at injection site Redness, swelling or induration >10% [ensure solution is at room temperature and inject into buttock]

	Flupenthixol decanoate (Fluanxol)	Fluphenazine decanoate (Modecate; Prolixin)	Haloperidol decanoate (Haldol LA)	Zuclopenthixol decanoate (Clopixol Depot)	Risperidone (Risperdal Consta)
Laboratory changes	Rarely leucopenia, eosinophilia	One case of jaundice reported in adults; rarely agranulocytosis; ECG changes seen in some patients	Rarely leucopenia, jaundice	Transient changes in liver function seen Rarely neutropenia, agranulocytosis	Within normal variation

* Important as indicator when maximum side effects will occur
** Useful for determining dosing interval; steady state will be reached in approximately 5 half-lives
*** Generally side effects are similar to oral drugs in same class

Antipsychotics (Neuroleptics)

Extrapyramidal Side Effects of Antipsychotics

	Acute Extrapyramidal Effects	Tardive Syndromes
Onset	Acute or insidious (up to 30 days)	After months or years of treatment, especially if drug dose decreased or discontinued
Proposed mechanism	Most EPS symptoms are due to dopamine (D₂ blockade	Supersensitivity of postsynaptic dopamine receptors induced by long-term blockade
Treatment	Respond to antiparkinsonian drugs See p. 165 Akathisia may be mediated by different mechanisms and is therefore more responsive to other treatments (e.g., benzodiazepines, β-blockers – see p. 165)	Antiparkinsonian agents drugs not effective and may exacerbate tardive dyskinesia Most treatments unsatisfactory; some are aimed at balancing dopaminergic and cholinergic systems Can mask symptoms temporarily by further suppressing dopamine with antipsychotics Novel antipsychotics are less likely to induce tardive dyskinesia and may have antidyskinetic effects see p. 154 Open and controlled studies suggest that branced-chain amino acids (Tarvil, 222 mg/kg tid) can reduce symptoms of tardive dyskinesia in adults and children

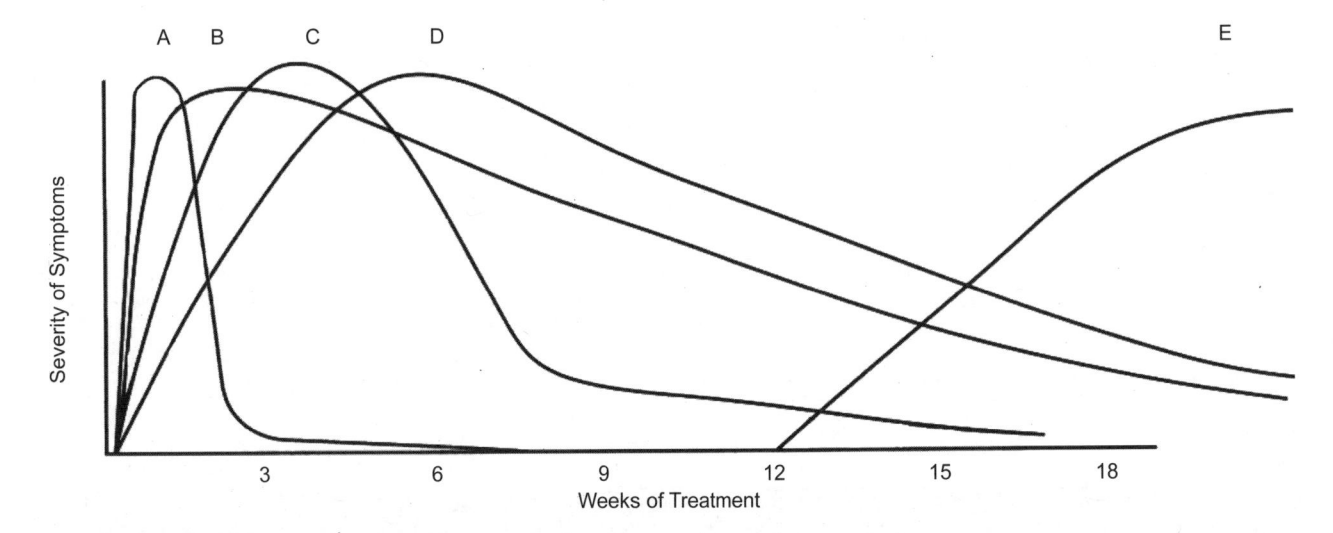

A: Dystonic reactions: uncoordinated spastic movements of muscle groups (e.g., trunk, tongue, face)
B: Akathisia: restlessness, pacing (may result in insomnia)
C: Akinesia: decreased muscular movements Rigidity: coarse muscular movement; loss of facial expression
D: Tremors: fine movement (shaking) of the extremities ("pill-rolling"); Pisa syndrome: can either be acute or tardive in nature (rare; occurs more commonly in people with brain damage/abnormality)
E: Tardive syndromes

Type	Physical (motor) symptoms	Psychological symptoms	Onset	Possible Risk Factors in Children and Adolescents	Clinical Course	Treatment	Differential diagnosis
Acute dystonias	Torsions and spasms of muscle groups; muscle spasms, e.g., oculogyric crisis, trismus, laryngospasm, torti/retro/anterocollis, tortipelvis, opisthotonus, blepharospasm	Anxiety, fear, panic, dysphoria Repetitive meaningless thoughts	Acute (usually within 24–48 h after first dose)	Common in young males Antipsychotic naive High potency conventional antipsychotics Rapid dose increase Lack of prophylactic antiparkinsonian medication Previous dystonic reaction/family history of dystonia Hypocalcemia, hyperthyroidism, hypoparathyroidism Recent cocaine use	Acute, painful, spasmodic; oculogyria may be recurrent Acute laryngeal/pharyngeal dystonia may be potentially life-threatening	Sublingual Lorazepam, IM benztropine, IM diphenhydramine To prevent recurrence: prophylactic antiparkinsonian agents Reduce dose or change antipsychotic	Seizures Catatonia Hysteria Malingering Hypocalcemia Tourette's Syndrome
Acute akathisia	Motor restlessness, fidgeting, pacing, swinging of leg, trunk rocking forward and backward, repeatedly crossing and uncrossing legs, shifting from foot to foot, inability to sit still Respiratory symptoms: dyspnea or breathing discomfort	Restlessness, irritability Agitation, violent outbursts, dysphoria Feeling "wound-up" or "antsy"; sensation of skin crawling Mental unease, irresistible urge to move	Acute to insidious (within hours to days)	Uncommon in children; occurs in adolescents High caffeine intake High potency conventional antipsychotics Anxiety Diagnosis of mood disorder (?) Microcytic anemia Low serum ferritin Risperidone	May continue through entire treatment Suggested that may contribute to suicide and/or violence	Antiparkinsonian agents drugs not very effective Diazepam, clonazepam, Lorazepam, β-blockers, cyproheptadine (preliminary reports) Reduce dose or change antipsychotic	Psychotic agitation/decompensation Severe agitation Anxiety Drug-seeking behavior/withdrawal
Acute pseudoparkinsonism	Stiffness, shuffling, mask-like face, "pillrolling"-type tremor (4–8 cycles per second; greater at rest and bilateral), akinesia, rigidity, stooped posture, postural instability, micrographia, bradykinesia, drooling, loss of arm swing	Slowed thinking Fatigue, anergia Cognitive impairment Depression	Acute to insidious (within 30 days)	High potency conventional antipsychotics Increased dose Concurrent neurological disorder Risperidone	May continue through entire treatment	Reduce dose or change antipsychotic Antiparkinsonian drug	Negative symptoms of schizophrenia Depression
Acute dyskinesias	Rapid involuntary movements; often involve the mouth and tongue	Distress (when talking, swallowing, eating)	Acute to insidious	Autism, mental retardation Use of conventional antipsychotics High doses or multiple antipsychotics Compromised brain function	May continue through entire treatment	Reduce dose or change antipsychotic Antiparkinsonian drug	Withdrawal dyskinesia Tardive dyskinesia Stereotypic behavior Tourette's Syndrome
Pisa Syndrome	Leaning to one side		Can be acute or tardive	Rare in children Compromised brain function	Often ignored by patients	Antiparkinsonian agents drug (higher doses)	

Extrapyramidal Side Effects of Antipsychotics (cont.)

Type	Physical (motor) symptoms	Psychological symptoms	Onset	Possible Risk Factors in Children and Adolescents	Clinical Course	Treatment	Differential diagnosis
Tardive dyskinesia	Involuntary choreoathetoid movements of face (e.g., tics, frowning, grimacing), lips (pursing, puckering, smacking), jaw (chewing, clenching), tongue ("fly-catcher," rolling, dysarthria), eyes (blinking, spasms), limbs (tapping, twitching), trunk (rocking, twisting), neck (nodding), respiratory (dyspnea, gasping, sighing, grunting, forceful breathing) Often coexists with parkinsonism and akathisia Abnormal movements disappear during sleep	Cognitive impairment Distress (when talking, swallowing, eating) and embarrassment	After 3 or more months of therapy Common early sign is "worm-like" movement of the tongue ("fly-catcher tongue")	Females Previous acute or persistent EPS Diabetes (?) Cognitive impairment/brain damage, lower IQ Autism Obstetrical complications at birth Alcohol/drug abuse may predispose to buccolingual masticatory symptoms Greater cumulative exposure to conventional antipsychotics May be associated with genetic variation of the D3 receptor gene	Persistent –discontinuation of antipsychotic early increases chance of remission Spontaneous remission in 14–24% after 5 years	SGA or TGA (clozapine reported to decrease blepharospasm) Suggestions for treatment include: Pyridoxine up to 400 mg/day Clonazepam 0.5–3 mg/day Tetrabenazine 25–50 mg/day Clonidine .05–.2 mg/day Branched-chain amino acids (Tarvil 222 mg/kg tid)	Spontaneous, acute, or withdrawal dyskinesia Stereotypic behavior Tourette's Syndrome Neurological conditions Movement disorder secondary to co-prescribed drug
Tardive dystonia	Sustained muscle contractions of face, eyes, neck, limbs, back or trunk (craniocervical area involved most frequently), e.g., blepharospasm, laryngeal dystonia, dysarthria, retroflexed hands		After months or years of therapy	Young male Genetic predisposition (?) Neurological disorder, mental retardation Coexisting tardive dyskinesia Akathisia	Persistent; discontinuation of antipsychotic early increases chance of remission	Switch to a SGA or TGA (clozapine reported to decrease blepharospasm) Suggestions for treatment include: Tetrabenazine 25–50 mg Benzodiazepines	Myoclonus Motor tics Idiopathic dystonia Meige syndrome
Tardive akathisia	Persistent symptoms of akathisia	As for akathisia	After months of therapy; after drug withdrawal	As for akathisia Coexisting tardive dyskinesia and dystonia	Persistent, discontinuation of antipsychotic early increases chance of remission Fluctuating course	Switch to a SGA or TGA Suggested treatments include: clonidine .05–.5mg / day; Benzodiazepines; β-blockers	As for akathisia

Switching Antipsychotics

ANTIPSYCHOTIC NONRESPONSE

- Ascertain diagnosis is correct and the role of antipsychotic in the child or adolescent is clear/correct
- Ascertain patient is adherent to therapy; determine and address any barriers to adherence
- Ensure there has been an adequate trial period (i.e., adequate dose given for adequate duration to see an effect)
- Ensure dosage prescribed is therapeutic (too low or excessive doses should be re-evaluated); see pp. 141–145 for usual dosage ranges of antipsychotics

Factors Complicating Response

- Concurrent drug abuse (alcohol, street drugs)
- Comorbid diagnoses (e.g., mental retardation, personality disorder)
- Concomitant use of metabolic enhancers (e.g., carbamazepine, cigarette smoking – see Drug Interactions pp. 124, 126, 129, 138, 142)
- Psychosocial factors that hinder response

Switching Antipsychotics

- If side effects limit dose or contribute to noncompliance, switching between classes is appropriate
- Evidence does not suggest a differential response between FGAs
- Switching from a FGA to a SGA may result in enhanced response in negative symptoms and cognition
- Switching from another SGA to clozapine may result in enhanced response

REASONS FOR SWITCHING

- Persistent positive symptoms – switch to another FGA or a SGA
- Persistent negative symptoms – switch to a SGA or lower the dose; consider aripiprazole
- Persistent cognitive or affective symptoms – consider a switch to a SGA
- Relapse despite compliance
- Non-compliance – consider a depot preparation (depending on reason for non-adherence)
- Persistent extrapyramidal side effects (EPS) despite dosage decrease
- Tardive dyskinesia (TD) – clozapine and quetiapine offer minimal risk
- Persistent/chronic side effects, e.g., galactorrhea, impotence, weight gain (see chart p. 149); metabolic side effects (see Endocrine Effects pp. 120, 128, 135) – consider a switch to an alternate SGA or TGA

Advantages of Switching

- Minimizes polypharmacy
- Second agent may be better tolerated
- Decreased potential for side effects and drug interactions
- Less costly

Disadvantages of Switching

- Risk of relapse due to time required to taper first drug, or need for washout
- Lose partial efficacy of first agent
- Delayed onset of action/response
- Risk that patient will end up on 2 agents if he/she improves during cross-taper
- May be difficult to distinguish withdrawal effects vs side effects vs symptoms of illness if cross-tapering

Switching Antipsychotics (cont.)

METHODS

- Four options:
  1) Withdraw the first drug gradually and begin the second drug following a washout period – preferred if patient is stable, but not clinically practical when patient is experiencing symptoms
  2) Stop the first drug and start the second drug at its usual initial dose; increase the dose over a 2–4 week period – not usually recommended unless the patient has had a serious adverse reaction to the first drug, as may result in drug withdrawal symptoms
  3) Maintain the first drug for 2–3 weeks while titrating the dose of the second drug; then withdraw the first drug over 1–2 weeks
  4) Decrease the dose of the first drug and start the second at a low dose; continue decreasing the dose of the first drug as the second one is increasing over a 2–4 week period. Be aware of additive or synergistic side effects of both drugs. Avoid, whenever possible, the ongoing use of two or more antipsychotics simultaneously for an indefinite period of time
- Rate of switching / cross-tapering should be slow in children and adolescents
- Consider (1) rebound or withdrawal effects of discontinued medication (especially if the drug is withdrawn abruptly, e.g., clozapine, quetiapine), (2) risk of relapse, (3) need for auxiliary medication (e.g., antiparkinsonian drug) during the conversion process, and (4) additive or synergistic effects of both drugs including side effects and potential for drug interactions

FGA to FGA

- For equivalent doses see chart pp. 143–145
- Consider side effects of each drug and the need for auxiliary medication such as antiparkinsonian agents

A. Low potency to high potency

- Rebound cholinergic and sedative effects are possible
- Taper first drug gradually as second drug is added

B. High potency to low potency

- Continue antiparkinsonian drug, if currently prescribed, until the changeover is complete to prevent the emergence of EPS, then withdraw the anti-parkinsonian drug gradually

FGA to SGA or TGA

- Decrease the FGA gradually while increasing the "second-generation" drug

SGA or TGA to FGA

- Taper first drug gradually as second drug is added
- Caution when switching from clozapine, as response to FGA and SGA seems to be less satisfactory following its use
- Clozapine and quetiapine withdrawal (especially abrupt withdrawal) has been associated with a high incidence of rebound psychosis in adults – may need to be withdrawn over several weeks

Antipsychotic Augmentation Strategies

As most data on augmentation strategies are uncontrolled, recommend that monotherapy first be optimized prior to use of augmentation strategies and those should not be continued unless clear clinical benefits are demonstrated.

Advantages of Augmentation	• May have a rapid onset • Response > 50% with most combinations • No need to taper first agent or have a washout
Disadvantages of Augmentation	• May have potentiation of side effects • Increased risk of drug interactions Increased cost • Potential for decreased adherence

REFRACTORY POSITIVE SYMPTOMS

Anticonvulsants	• E.g., valproate, lamotrigine; reviews and meta-analysis suggest no significant benefit with carbamazepine in adults • Animal studies suggest that valproate augments prefrontal cortical dopamine release of antipsychotics; lamotrigine augments antipsychotics by antagonizing overactive kainate glutamate receptor • May be useful in patients with excitation, aggressive or impulsive behavior or EEG abnormalities • Valproate can increase antipsychotic plasma levels (see Drug Interactions p. 124)
Lithium	• Plasma level: 0.8–1.2 mmol/l • Contradictory data as to efficacy reported • Review of double-blind studies suggests that lithium can be of benefit in treatment-refractory patients with concomitant mood symptoms (e.g., schizoaffective) or conduct disorder • Clinical improvement may be evident in the first week • May also decrease the rate of relapse in chronic patients • Monitor side effects, including neurotoxicity, especially if the antipsychotic is prescribed in higher dose
Benzodiazepines	• See benzodiazepines (p. 169) for recommended dosages and side effects • Useful in agitated, anxious, acutely psychotic patients (e.g., lorazepam) • Noted to decrease hallucinations and delusions • Improvement may be modest and short-lived • Monitor for disinhibition; more often seen in children who have autism or are mentally challenged

Antipsychotics (Neuroleptics)

Antipsychotic Augmentation Strategies (cont.)

Combining Two Antipsychotics	• There are few controlled studies that evaluate the efficacy of combining two antipsychotics; and no convincing evidence in favor of this strategy; the risk of side effects, drug interactions as well as cost are increased; some data supports adjunctive (low-dose) FGA augmentation of clozapine in treatment-refractory patients • Generally discouraged as risk of D_2-related side effects are increased with such combinations, including acute EPS, elevated prolactin and tardive dyskinesia
Electroconvulsive Therapy	• Little data in children and adolescents • Of benefit in acute schizophrenia, especially if catatonic or affective symptoms present • Some reports suggest superiority with bilateral treatment; usually 12–20 treatments required for schizophrenia in adults • Symptoms that improve include: delusions, hallucinations, agitation, hostility and depression • Modest evidence of efficacy in treatment-refractory patients and benefits appear short-lived • Lack of guidelines regarding maintenance ECT in those who have responded
Ethyleicosapentamoate (E-EPA)	• Suggested to exert augmenting effect by decreasing phospholipase-A2 which is overactive in schizophrenia • Review of double-blind trials suggests 2 g/day is useful in adult patients refractory to clozapine; beneficial in decreasing TD and triglycerides
REFRACTORY NEGATIVE SYMPTOMS	It is important to distinguish primary and secondary negative symptoms. Secondary negative symptoms should be treated, as necessary There are no treatments with proven efficacy for primary negative symptoms
Dopamine Agonists	• Short-term improvement only noted with use of D_2 agonists such as bromocriptine and apomorphine
Stimulants	• E.g., dextroamphetamine, methylphenidate • Transient improvement in negative symptoms and cognitive function reported in children with comorbid ADHD; exacerbation of positive symptoms can occur
Antidepressants	• TCAs, SSRIs, mirtazapine, and nefazodone reported to decrease negative symptoms or co-morbid depression, and improve poor social or work functioning some patients (caution regarding interactions). Benefit may be due to improvement in secondary vs primary negative symptoms

- AACAP (2001). Practice parameters for the assessment and treatment of children and adolescents with schizophrenia. *Journal of the American Academy of Child and Adolescent Psychiatry 40 (2, Suppl.),* 4S–23S.
- Aman, M.G. Gharabawi, G.M. (2004). Treatment of behavior disorders in mental retardation: report on transitioning to atypical antipsychotics with an emphasis on risperidone. *Journal of Clinical Psychiatry 65(9),*1197–1210
- American Psychiatric Association (1997). Practice guidelines for the treatment of patients with schizophrenia. *American Journal of Psychiatry 154(4) (Apr. Suppl.),* 1–63.
- Amou, M.G., Gharabawi, G.M. (2004). Treatment of behavior disorders in mental retardation: Report on transitioning to atypical antipsychotics with an emphasis on risperidone. *Journal of Clinical Psychiatry 65(9),* 1197–1210.
- Blin, O., Micallef, J. (2001). Antipsychotic-associated weight gain and clinical outcome parameters. *Journal of Clinical Psychiatry 62 (Suppl. 7),* 11–21.
- Buck, M.L. (2001). Use of the atypical antipsychotic agents in children and adolescents. *Medscape Pediatric Pharmacotherapy 7(8),* 1–6.
- Cheng-Shannon, J., McGough, J.J., Pataki, C. et al. (2004). Second-generation antipsychotic medications in children and adolescents. *Journal of Child and Adolescent Psychopharmacology 14(3),* 372–394.
- Correll, C.U., Leucht, S., Kane, J.M. (2004). Lower risk for tardive dyskinesia associated with second-generation antipsychotics: A systematic review of 1-year studies. *American Journal of Psychiatry 161,* 414–425.
- Czekalla, J., Kollack-Walker, S., Beasley, C.M. (2001). Cardiac safety parameters of olanzapine: Comparison with other atypical and typical antipsychotics. *Journal of Clinical Psychiatry 62 (Suppl. 2),* 35–40.
- DelBello, M., Grcevich, S. (2004). Phenomenology and epidemiology of childhood psychiatric disorders that may necessitate treatment with atypical antipsychotics. *Journal of Clinical Psychiatry 65(Suppl.6),* 12–19.
- Ernst, C.L., Goldberg, J.F. (2002). The reproductive safety profile of mood stabilizers, atypical antipsychotic, and broad-spectrum psychotropics. *Journal of Clinical Psychiatry 63 (Suppl. 4),* 42–55.
- Expert Consensus Guideline Series (2003). Optimizing pharmacologic treatment of psychotic disorders. *Journal of Clinical Psychiatry 64 (Suppl. 12),* 1–100.
- Findling, R.L., McNamara, N.K. (2004). Atypical antipsychotics in the treatment of children and adolescents: Clinical applications. *Journal of Clinical Psychiatry 65(Suppl.6),* 30–44.
- Findling, R.L., Steiner, H., Weller, F.B. (2005). Use of antipsychotics in children and adolescents. *Journal of Clinical Psychiatry 66 (Suppl. 17),* 29–40.
- Findling, R.L. (2003). Dosing of atypical antipsychotics in children and adolescents. Primary care companion. *Journal of Clinical Psychiatry 5(Suppl. 6),* 10–13.
- Gardner D.M., Baldessarini R.J., Waraich P. (2005). Modern antipsychotic drugs: A critical overview. *Canadian Medical Association Journal 172(13),* 1703–1711
- Grundy, S.M., Cleeman, J.I., Daniels, S.R. et al. (2005). Diagnosis and management of the metabolic syndrome. An American Heart Association/National Heart, Lung, and Blood Institute Scientific Statement Circulation.112, 2735–2752.

Antipsychotics (Neuroleptics)

References and Selected Readings (cont.)

- Kinon, B.J., Basson, B.R., Gilmore, J.A. et al. (2000). Strategies for switching from conventional antipsychotic drugs or risperidone to olanzapine. *Journal of Clinical Psychiatry 61,* 833–840.
- Lewis, R. (1998). Typical and atypical antipsychotics in adolescent schizophrenia: Efficacy, tolerability, and differential sensitivity to extrapyramidal symptoms. *Canadian Journal of Psychiatry 43,* 596604.
- Lieberman, J.A., Strong, T.S., McEvoy, J.P. et al. (2005). Effectiveness of antipsychotic drugs in patients with chronic schizophrenia. *New England Journal of Medicine 353(12),* 1209–1223
- Lindenmayer, J.-P., Natham, A.-H., Smith, R.C. (2002). Hyperglycemia associated with the use of atypical antipsychotics. *Journal of Clinical Psychiatry 62 (Suppl. 23),* 30–38.
- Marder, S.R., Essock, S.M., Miller, A.L. et al. (2004). Physical health monitoring of patients with schizophrenia. *American Journal of Psychiatry 161(8),* 1334–1349.
- McConville, B.J., Sorter, M.T. (2004). Treatment challenges and safety considerations for antipsychotic use in children and adolescents with psychosis. *Journal of Clinical Psychiatry 65(Suppl. 6),* 20–29.
- Potenza, M.N., McDougle, C.J. (1998). Potential of atypical antipsychotics in the treatment of nonpsychotic disorders. *CNS Drugs 9(3),* 213–232.
- Pres, R.W. (2002). Pharmacological approaches to psychotropic-induced weight gain. *International Drug Therapy Newsletter 37(7),* 49–53.
- Richelson, E. (1999). Receptor pharmacology of neuroleptics: Relation to clinical effects. *Journal of Clinical Psychiatry 60 (Suppl. 10),* 5–14.
- Sacks, F.M. (2004). Metabolic syndrome: Epidemiology and consequences. *Journal of Clinical Psychiatry 65(Suppl. 6),* 3–12.
- Schooler, N., Rabinowitz, J., Davidson, M. (2005). Risperidone and haloperidol in first-episode psychosis: A long-term randomized trial. *American Journal of Psychiatry 162(5),* 947–953.
- Seeman, M.V., Seeman, P. (2002). Choosing an antipsychotic and why. *Clinical Update, Medscape CME,* article 441135.4, Sept. 16.
- Silva, R.R., Munoz, D.M., Alpert M. et al. (1999). Neuroleptic malignant syndrome in children and adolescents. *Journal of the American Academy of Child and Adolescent Psychiatry 38(2),* 187–194.
- Stahl, S. (2001). "Hit-and-run" actions at dopamine receptors, Part 1 and Part 2. *Journal of Clinical Psychiatry 62(9),* 670–671 and *62(10),* 747–748.
- Thase, M.E. (2002). What role do atypical antipsychotic drugs have in treatment-resistant depression? *Journal of Clinical Psychiatry 63(2),* 95–103.
- Toren, P., Ratner, S., Laor, N., Weizman, A. (2004). Benefit-risk assessment of atypical antipsychotics in the treatment of schizophrenia and comorbid disorders in children and adolescents. *Drug Safety* 27(14):1135–1156.
- Wirshing, D.A. (2004). Schizophrenia and obesity: Impact of antipsychotic medications. *Journal of Clinical Psychiatry 65 (suppl.8),* 13–26.
- Wirshing, W.C. (2001). Movement disorders associated with neuroleptic treatment. *Journal of Clinical Psychiatry 62 (Suppl. 21),* 15–18.

AGENTS FOR TREATING EXTRAPYRAMIDAL SIDE EFFECTS

PRODUCT AVAILABILITY

Chemical Class	Generic Name	Trade Name[A]	Dosage Forms and Strengths	Monograph Statements
Dopamine agonist[E]	Amantadine	Symmetrel	Capsules: 100 mg Oral syrup: 50 mg/5 ml	Dosage recommendations available for children over age 1
Antihistamine[E]	Diphenhydramine	Benadryl	Tablets/Capsules: 25 mg, 50 mg Chewable tablets[C]: 12.5 mg Oral disintegrating (Thin strips)[C]: 12.5 mg, 25 mg Oral solution: 6.25 mg/5 ml, 12.5 mg/5 ml Injection: 50 mg/ml	Dosage recommendations available for infants and children
	Orphenadrine[D]	Norflex	–	–
β-blocker	Propranolol	Inderal	Tablets: 10 mg, 20 mg, 40 mg, 60 mg[B], 80 mg, 90 mg[B], 120 mg[C] Solution[B]: 4 mg/ml, 8 mg/ml Oral concentrate[B]: 80 mg/ml Injection: 1 mg/ml	Dosage recommendations available for children
		Inderal LA	Sustained-release capsules: 60 mg, 80 mg, 120 mg, 160 mg	LA: experienced limited in children under age 12
Benzodiazepine	Clonazepam	Rivotril[C], Klonopin[B]	Tablets: 0.25mg, 0.5 mg, 1 mg, 2 mg	Dosage recommendations available for infants and children
	Diazepam	Valium	Tablets: 2 mg, 5 mg, 10 mg Oral solution: 5 mg/5ml, 5 mg/ml[B] Injection: 5 mg/ml	Dosage recommendations available for infants and children
		Diazepam Intensol[B] Diastat Diazemuls[C]	Oral concentrate[B]: 5 mg/ml Rectal gel: 5 mg/ml Emulsion injection (IV/IM)[C]: 5 mg/ml	
	Lorazepam	Ativan	Tablets: 0.5 mg, 1 mg, 2 mg Sublingual tablets[C]: 0.5 mg, 1 mg, 2 mg Injection: 2 mg/ml[B], 4 mg/ml	Oral: efficacy not established in children under age 12 Injection: not recommended in children under age 18
		Lorazepam Intensol[B]	Oral Concentrate[B] 2 mg/ml	
Anticholinergic agent[E]	Benztropine	Cogentin	Tablets: 0.5 mg, 1 mg, 2 mg Solution[C]: 2 mg/5 ml Injection: 1 mg/ml	Contraindicated in children under age 3; use cautiously in older children
	Biperiden[B]	Akineton	Tablets: 2 mg	Side effects not established in children
	Ethopropazine[C][D]	Parsitan	–	–
	Procyclidine	Kemadrin	Tablets: 2.5 mg[C], 5 mg Oral solution[C]: 2.5 mg/5 ml	Safety and efficacy not established in children
	Trihexyphenidyl	Artane	Tablets: 2 mg, 5 mg Oral solution[B]: 2 mg/5 ml	Safety and efficacy not established in children

[A] Generic preparations may be available, [B] Not marketed in Canada, [C] Not marketed in USA, [D] Not generally used in children – not reviewed in this chapter, [E] Antiparkinsonian agent

Agents for Treating Extrapyr. Side Effects

Agents for Treating Extrapyramidal Side Effects (cont.)

INDICATIONS

Certain anticholinergic and antihistaminic agents are indicated to relieve the neurological (muscular) side effects induced by antipsychotics (see pp. 166–167 for comparison of drugs): None are approved for this use in children and adolescents

Approved (for Adults)

- Acute dyskinesias, dystonias
- Pseudoparkinsonian effects (tremor, rigidity, shuffling)
- Akathisia (restlessness)
- Akinesia (decreased muscle movement)

GENERAL COMMENTS

- Use caution when giving children anticholinergic agents due to concern over cognitive impairment
- No clear evidence that one drug is more efficacious than another; individual patients may respond better, or tolerate one drug over another
- Used infrequently with "second-generation" antipsychotics unless higher doses used (e.g., risperidone > 4 mg)
- Controversy exists whether antiparkinsonian agents should be given prophylactically to children and adolescents at risk of developing EPS with antipsychotic drugs, or whether they should be used only when EPS develops; mostly used as needed
- Akathisia may only respond to treatment with anticholinergic agents when symptoms of parkinsonism are also present; akathisia may respond better to β-blockers

PHARMACOLOGY

- Centrally-active anticholinergic drugs cross the blood-brain barrier, block excitatory cholinergic pathways in the basal ganglia, and restore the dopamine/acetylcholine balance disrupted by neuroleptic drugs, thus treating EPS
- Muscarinic receptors are subclassified into M_1 (predominate in the striatum) and M_2 (predominate in cardiac ventricles) subtypes. Antiparkinsonian agents drugs show a range of selectivity on M_1 vs M_2 as follows: biperiden > procyclidine > trihexyphenidyl > benztropine. M_1 selectivity predicts lower peripheral side effects
- Anticholinergic drugs also block presynaptic reuptake of dopamine (primarily benztropine), norepinephrine (primarily diphenhydramine), and serotonin (weakly)
- Amantadine has moderate NMDA (n-methyl-D-aspartate) receptor blocking properties and exerts its activity by increasing dopamine at the receptor

DOSING

- See chart pp. 166–167
- Dosage increases must be balanced against the risk of evoking anticholinergic side effects

ADVERSE EFFECTS OF ANTIPARKINSONIAN AGENTS

CNS Effects

- CNS effects: seen at high doses; include stimulation, disorientation, confusion, hallucinations, restlessness, weakness, incoherence, headache; cognitive impairment including decreased memory and distractibility
- Excess use/abuse of these drugs may lead to an anticholinergic (toxic) psychosis with symptoms of disorientation, confusion, euphoria

(see Toxicity), in addition to physical signs such as dry mouth, blurred vision, dilated pupils, dry flushed skin

- Dopamine-agonist activity of amantadine can cause worsening of psychotic symptoms, nightmares, insomnia, and mood disturbances

Anticholinergic Effects

- Related to anticholinergic potency: atropine > trihexyphenidyl > benztropine > biperiden > procyclidine > diphenhydramine
- Common: dry mouth, blurred vision, constipation, dry eyes, flushed skin
- Occasional: delayed micturition, urinary retention, sexual dysfunction
- Excess doses can suppress sweating, resulting in hyperthermia

Cardiovascular Effects

- Palpitations, tachycardia; high doses can cause arrhythmias

GI Effects

- Nausea, vomiting

PRECAUTIONS

- Use cautiously in patients with conditions in which excess anticholinergic activity could be harmful, e.g., prostatic hypertrophy, urinary retention, narrow-angle glaucoma, myasthenia gravis
- May decrease sweating; use cautiously in hot weather to prevent hyperthermia
- Use with caution in patients with respiratory difficulties, as anticholinergics can dry bronchial secretions and make breathing more difficult
- If antiparkinsonian agent is withdrawn abruptly may result in restlessness, anxiety, dyskinesia, dysphoria, sweating and diarrhea; akinetic depression reported
- Euphorigenic and hallucinogenic properties may lead to abuse of anticho-linergic agents
- Use of antiparkinsonian agents in patients with existing TD can exacerbate the movement disorder and may unmask latent TD

TOXICITY OF ANTIPARKINSONIAN AGENTS

- Can occur following excessive doses, with combination therapy, or with drug abuse
- Autonomic signs: dilated pupils, dry flushed skin, thirst, tachycardia, urinary retention, constipation, paralytic ileus, anorexia, staggering gait
- Mental signs: clouded sensorium, dazed, perplexed or fearful countenance, insomnia, euphoria, irritability, excitation, disorientation in time and space, difficulties in thinking and concentration, exacerbation of psychotic behavior, visual hallucinations (grasping at air), and tactile hallucinations (picking objects from skin)

Management

- If toxicity is suspected, stop all drugs with anticholinergic activity; symptoms should abate within 24–48 h
- Physostigmine 1–3 mg IM has been used to reverse both central and peripheral effects; use of this drug is not currently recommended as it can cause seizures, cardiac effects, and excessive cholinergic effects

USE IN PREGNANCY

- A possible association found between use of anticholinergic antiparkinsonian drugs and minor malformations; prophylactic use of these drugs during pregnancy is not recommended
- Amantadine contraindicated during first trimester
- Propranolol use in second/third trimester associated with decreased fetal and placental weight
- For benzodiazepines see p. 169
- Diphenhydramine: data suggests it is safe to use in pregnancy

Breast Milk

- No specific data available; however, infants are sensitive to anticholinergic effects of drugs
- Anticholinergic properties may inhibit lactation

NURSING IMPLICATIONS

- Antiparkinsonian drugs should be given only to relieve extrapyramidal side effects of antipsychotics; excess use or abuse can precipitate a toxic psychosis

Agents for Treating Extrapyr. Side Effects

Agents for Treating Extrapyramidal Side Effects (cont.)

- Some side effects of these drugs (i.e., anticholinergic) are additive to those of antipsychotics; observe patient for signs of side effects or toxicity
- Monitor patient's intake and output. Urinary retention can occur; bethanechol (Urecholine) can be used to reverse this problem
- To help prevent gastric irritation, administer drug after meals
- Relieve dry mouth by giving patient cool drinks, ice chips, sugarless chewing gum, or hard, sour candy. Suggest frequent rinsing of the mouth, and teeth should be brushed regularly. Patients should avoid calorie-laden beverages and sweet candy as they not only increase the likelihood of dental caries, but also promote weight gain. May predispose patient to monilial infections. Products that promote or replace salivation (e.g., MoiStir, Saliment) may be of benefit
- Blurring of near vision is due to paresis of the ciliary muscle. This can be helped by wearing suitable glasses or reading by a bright light
- Dry eyes may be of particular difficulty to those wearing contact lenses. Artificial tears or contact lens wetting solutions may be of benefit in dealing with this problem
- Anticholinergics reduce peristalsis and decrease intestinal secretions, leading to constipation. Increasing fluids and bulk (e.g., bran, salads) as well as fruit in the diet is beneficial. If necessary, bulk laxatives (e.g., Metamucil, Prodiem) or a stool softener (e.g., docusate) can be used; lactulose may be used for chronic constipation
- Warn the patient about combined sedative effects and not to operate machinery until response to the drug has been determined
- Appropriate patient education regarding medication and side effects is necessary prior to discharge
- If akathisia does not respond to standard antiparkinsonian agents, diphenhydramine, propranolol, lorazepam, clonazepam, or diazepam can be tried

PATIENT INSTRUCTIONS
- Detailed instructions for patients and caregivers are provided in the Information Sheet on p. 318

DRUG INTERACTIONS
- Clinically significant interactions are listed below (for benzodiazepines, see pp. 175–177)

Class of Drug	Example	Interaction Effects
Adsorbent	Activated charcoal, antacids, kaolin-pectin (attapulgite), cholestyramine	Oral absorption decreased when used simultaneously
Antiarrhythmic	Quinidine	Inhibited renal clearance of amantadine (in males)
Anticholinergic	Antidepressants, antihistamines, antipsychotics (especially low-potency)	Increased atropine-like effects causing dry mouth, blurred vision, constipation, etc. May produce inhibition of sweating and may lead to paralytic ileus High doses can bring on a toxic psychosis
Antidepressant SSRI	Paroxetine, fluoxetine	Case reports of reversal of antidepressant and antibulimic effects when cyproheptadine (a serotonin antagonist) was added to fluoxetine and paroxetine therapy Increased plasma level of procyclidine (by 40%)
Antihypertensive	Hydrochlorothiazide, triamterene	Reduced renal clearance of amantadine resulting in drug accumulation and possible toxicity

Class of Drug	Example	Interaction Effects
Antiinfective	Co-trimoxazole (Trimethoprim/Sulfamethoxazole)	Competition for renal clearance resulting in elevated plasma level of amantadine
Antipsychotic	Haloperidol, trifluoperazine	May aggravate tardive dyskinesia or unmask latent TD May increase or decrease plasma level of antipsychotic Potential additive hypotensive effects if combined with β-blockers Increased anticholinergic effects
Caffeine		May offset beneficial effects by increasing tremor and akathisia
Digoxin		Increased bioavailability of digoxin tablets (not capsules or liquids) Increased plasma level of digoxin due to decreased gastric motility
Quinine		Increased plasma level of amantadine due to inhibited renal clearance (by 27% in males) – of limited significance

Effects on Extrapyramidal Symptoms

Agent	Tremor	Rigidity	Dystonia	Akinesia	Akathisia
Amantadine (Symmetrel)	++	++	+	+++	++
Benztropine (Cogentin)	++	+++	+++	++	++
Biperiden (Akineton)	++	++	++	+++	++
β-Blockers (e.g., propranolol, nadolol)	+	–	–	–	+++
Clonazepam (Rivotril, Klonopin)	–	+	++	–	+++
Diazepam (Valium)	+	+	++	–	+++
Diphenhydramine (Benadryl)	+	+	+++	–	+++
Lorazepam (Ativan)	+	+	+++	–	+++
Procyclidine (Kemadrin)	++	++	++	++	++
Trihexyphenidyl (Artane)	++	++	++	++	++

Based on literature in adults and on clinical observations: – effect not established, + some effect (20% response), ++ moderate effect (20–50% response), +++ good effect (> 50% response)

Agents for Treating Extrapyr. Side Effects

Comparison of Agents for Treating Extrapyramidal Side Effects

Antiparkinsonian Agents	Therapeutic Effects	Adverse Effects	Dose	CYP-450 Metabolizing Enzymes[a]	CYP-450 Inhibition[b]
Amantadine (Symmetrel)	May improve akathisia, akinesia, rigidity, acute dystonia, parkinsonism, and tardive dyskinesia; may enhance the effects of other antiparkinsonian agents Tolerance to fixed dose may develop after 1–8 weeks Found effective in treating antipsychotic and SSRI-induced sexual dysfunction May reverse symptoms of galactorrhea Early data suggest a possible role in ADHD, impulsive and aggressive behavior in children with developmental disabilities or conduct disorder, autistic disorder, and in treating cocaine craving and use	Common: indigestion, excitement, insomnia, difficulty in concentration, dizziness Less often: peripheral edema, skin rash, livido reticularis (mottled skin discoloration), tremors, slurred speech, ataxia, depression, and lethargy (these are dose-related and disappear on drug withdrawal) Confusion, hallucinations and seizures reported in patients with renal insufficiency Less anticholinergic than other agents; safe to use low doses in glaucoma	Orally: Children: 2.5 mg/kg per day Up to 300 mg/day (3.7–8.2 mg/kg/day) used in children with autistic disorder Dose adjustment required in presence of impaired renal function	—[c]	—[c]
Antihistamines Diphenhydramine (Benadryl)	Has effect on acute dystonia Sedative effect may benefit tension and excitation; may enhance the effects of other antiparkinsonian agents	Somnolence, confusion, cognitive impairment, dizziness, dry mouth, constipation	Orally: Age 2–5 years: 6.25 mg up to qid Age 6–12 years: 12.5–15 mg up to qid Over age 12: 25–50 mg up to qid IM/IV: 10–50 mg for dystonia	2D6	2D6
β-Blockers (Propranolol)	Very useful for akathisia and tremor Also used in aggression, self-abuse, and agitation Alternative to antipsychotics for aggression in developmentally delayed children	Monitor pulse and blood pressure; do not stop high dose abruptly due to rebound tachycardia, hypertension Bronchospasms	Orally: 2–8 mg/kg or 10 mg tid up to 60 mg daily	IA2, 2D6, 2C19, 3A4	2D6
Benzodiazepines Diazepam (Valium, etc.)	Beneficial effect on akathisia and acute dystonia Muscle relaxant Effect on agitation, anxiety	Drowsiness, lethargy, confusion Disinhibition, withdrawal actions Risk of abuse and dependence	Orally: begin at 1–2.5 mg 3–4 times/day and increase gradually as needed and tolerated Parenterally as sedative and muscle relaxant at 0.2 mg/kg	3A4, 2C19, 2B6	3A4[d]

Antiparkinsonian Agents	Therapeutic Effects	Adverse Effects	Dose	CYP-450 Metabolizing Enzymes[a]	CYP-450 Inhibition[b]
Lorazepam (Ativan)	Beneficial effect on akathisia Excellent for acute dyskinesia (sublingual works quickest) Severe agitation, anxiety, insomnia	As above	Ages 5–13: Orally or sublingual: 0.5–4 mg/day (0.05mg/kg/day) IM: 0.025–0.05 mg/kg/dose	–	–
Clonazepam (Rivotril, Klonopin)	Useful for akathisia Anxiety, severe agitation, insomnia	As above	Orally: 0.25–3 mg/day	3A4	–
Benztropine (Cogentin)	Beneficial effect on rigidity, dystonia, tremor May decrease sialorrhea and drooling Powerful muscle relaxant; sedative action Cumulative and long-acting; once-daily dosing can be used (preferably in the morning) IM/IV: dramatic effect on dystonic symptoms	Dry mouth, blurred vision, urinary retention, constipation Increases intraocular pressure Toxic psychosis when abused or overused	Orally: 0.5–3 mg/day, up to 6 mg/day IM/IV: 1–2 mg; may repeat once in 30 min in adolescents	2D6	
Biperiden (Akineton)	Has effect against rigidity and akinesia	Less likely to cause peripheral anticholinergic effects May cause euphoria, confusion, sedation, and increased tremor	Orally: 2–8 mg daily	?	?
Procyclidine (Kemadrin)	Similar to trihexyphenidyl Milder and questionable effect on tremor	Less pronounced side effects than with trihexyphenidyl; blurred vision, dry mouth Stimulation and giddiness in some patients Can be abused	Orally: 2.5 mg bid May need up to 20 mg/day	?	2D6
Trihexyphenidyl (Artane)	Mild to moderate effect against rigidity and dystonia Tremor alleviated to a lesser degree; as a result of relaxing muscle spasm, more tremor activity may be noted Stimulating – can be used during the day for sluggish, lethargic, and akinetic patients	Dry mouth, blurred vision, GI distress Less sedating potential Severe and persistent mental confusion, cognitive impairment may occur; must recognize this as a toxic state At toxic doses: restlessness, delirium, hallucinations; these disappear when the drug is discontinued (most anticholinergic of the antiparkinsonian agents – liable to be abused as a euphoriant)	Orally: 2–10 mg daily, up to 30 mg tolerated in younger patients Doses up to 80 mg have been used in the treatment of dystonias	?	?

[a] Cytochrome P-450 isoenzymes involved in liver metabolism of drug (data not consistent among references), [b] Cytochrome P-450 isoenzymes inhibited by drug, [c] Undergoes little metabolism; 90% of dose recovered unchanged in the urine; does not affect the metabolism of other drugs, [d] Pertains to metabolite (Data regarding CYP-450 isoenzymes not consistent among references)

Agents for Treating Extrapyr. Side Effects

Agents for Treating EPS – References and Selected Readings

- Fernandez, H.H., Friedman, J.H. (2003). Classification and treatment of tardive syndromes. *Neurology 9(1)*, 16–27.
- Halliday, J., Farrington, S., Macdonald, S. et al. (2002). Nithsdale Schizophrenia Surveys 23: Movement disorders. 20 year review. *British Journal of Psychiatry 181*, 422–427.
- Mamo, D.C., Sweet, R.A., Keshavan, M.S. (1999). Managing antipsychotic-induced parkinsonism. *Drug Safety 20(3)*, 269–275.
- Miller, C.H., Fleischhacker, W.W. (2000). Managing antipsychotic-induced acp-0ute and chronic akathisia. *Drug Safety 22(1)*, 73–81.
- Rodnitzky R.L. (2005). Drug-induced movement disorders in children and adolescents. *Expert Opinion in Drug Safety 4(1)*, 91–102.

ANXIOLYTIC AGENTS

CLASSIFICATION

- Anxiolytic agents can be classified as follows:

Chemical Class	Agent	Page
Antidepressant	SSRI, SNRI	See pp. 41 and 58
Antihistamine[A]	Example: Hydroxyzine[A] (Atarax, Vistaril)	See below (A) and p. 188
Azaspirodecanedione (Azaspirone)	Buspirone	See p. 184
Barbiturate[B]	Examples: Phenobarbital (Luminal)[C]	See below (B)
Benzodiazepine	Examples: lorazepam, clonazepam	See below

[A] H_1 antagonist with few side effects; used primarily for itching of psychogenic origin. Dose: 10–400 mg/day. Tolerance to sedative effects will develop over several weeks. Has been used in children as anxiolytic, but clinical efficacy not substantiated and adverse effects may be troublesome (including drowsiness, affective and cognitive symptoms).

[B] Act as CNS depressants; seldom used as anxiolytics, because they are habit-forming, causing physical dependence; they can have severe withdrawal symptoms; tolerance develops quickly, requiring increased dosage; they have a low margin of safety (therapeutic dose close to toxic dose); they are involved in many drug interactions (induce metabolizing enzymes); they can evoke behavioral disturbances (e.g. hyperactivity) and depression in children.

[C] Phenobarbital has been used as an anxiolytic for those unable to benefit from benzodiazepines or buspirone

Benzodiazepines

CLASSIFICATION

- Benzodiazepines can be categorized as follows:

		Anxiolytic	Sedative/Hypnotic	Anticonvulsant	Potency
Short-acting	Midazolam (Versed)[A]	+	+++		high
	Triazolam (Halcion)	+	+++		high
Intermediate	Alprazolam (Xanax)	++	+	+	high
	Bromazepam (Lectopam)[C]	++	+		high
	Estazolam (ProSom)[B][D]	+	+++	+	high
	Lorazepam (Ativan)	+++	++	++	high
	Oxazepam (Serax)	++	++		low
	Temazepam (Restoril)	+	+++	+	low

Benzodiazepines (cont.)

		Anxiolytic	Sedative/Hypnotic	Anticonvulsant	Potency
Long-acting	Chlordiazepoxide (Librium)	++			low
	Clobazam[E]	–	–	+++	high
	Clonazepam (Rivotril, Klonopin)	++	+	+++	high
	Clorazepate (Tranxene, Tranxilene)	++			medium
	Diazepam (Valium)	+++	++	++	medium
	Flurazepam (Dalmane)	+	+++		medium
	Nitrazepam (Mogadon)[C]	+	+++	++	high
	Quazepam (Doral)[B][D]	+	+++	+	medium

Activity: + weak, ++ moderate, +++ strong, [A] Acute use only, [B] Not marketed in Canada, [C] Not marketed in the USA, [D] Not generally used in children – not included in this chapter, [E] Not used in anxiety disorders and not reviewed in this chapter

PRODUCT AVAILABILITY

Generic Name	Trade Name[A]	Dosage Forms and Strengths	Monograph Statement
Alprazolam	Xanax Xanax TS[C] Xanax XR[B] Niravam [B]	Tablets: 0.25 mg, 0.5 mg, 1 mg, 2 mg[B] Oral concentrate 1 mg/ml Triscored tablets[C]: 2 mg Extended-release tablets [B] 0.5 mg, 1 mg, 2 mg, 3 mg Oral disintegrating tablets[B] 0.25 mg, 0.5 mg, 1 mg, 2 mg	Safety and efficacy not established in children under age 18
Bromazepam[C]	Lectopam	Tablets: 1.5 mg, 3 mg, 6 mg	Safety and efficacy not established in children under age 18
Chlordiazepoxide	Librium Libritabs [B]	Capsules: 5 mg, 10 mg, 25 mg Tablets: 5 mg, 25 mg	Not recommended for children under age 6
Clonazepam	Rivotril[C], Klonopin[B] Klonopin Wafers [B]	Tablets: 0.25 mg, 0.5 mg, 1 mg, 2 mg Oral disintegrating tablets[B] 0.125 mg, 0.25 mg, 0.5 mg, 1 mg, 2 mg	Not studied in psychiatric disorders for children under age 18; dosage recommendations available for seizure disorders
Clorazepate	Tranxene[C], Tranxilene[B] Tranxene SD[B]	Tablets: 3.75 mg, 7. 5 mg, 15 mg Tablets: 11.25 mg, 22.5 mg	Not recommended for children under age 9
Diazepam	Valium Diazepam Intensol[B] Diastat Diazemuls [C]	Tablets: 2 mg, 5 mg, 10 mg Oral Solution: 5 mg/5 ml, 5 mg/ml[B] Injection:5 mg/ml Oral concentrate[B]: 5 mg/ml Rectal gel: 5 mg/ml Emulsion injection (IM/IV) [C]: 5 mg/ml	Dosage recommendations available for infants and children
Estazolam[B][D]	ProSom		–

Generic Name	Trade Name[A]	Dosage Forms and Strengths	Monograph Statement
Flurazepam	Dalmane	Capsules: 15 mg, 30 mg	Safety and efficacy not established in children under age 15
Lorazepam	Ativan	Tablets: 0.5 mg, 1 mg, 2 mg Sublingual tablets[C]: 0.5 mg, 1 mg, 2 mg Oral solution[B]: 0.5 mg/5 ml Injection: 2 mg/ml[B], 4 mg/ml	Oral: Safety and efficacy not established in children under age 12 Injection: Not recommended in children under age 18
Midazolam	Versed	Syrup[B]: 2 mg/ml Injection: 1 mg/ml, 5 mg/ml	Dosage recommendations available for infants and children
Nitrazepam[C]	Mogadon	Tablets: 5 mg, 10 mg	Safety and efficacy not established in children under age 18
Oxazepam	Serax	Tablets: 10 mg[C], 15 mg, 30 mg[C] Capsules[B]: 10 mg, 15 mg, 30 mg	Safety and efficacy not established in children under age 6
Quazepam[B][D]	Doral		–
Temazepam	Restoril	Capsules: 7.5 mg[B], 15 mg, 22.5 mg[B], 30 mg	Safety and efficacy not established in children under age 18
Triazolam	Halcion	Tablets: 0.125 mg, 0.25 mg	Safety and efficacy not established in children under age 18

[A] Generic preparations may be available, [B] Not marketed in Canada, [C] Not marketed in USA, [D] Not generally used in children – not included in this chapter

INDICATIONS

| Approved in Children and Adolescents | • Some benzodiazepines approved for the treatment of anxiety in children over 6 years of age (e.g., chlordiazepoxide, diazepam); used primarily for conditions resistant to behavior management or to alternate pharmacotherapy. |

Approved (for Adults)

- Management of mild to moderate anxiety, tension, excitation and agitation
- Generalized anxiety disorder
- Management of acute and chronic alcohol withdrawal syndromes
- Tetanus (diazepam)
- Convulsions: status epilepticus, absence seizures, infantile spasms, simple-partial and complex-partial seizures
- Insomnia
- Panic disorder with or without agoraphobia (alprazolam, clorazepate)
- Muscle spasms, dystonia, "restless legs" syndrome
- Sedation prior to dental procedures or surgery, endoscopy and bronchoscopy, enhancement of analgesia during labor and delivery

Benzodiazepines (cont.)

Other Uses in Children and Adolescents	• Akathisia due to antipsychotic agents • Night terrors, somnambulism • In mania used concomitantly with antipsychotic or lithium to control agitation • Mania and bipolar disorder prophylaxis (clonazepam) • In schizophrenia used with antipsychotic to control agitation; may potentiate their effect and decrease dosage requirements • Adjustment disorder, social phobia, separation anxiety disorder • Catatonia (parenteral and sublingual lorazepam; diazepam, clonazepam) • Myoclonus, Tourette's syndrome (clonazepam) • Acute dystonia (SL or IM lorazepam) • Premenstrual dysphoric disorder (alprazolam) • Control of violent outbursts, assaultive behavior (lorazepam, clonazepam) – reduce agitation and behavioral problems associated with severe over-arousal or anxiety; used also in combination with mood stabilizers, anti-psychotics, or β-blockers
PHARMACOLOGY	• Causes CNS depression at the levels of the limbic system, the brain-stem reticular formation, and the cortex • Benzodiazepines bind to the "benzodiazepine"-GABA-chloride receptor complex, facilitating the action of GABA (an inhibitory neurotransmitter) on CNS excitability. Intensity of action depends on degree of receptor occupancy. In children the GABA receptor also has an excitatory role; this may explain the disinhibiting effects of benzodiazepines in young children and those who have organic brain syndromes • Clonazepam has 5-HT-potentiating properties
GENERAL COMMENTS	• Benzodiazepines are suggested to relieve behavioral and somatic manifestations of anxiety, but may have little effect on cognitive or psychic symptoms • Benzodiazepines are considered adjunctive agents mostly for short-term use in children and adolescents; may be most helpful during the beginning phase of treatment and are not recommended long-term. • Benzodiazepines should be avoided where possible in children with aggressive, impulsive tendencies, as their disinhibitory effects can aggravate these conditions. In general they should be used in children and adolescents without comorbid substance abuse or major depression who require relief from moderate to severe anxiety or manic symptoms • Chronic use in children should be carefully evaluated to prevent possible adverse effects on physical and mental development (cognition)
DOSING	• See pp. 178–183 for individual agents • Benzodiazepines are metabolized faster in children than in adults; may require small divided doses to maintain blood level • Concerns of dependence and abuse limit their usefulness

- Following IV administration of diazepam or chlordiazepoxide, local pain and thrombophlebitis may occur due to precipitation of the drug, or due to an irritant effect of propylene glycol; IV diazepam emulsion (Diazemuls) is less likely to cause this problem
- IM use is discouraged with chlordiazepoxide and diazepam as absorption is slow, erratic, and possibly incomplete; local pain often occurs. Lorazepam IM is adequately absorbed (although sometimes erratic)

PHARMACOKINETICS

- See pp. 178–183 for individual agents
- Marked interindividual variation (up to 10-fold) is found in all pharmacokinetic parameters. Age, smoking, liver disease, physical disorders, as well as concurrent use of other drugs may influence parameters by changing the volume of distribution and elimination half-life of these drugs
- Well absorbed from GI tract after oral administration; food can delay the rate, but not the extent of absorption; onset of action is determined by rate of absorption and lipid solubility
- Lipid solubility denotes speed of entry into (lipid) brain tissue, followed by extensive redistribution to adipose tissue (children typically have little adipose tissue; this can result in a shorter duration of action). Benzodiazepines, as a class, have a high volume of distribution (i.e., the tissue drug concentration is much higher than the blood drug concentration)
- The duration of action is determined mainly by the distribution and not by elimination half-life (except for ultra-short half-life drugs like midazolam and triazolam)
- In general, high-potency benzodiazepines tend to have shorter half-lives
- The potency of a benzodiazepine is the affinity of the parent drug, or its active metabolites, for benzodiazepine receptors, in vivo.
- Benzodiazepines with long $T_{1/2}$ are more likely to negatively impact daytime functions (e.g., hangover, sedation) than short $T_{1/2}$ agents drugs with short $T_{1/2}$ are more likely to result in symptoms of withdrawal, anxiety between doses (rebound), and anterograde amnesia than agents with long $T_{1/2}$
- The major pathways of metabolism are hepatic microsomal oxidation and demethylation. Conjugation to more polar (water-soluble) glucuronide derivatives allows for excretion. Biotransformation by oxidation can be impaired by disease states (e.g., hepatic cirrhosis), by age or by drugs that impair the metabolism. Drugs undergoing conjugation only (e.g., oxazepam) are not so affected

ADVERSE EFFECTS

- Are few, and often disappear with dosage adjustments

CNS Effects

- Most common are extensions of the generalized sedative effect, e.g., fatigue, drowsiness
- Impaired mental speed, central cognitive processing ability, memory and perceptomotor performance (dose-related) – have been seen in adults; limited data in pediatric patients
- Anterograde amnesia (more likely with high potency agents or higher doses)
- Behavior dyscontrol or paradoxical agitation (in up to 40% of children – especially with organic brain disorder or aggressive/impulsive tendencies); this can be manifested in the form of irritability, tantrums, aggression, insomnia, nightmares, overexcitability, hyperactivity, rage spells, hallucinations or oppositional behavior
- Case reports of psychotic symptoms in children given low doses
- Confusion and disorientation
- Treatment-emergent depression (13% incidence with clonazepam)
- Excessive doses (parenterally) can result in respiratory depression and apnea; can interact with some other sedative agents and with alcohol (see Interaction pp. 175–177)
- Muscle weakness, incoordination, ataxia, slurred speech
- Headache

Benzodiazepines (cont.)

Other Adverse Effects	• Anticholinergic effects, e.g., blurred vision (mild), dry mouth (uncommon) • Dizziness • Increased salivation (clonazepam); troublesome hypersecretion in children with chronic respiratory disease • Few documented allergies to benzodiazepines; rarely reported skin reactions include rashes, fixed drug eruption, photosensitivity reactions, pigmentation, alopecia, bullous reactions, exfoliative dermatitis, vasculitis, erythema nodosum, thrombocytopenia and purpura in adults

DISCONTINUATION SYNDROME	• Benzodiazepines present different risks of physiological dependence at therapeutic doses, depending on the individual as well as the drug's potency and its elimination half-life; very little data on the development of tolerance or dependence in children
	• Discontinuation of a benzodiazepine can produce:
	  – Withdrawal: occurs 1–2 days (short-acting) to 5–10 days (long-acting) following any drug discontinuation. Common symptoms include insomnia, agitation, anxiety, perceptual changes, dysphoria, headache, muscle aches, twitches, tremors, loss of appetite, metallic taste, and GI distress. Severe reactions can occur such as delirium, psychotic states, tonic-clonic or absence seizures, and coma
	  – Rebound: occurs hours to days after drug withdrawal; symptoms (of anxiety) are similar but more intense than those reported originally
	  – Relapse: symptoms occur weeks to months after drug withdrawal and are similar to original symptoms of anxiety
	• Pseudowithdrawal is a psychological withdrawal as a result of the patient's apprehension about discontinuing the drug – consists of anxiety symptoms accompanied by true withdrawal symptoms

Management	• To withdraw a patient from a benzodiazepine, taper dose by 25% every 5 days – may need to go slower if patient has been using the benzodiazepine for an extended time period (several months). Some clinicians use lower dosage reduction during the latter part of the taper period and/or convert to an equivalent dose of diazepam (see pp. 178–183).
PRECAUTIONS	• Do not use in patients with sleep apnea • Administer with caution to children with respiratory disease (e.g., asthma, COPD), liver disease, and to patients performing hazardous tasks requiring mental alertness or physical coordination • Benzodiazepines may diminish the therapeutic efficacy of electroconvulsive therapy (ECT) by raising the seizure threshold • Anxiolytics lower the tolerance to alcohol, and high doses may produce mental confusion similar to alcohol intoxication • Can cause physical and psychological dependence, tolerance, and withdrawal symptoms – correlated to dose and duration of use • Benzodiazepines are at risk of being abused by susceptible individuals (e.g., habitual polydrug users); they prefer agents with rapid peak drug effects (e.g., diazepam, lorazepam, alprazolam) • Withdrawal symptoms resemble those of alcohol and barbiturates. Abrupt withdrawal following prolonged use of high doses can produce seizures (especially with alprazolam)
TOXICITY	• Rarely if ever fatal when taken alone; may be lethal when taken in combination with other drugs, such as alcohol and barbiturates • Symptoms of overdose include hypotension, depressed respiration, and coma
Management	• Flumazenil injection (a benzodiazepine antagonist) reverses the hypnotic-sedative effects of benzodiazepines. Repeated doses may be required due to the short duration of action of flumazenil

USE IN PREGNANCY

- Benzodiazepines and metabolites freely cross the placenta and accumulate in fetal circulation
- Some studies suggest an association between benzodiazepine use in the first trimester and teratogenicity; data contradictory; 0.4–0.7% incidence of cleft palate – suggest ultrasound screening of fetus
- High doses or prolonged use by mother in third trimester may precipitate fetal benzodiazepine syndrome: including floppy infant syndrome, impaired temperature regulation and withdrawal symptoms in newborn

Breast Milk

- Benzodiazepines are excreted into breast milk in levels sufficient to produce effects in the newborn, including sedation, lethargy, and poor temperature regulation; e.g., infant can receive up to 13% of maternal dose of diazepam and 7% of lorazepam dose
- Metabolism of benzodiazepines in infants is slower especially during their first 6 weeks; long-acting agents can accumulate
- American Academy of Pediatrics considers benzodiazepines as drugs "whose effect on nursing infants is unknown but may be of concern"

NURSING IMPLICATIONS

- Assess the anxiety level of patients on these drugs to determine if anxiety control has been accomplished or if over-sedation has occurred
- Inform patients that activities requiring mental alertness should not be performed after taking drug (e.g., driving or operating machinery)
- Caution patients not to use other CNS depressant drugs (e.g., antihistamines or alcohol) without consulting the doctor
- Excessive consumption of caffeinated beverages or stimulants will counteract the effects of anxiolytics
- Grapefruit juice can increase the blood level of alprazolam and triazolam
- Tolerance and physical addiction can occur; withdrawal symptoms can be produced with abrupt discontinuation after prolonged use
- Watch for signs of behavioral disinhibition or paradoxical reactions; may need to discontinue the benzodiazepine
- Alprazolam XR should be administered at a consistent time of day, once daily (preferably in the morning); it should not be broken, crushed, or chewed, but should be swallowed whole
- PRN use of short acting agents should be limited to < 1 week

PATIENT INSTRUCTIONS

- Detailed instructions for patients and caregivers are provided in the Information Sheet on p. 320

DRUG INTERACTIONS

- Many interactions; only clinically significant ones are listed below

Class of Drug	Example	Interaction Effects
Allopurinol		Decreased metabolism and increased half-life of benzodiazepines that are metabolized by oxidation (see charts pp. 178–183), leading to increased drug effect
Anesthetics	Ketamine Volatile (e.g., halothane)	Prolonged recovery with diazepam due to decreased metabolism Decreased protein binding of diazepam resulting in increased pharmacological effects
Antiarrhythmic	Amiodarone	Reduced metabolism and increased plasma level of midazolam

Anxiolytic Agents

Benzodiazepines (cont.)

Class of Drug	Example	Interaction Effects
Antibiotic	Erythromycin, clarithromycin, troleandomycin	Decreased metabolism and increased plasma levels of benzodiazepines metabolized by CYP3A4, including midazolam (by 54%), triazolam (by 52%), alprazolam (by 60%), estazolam, and diazepam; no interaction with azithromycin
	Chloramphenicol	Decreased metabolism of benzodiazepines that are metabolized by oxidation
	Quinolones: ciprofloxacin, enoxacin	Decreased metabolism of diazepam
	Quinupristin/dalfopristin	Decreased metabolism of midazolam and diazepam via CYP3A4
Anticoagulant	Warfarin	Decreased PT ratio or INR response with chlordiazepoxide
Anticonvulsant	Carbamazepine, barbituates	Increased metabolism and decreased plasma level of benzodiazepines metabolized by CYP3A4, including alprazolam (>50%) and clonazepam (19–37%), diazepam Additive CNS effects
	Phenytoin	Variable effects on phenytoin plasma level reported with clonazepam Increased phenytoin level and toxicity reported with diazepam and chlordiazepoxide
	Valproate	Displacement by diazepam from proteinbinding resulting in increased plasma level Decreased metabolism and increased pharmacological effects of clonazepam and lorazepam

Antidepressant
  Cyclic
  SSRI
	Desipramine, imipramine
	Fluoxetine, fluvoxamine, sertraline
		Increased plasma levels of desipramine and imipramine with alprazolam (by 20% and 31%, respectively)
		Decreased metabolism and increased plasma level of benzodiazepines metabolized by CYP3A4, including alprazolam (by 100% with fluvoxamine and 46% with fluoxetine) and diazepam (13% decrease with sertraline)

Antifungal	Itraconazole, ketoconazole fluconazole	Decreased metabolism and increased half-life of chlordiazepoxide and midazolam; decreased metabolism of triazolam (6–7 fold); reduce dose by 50–75%; AUC of alprazolam increased up to 4 fold
Antipsychotic	Clozapine	Marked sedation, increased salivation, hypotension (collapse), delirium, and respiratory arrest reported; more likely to occur early in treatment when clozapine is added to benzodiazepine regimen
	Olanzapine	Synergistic increase in somnolence when lorazepam given with IM olanzapine. Recommend lorazepam be given at least 1 h after IM olanzapine
Antituberculosis therapy	Isoniazid	Decreased metabolism of benzodiazepines that are metabolized by oxidation (triazolam clearance decreased by 75%)
	Rifampin	Increased metabolism of benzodiazepines that are metabolized by oxidation due to enzyme induction of CYP3A4 (diazepam by 300%, midazolam by 83%, estazolam)
β-Blocker	Propranolol	Increased half-life and decreased clearance of diazepam and bromazepam (no interaction with alprazolam, lorazepam, or oxazepam)
Caffeine		May counteract sedation and increase insomnia
Ca-channel Blocker	Diltiazem	Decreased metabolism and increased plasma level of benzodiazepines metabolized by CYP3A4 including triazolam (by 100%), and midazolam (by 105%)
	Verapamil	Increased plasma level of midazolam by 97% due to inhibited metabolism via CYP3A4

Class of Drug	Example	Interaction Effects
CNS depressant	Barbiturates, antihistamines Alcohol	Increased CNS depression; with high doses coma and respiratory depression can occur Alprazolam reported to increase aggression in moderate alcohol drinkers Brain concentrations of various benzodiazepines altered by ethanol: triazolam and estazolam concentrations decreased, diazepam concentration increased, no change with chlordiazepoxide
Digoxin		Decreased metabolism and elimination of digoxin
Disulfiram		Decreased metabolism of benzodiazepines that are metabolized by oxidation
Grapefruit juice		Increased absorption of diazepam and triazolam due to inhibition of CYP3A4 in the gut by grapefruit juice Decreased metabolism of alprazolam, midazolam, diazepam, and triazolam via CYP3A4 resulting in increased peak concentration and bioavailability
H$_2$ antagonist	Cimetidine	Decreased metabolism of benzodiazepines that are metabolized by oxidation (no effect with ranitidine, famotidine or nizatidine); peak plasma concentration of alprazolam increased by 86%
Hormone	Estrogen, oral contraceptives	Decreased metabolism of benzodiazepines that are metabolized by oxidation, e.g., diazepam, chlordiazepoxide, nitrazepam; increased half-life of alprazolam by 29% Clearance of combined oral contraceptives may be reduced with diazepam
Immunosuppressant	Cyclosporin	Decreased metabolism of cyclosporin with midazolam via CYP3A4
Kava Kava		May potentiate CNS effects causing increased side effects and toxicity
Lithium		Increased incidence of sexual dysfunction (up to 49%) when combined with clonazepam
L -Dopa		Benzodiazepines can reduce the effcacy of l-dopa secondary to the GABA agonist effect
Omeprazole		Increased ataxia and sedation due to decreased metabolism of benzodiazepines metabolized by oxidation (no effect with lansoprazole)
Pomegranate Juice		May decrease metabolism benzodiazepines that are metabolized by oxidation via CYP3A4 (e.g., triazolam, alprazolam)
Probenecid		Decreased clearance of lorazepam (by 50%)
Propoxyphene		Increased half-life of alprazolam (by 58%) due to inhibited hydroxylation
Protease inhibitors	Ritonavir, Indinavir	Increased plasma level of benzodiazepines that are metabolized by oxidation via CYP3A4 (e.g., triazolam, alprazolam)
Smoking – cigarettes		Increased clearance of diazepam and chlordiazepoxide due to enzyme induction Alprazolam concentration reduced by up to 50%
St. John's Wort		Decreased half-life of alprazolam by 50% due to induced metabolism via CYP3A4

Anxiolytic Agents

Comparison of the Benzodiazepines

Drug	Suggested Dosages in Children	Compara-tive Dose (mg) in Adults**	Peak Plasma Level PO C_{max}	Lipid Solubility [c]	Elimination Half-life	Metabolites*** (m = main metabo-lite)	Comments	Use in Renal and Hepatic Disorders	Clinical Considerations
Alprazolam	Doses not well established in children Up to 3.5 mg/day have to be used in studies Max. dose: 0.04 mg/kg/day	0.5	Oral tablet = 1–2 h XR = 5–11 h (high fat meal increases C_{max} by 25% and decreases max by about 30%) Reported to reach higher C_{max} in Asians	Moderate	Oral tablet = 9–20 h XR = 11–16 h (mean: 11 h) Half-life increased in obese patients and in Asians	Metabolized by oxidation: 29 metabolites; principal ones are: a-hydroxyalprazolam [m] desmethylalprazolam 4-hydroxyalprazolam Metabolized by CYP3A4[p] and 1A2 Metabolites and parent compound excreted in urine	Rapidly and com-pletely absorbed orally and sublingually Absorption rate for XR preparation differs significantly, depend-ing on time of day administered 80% protein bound Plasma level of alpra-zolam may correlate with efficacy in panic disorder Plasma level decreased in smokers by up to 50%	*Renal:* increased plasma level of free (unbound) alprazolam and possible decreased clear-ance *Hepatic:* half life increased	Use: anxiolytic sedative generalized anxiety panic attack pro-phylaxis adjunct in depres-sion tid dosing recom-mended Increases stage 2, and decreases stages 1 and 4 and REM sleep; caution on withdrawal Low degree of seda-tion Case reports of be-havioral side effects including mania XR preparation may prolong side effects such as sedastion
Bromazepam[b]	Up to 6 mg/day	3.0	0.5–4 h	Low	8–30 h	Metabolized by oxidation: 3-hydroxy-bromazepam Metabolized by CYP3A4	Metabolite reported to have anxiolytic activity; does not accumulate on chronic dosing		Use: anxiolytic sedative

Drug	Suggested Dosages in Children	Comparative Dose (mg) in Adults**	Peak Plasma Level PO C_{max}	Lipid Solubility (c)	Elimination Half-life	Metabolites*** (m = main metabolite)	Comments	Use in Renal and Hepatic Disorders	Clinical Considerations
Chlordiaz-epoxide	Over age 6: 5 mg 2–4 times daily; may be increased in some patients up to 10 mg (given 2–3 times daily) or 0.5 mg/kg/day	25.0	1–4 h	Moderate	4–29 h (parent drug) 28–100 h (metabolites)	Metabolized by oxidation: desmethyl-chlordiazepoxide (m) oxazepam desmethyldiazepam Metabolized by CYP3A4 and 2C19(m)	Onset of activity may be delayed; parent compound less potent than metabolites Metabolites accumulate on chronic dosing IM drug erratically absorbed Decrease dose by 50% in patients with CrCl < 10 ml/min	*Renal:* decrease dose by 50% in patients with creatinine clearance <10 ml/min *Hepatic:* 2- to 3-fold increase in half-life seen in patients with cirrhosis	Use: anxiolytic sedative alcohol withdrawal Antacids* decrease absorption in GI tract, but do not influence completeness of absorption Moderate degree of sedation
Clonazepam	Children < 30 kg: initial dose = 0.01–0.03 mg/kg given in 2–3 divided doses Adolescents and children > 30 kg: initial dose = 0.5–1 mg/day and can be increased by 0.5–1 mg q 2–3 days to a maximum of 3 mg/day	0.25	1–4 h	Low	Children: 22–33 h Adults: usual = 30–40 h, range = 19–60 h	Metabolized by oxidation: no active metabolite Metabolized primarily by CYP3A4(p) Less than 2% of drug excreted unchanged	Well absorbed; slow onset of activity (20–60 min) 85% protein bound Duration of action: young children = 6–8 h, adults: = up to 12 h	*Renal:* no change *Hepatic:* increase in free (unbound) clonazepam in patients with cirrhosis	Use: anticonvulsant anxiolytic separation anxiety disorder panic attack prophylaxis prophylaxis of BD manic episode of BD akathisia aggressive behavior Tourette's Syndrome Sedation, irritability, disinhibition, and opposition behavior reported

Comparison of the Benzodiazepines (cont.)

Drug	Suggested Dosages in Children	Comparative Dose (mg) in Adults**	Peak Plasma Level PO C_{max}	Lipid Solubility [c]	Elimination Half-life	Metabolites*** (m = main metabolite)	Comments	Use in Renal and Hepatic Disorders	Clinical Considerations
Clorazepate Dipotassium	Age 9–18: start at 3.75–7.5 mg 1–2 times/day; may increase by 3.75–7.5 mg q week to a maximum of 60 mg/day Usual dose: 0.5–1 mg/kg/day	10.0	0.5–2 h	High	1.3–120 h (variable due to metabolites)	Metabolized by oxidation: N-desmethyl-diazepam Oxazepam	Hydrolyzed in the stomach to active metabolite (parent compound inactive) Rate of hydrolysis depends on gastric acidity, therefore absorption is unreliable (one study disputes this) Metabolite accumulates on chronic dosing	*Renal:* clearance of metabolite impaired *Hepatic:* ?	Use: anxiolytic alcohol withdrawal Antacids and sodium bicarbonate reduce the rate and extent of appearance of active metabolite in the blood Fast onset of action (< 30 min) Moderate degree of sedation
Diazepam	1–2.5 mg 3–4 times daily (0.1–0.8 mg/kg/day in divided doses) Preoperative sedation: IV: 0.1 mg/kg/dose Oral: 0.1–0.5 mg/kg/day (up to 20 mg max)	5	1–2 h	High	< 2 years: 40–50 h Age 2–12: 15–21 h Age 12–16: 18–20 h Half-life of n-desmethyl-diazepam is up to 150 h Males have shorter half-life and higher clearance rates than females	Metabolized by oxidation: N-desmethyldiazepam [m] oxazepam 3-hydroxydiazepam temazepam Metabolized by CYP3A4, 2C19, and 2B6	Protein binding: neonates = 85%, adults = 98% Rapid onset of action (< 30 min) followed by a redistribution into adipose tissue IM drug erratically absorbed Smoking: associated with higher diazepam clearance Do not mix injection with other medication; protect from light	*Renal:* increased plasma level of free (unbound) diazepam and decreased clearance *Hepatic:* 2- to 3-fold increase in half-life in patients with cirhosis	Use: anxiolytic sedative anticonvulsant (status epilepticus) alcohol withdrawal panic disorder sleep terror disorder skeletal muscle relaxant preoperative sedation Increases stage 2, and decreases tages 1 and 4 and REM sleep High degree of sedation

Drug	Suggested Dosages in Children	Comparative Dose (mg) in Adults**	Peak Plasma Level PO C_{max}	Lipid Solubility (c)	Elimination Half-life	Metabolites*** (m = main metabolite)	Comments	Use in Renal and Hepatic Disorders	Clinical Considerations
Flurazepam	15 mg at bedtime	15	0.5–1 h	High	0.3–3 h (parent drug) 40–250 h (metabolites)	Metabolized by oxidation: N-desalkylflurazepam (m) OH-ethylflurazepam flurazepam aldehyde Metabolized by CYP2C, 2D6, and 3A4	Fast onset of action (< 30 min) Rapidly metabolized to active metabolite	*Renal:* ? *Hepatic:* metabolism impaired	Use: hypnotic Decreases stage 1 and increases stage 2 sleep; no effect on REM Increase in daytime sedation over time; hangover
Lorazepam	Sedative dose: 0.02–0.09 mg/ kg/dose given q 4–8 h Preoperative dose: SL: 0.05 mg/kg/dose(max of 4 mg)	1–1.5	Oral: 1–6 h IM: 45–75 min IV: 5–10 min SL: 60 min	Moderate	Children: 6–17 h Adolescents and adults: 10–20 h	Conjugated to form lorazepam glucuronide	Slow onset of action: oral = 60 min, IM = 30–60 min Well absorbed sublingually 85% protein bound Give at least twice daily to maintain steady state levels Metabolite not pharmacologically active Not involved in metabolism interactions via CYP enzymes	*Renal:* half-life of metabolite increased *Hepatic:* half-life and Vd doubled in patients with cirrhosis	Use: anxiolytic sedative preoperative sedation muscle relaxant catatonia manic phase of BAD akathisia acute dystonia Produces anterograde amnesia Blood levels fall quickly on discontinuation; withdrawal symptoms appear sooner than with long-acting drugs Decreases stage 1 and REM

Comparison of the Benzodiazepines (cont.)

Drug	Suggested Dosages in Children	Compara-tive Dose (mg) in Adults**	Peak Plasma Level PO C_{max}	Lipid Solubility [c]	Elimination Half-life	Metabolites*** (m = main metabolite)	Comments	Use in Renal and Hepatic Disorders	Clinical Considerations
Midazolam	IV dose based on age and body weight (see product monograph) IM dose: 0.1–0.15 mg/kg up to 0.5 mg/kg in severe anxiety (max of 10 mg) Oral: 0.25–1.0 mg/kg/dose (max of 20 mg)	Acute use only	IV = 0.5–1 min IM = 30 min Oral = 10–160 min	High	IV children: 0.78–3.3 h Oral: 2.2–6.8 h	Metabolized by oxidation: 1-OH-methylmidazolam 4-OH-midazolam Metabolized primarily by CYP3A4	Dose is based on ideal body weight; children under age 6 may require higher doses than older children Fast onset of action Metabolittes active	*Renal:* decrease dose by 50% in patients with creatinine clearance <10 ml/min *Hepatic:* metabolism significantly impaired in patients with cirrhosis	Use: preoperative sedative, anxiolytic, IV or IM induction of anesthesia May produce hypotension, hypoventilation and apnea in children Produces anterograde amnesia Withdrawal reactions reported following high dose use (total dose > 60 mg/kg)
Nitrazepam[b]	Starting dose: 0.25 mg/kg/day Can increase gradually to 1.2 mg/kg/day	2.5	0.5–7 h	Low	15–48 h	Metabolized by nitroreduction by 2D6, CYP2E1 No active metabolites	Excreted as amino and acetamide analogs Accumulates with chronic use	*Renal:* ? *Hepatic:* metabolism impaired	Use: sedative Decreases REM sleep
Oxazepam	Dose not established up to age 12 > 12 years: 7.5–15mg at bedtime; up to 30 mg/day	15	1–4 h	Low	3–25 h	Conjugated to oxazepam glucuronide	Slow onset of action Give at least twice daily to maintain steady state Metabolites not pharmacologically active Half-life and plasma clearance not affected much by age or sex No metabolic interactions	*Renal:* prolonged half-life *Hepatic:* no effect	Use: anxiolytic sedative alcohol withdrawal muscle relaxant

Drug	Suggested Dosages in Children	Compara-tive Dose (mg) in Adults**	Peak Plasma Level PO C_{max}	Lipid Solubility [c]	Elimination Half-life	Metabolites*** (m = main metabo-lite)	Comments	Use in Renal and Hepatic Disorders	Clinical Considerations

Temazepam	0.3–0.5 mg/kg	10	2.5 h mean	Moderate	3–25 h	Conjugated Metabolized by 2B6[p], 3A4	Hard gelatin capsule; variable rate of absorption depending on formulation; 5% excreted as oxazepam in the urine; plasma concentration too low to detect
							No accumulation with chronic use; no meta-bolic interactions
								Renal: ?
								Hepatic: no effect
									Use:
									  anxiolytic
									  sedative
									On doses of 30 mg/day or more, may cause hang-over, morning nausea, headache, drowsiness, and vivid dreaming
									Decreases sleep stages 3 & 4 Rebound insomnia has been reported

Triazolam	< 18 years of age: doses not well established; suggested dose: 0.005–0.025 mg/kg	0.25	1–2 h	Moderate	1.5–6 h	Metabolized by oxi-dation: 7-α-hydroxy-derivative Metabolized by CYP3A4[p]	Well absorbed sublin-gually
							Fast onset of action (< 30 min)
							89 % protein bound Metabolite inactive; negligible accumula-tion of drug due to high hepatic clear-ance (dependent on hepatic blood flow and microsomal oxidizing capacity)
							Although half-life is short, clinical effects have been observed up to 16 h after a single dose
								Renal: no change
								Hepatic: reduced clear-ance
									Use:
									  sedation prior to
									   dental procedure
									  hypnotic
									Decreases stage 1, and increases stage 2 sleep; significantly increases latency to REM compared with baseline; re bound insomnia and anxiety reported
									Dose-related ataxia, diplopia, and an-terograde amnesia reported, especially in doses above 0.025 mg/kg daily; reports of rage, automatism
									Avoid in pregnancy

* Apply to all benzodiazepines except where noted, ** Doses pertain to adults and are approximate; they can be used as conversion doses when switching among various benzodiazepines, especially dur-ing the withdrawal process; consultation with an expert is advised, *** See comments under Pharmacokinetics p. 147 [a] Not marketed in Canada, [b] Not marketed in USA, [c] High lipid solubility denotes fast entry into (lipid) brain tissue, rapid onset and increased risk of memory impairment [p] Primary route of metabolism, where known

Buspirone

PRODUCT AVAILABILITY

Chemical Class	Generic Name	Trade Name[A]	Dosage Forms and Strengths	Monograph Statement
Azaspirone	Buspirone	Buspar	Tablets: 5 mg[B], 7.5 mg[B] 10 mg, 15 mg[B], 30 mg[B]	Safety and efficacy not established in children under age 18

[A] Generic preparations may be available, [B] Not marketed in Canada

INDICATIONS

No approved indications in children and adolescents

Approved (for Adults)

- Anxiolytic, useful in:
  - Chronic anxiety, GAD
  - Situations where sedation or psychomotor impairment may be dangerous
  - Patients with a history of substance abuse or alcohol abuse

Other Uses

- Treatment of obsessive compulsive disorder; may potentiate effects of SSRIs or clomipramine on obsessions
- Preliminary reports show some efficacy in reducing anxiety, flashbacks and insomnia in posttraumatic stress disorder and in the treatment of body dysmorphic disorder
- Separation anxiety disorder unresponsive to other treatment
- Open studies suggest efficacy in the treatment of anxiety, hyperactivity, aggression, and irritability in pervasive developmental disorders (autism) and ADHD
- Contradictory evidence as to efficacy in GAD and social phobia; may be useful as an augmenting agent in partial responders to SSRIs

GENERAL COMMENTS

- Buspirone (Buspar) is a selective anxiolytic of the azaspirone class; unlike the benzodiazepines, it has no anticonvulsant or muscle-relaxant properties
- Not suitable for emergency use due to slow onset of action
- Patients may find it less effective or acceptable if given subsequent to benzodiazepine use (inconsistent results in studies)
- Recent data suggest lack of efficacy for generalized anxiety disorder in children aged 6–17 years, at doses recommended for adults
- Tolerance to effects of buspirone has not been reported; no withdrawal symptoms reported
- Has a low potential for abuse or addiction and is less sedating than benzodiazepines
- Lack of effect on respiration may make it useful in patients with pulmonary disease or sleep apnea – may actually stimulate respiration
- Minimal effect on cognition, memory or driving performance
- May have a preferential effect for psychic symptoms of anxiety, irritability and aggression with little effect on behavioral manifestations

PHARMACOLOGY

- Unlike the benzodiazepines, buspirone does not bind to the GABA-"benzodiazepine" receptor complex, but has a marked effect on serotonin transmission and affects nonadrenergic and dopaminergic activity
- A partial 5-HT^{1A} agonist; chronic administration causes downregulation of 5-HT^2 receptors. A major metabolite (1-(2-pyrimidinyl)-piperazine) enhances norepinephrine release

DOSAGE

- Start with 2.5–5 mg bid and increase weekly by 5 mg to a maximum of 30 mg/day; usual range: 5–30 mg daily in divided doses
- Decrease dose by 25–50% in patients with creatinine clearance < 10 ml/min
- A lag time of 1–2 weeks may be needed for the anxiolytic effect to occur; rarely doses up to 40 mg daily are required
- ☞ **Not effective on a prn basis**

PHARMACOKINETICS

- Absorption is virtually complete; first-pass effect reduces bioavailability to about 4%
- Food may delay oral absorption and decrease the extent of first-pass effect and therefore increase oral bioavailability; C_{max} increased up to 116%
- Highly bound to plasma proteins (86–95%)
- Peak plasma level: 0.7–1.5 h; C_{max} and AUC of drug and active metabolite are equal to or higher in children and adolescents than in adults
- Onset of action takes days to weeks; maximum effect seen in 3–4 weeks
- Elimination half-life: 2–11 h. Metabolite: 1-(2-pyrimidinyl) piperazine (active); parent drug metabolized by CYP3A4 and 2C19; metabolite metabolized by 2D6
- Clearance decreased in renal and hepatic impairment

ADVERSE EFFECTS

- Drowsiness more common in children than in adults
- Headache, dizziness, lightheadedness, nervousness, restlessness, excitement, fatigue, sedation, paresthesia, numbness, GI upset, rash urticaria
- Behavior activation, euphoria, increased aggression and psychosis reported in children
- Due to its effect on dopamine, the possible risk of neurological effects has been a concern; however, buspirone does not lead to postsynaptic dopamine receptor hypersensitivity since it binds only to presynaptic dopamine auto-receptors; when combined with antipsychotic, increases in extrapyramidal reactions (including dyskinesias) have been reported
- Cases of possible psychotic deterioration reported in pediatric patients
- Dose-dependent increase in prolactin and growth hormone levels reported

DISCONTINUATION SYNDROME

- Withdrawal effects have not been reported

Anxiolytic Agents

Buspirone (cont.)

PRECAUTIONS

- Has no cross-tolerance with benzodiazepines and will not alleviate benzodiazepine withdrawal; when switching, taper benzodiazepine dose while adding buspirone to the regimen
- Caution in patients with seizure disorder as drug has no anticonvulsant activity
- Do not use concurrently with MAOIs or within 10 days of an MAOI

TOXICITY

- Excessive doses produce extension of pharmacological effects including dizziness, nausea, and vomiting; monitor respiration, BP, and pulse, and give symptomatic and supportive therapy

USE IN PREGNANCY

- Safety in pregnancy has not yet been determined; Category B drug, no teratogenicity in animal studies

Breast Milk

- Buspirone and metabolites are excreted in human milk; no data on safety

NURSING IMPLICATIONS

- The effect of buspirone is gradual; improvement may be seen as early as 7–10 days after starting therapy, but typically require more than 2 weeks
- As an immediate response does not occur, buspirone should be taken consistently, not on a PRN basis
- When switching from a benzodiazepine to buspirone it is important to gradually taper the benzodiazepine to avoid precipitating a withdrawal reaction
- Administer in a consistent manner in relation to food (i.e., always with or without food)

PATIENT INSTRUCTIONS

- Detailed instructions for patients and caregivers are provided in the Information Sheet on p. 322.

DRUG INTERACTIONS

- Clinically significant interactions are listed below

Class of Drug	Example	Interaction Effect
Antibiotic	Erythromycin	Increased plasma level of buspirone (5-fold) due to inhibited metabolism via CYP3A4
Antidepressant SSRI	Fluoxetine, fluvoxamine	May potentiate anti-obsessional effects of the antidepressants Increased plasma level of buspirone (3-fold with fluvoxamine) Case reports of serotonin syndrome, euphoria, seizures or dystonia with combination
SARI	Trazodone	Case of serotonin syndrome with high dose of trazodone
Irreversible MAOI	Phenelzine, tranylcypromine	Elevated blood pressure reported

Class of Drug	Example	Interaction Effect
Antifungal	Itraconazole	Increased plasma level of buspirone (13-fold) due to inhibited metabolism via CYP3A4
Antipsychotic	Haloperidol	Increased plasma level of haloperidol by 26% due to inhibited metabolism
Antitubercular drug	Rifampicin	Decreased peak plasma concentration and half-life of buspirone due to induced metabolism via CYP3A4
Benzodiazepine	Diazepam	Increased serum level of benzodiazepine
Calcium-channel blocker	Verapamil, diltiazem	Increased peak plasma level of buspirone (3–4-fold) due to inhibited metabolism via CYP3A4
Digoxin		Effects of digoxin may be increased
Grapefruit juice		Increased peak plasma level of buspirone (up to 15-fold), AUC (up to 20-fold) and half-life (1.5-fold) due to inhibited metabolism via CYP3A4
Immunosuppressant	Cyclosporin A	Increased serum level of cyclosporin A with possible renal adverse effects
St. John's Wort		Case report of possible serotonin syndrome (see p. 46)

Anxiolytics – References and Selected Readings

- American Academy of Child and Adolescent Psychiatry Official Action (1997). Practice parameters for the assessment and treatment of children and adolescents with anxiety disorders. *Journal of the American Academy of Child and Adolescent Psychiatry 36(10),* 695–845.
- Culpepper, L. (2003). Use of algorithms to treat anxiety in primary care. *Journal of Clinical Psychiatry 64(Suppl. 2),* 30–33.
- Fulton, B., Brogden, R.N. (1997). Buspirone: An updated review of its clinical pharmacology and therapeutic applications. *CNS Drugs 7(1),* 68–88.
- Goddard, A.W., Shekhar, A., Anand, A. et al. (2002). Psychopharmacology of pediatric anxiety disorders. *International Drug Therapy Newsletter 37(12),* 89– 94.
- Goodman, W.K. (2004). Selecting pharmacotherapy for generalized anxiety disorder. *Journal of Clinical Psychiatry 65(Suppl. 13),* 8–13.
- Labellarte, M.J., Ginsburg, G.S., Walkup, J.T. et al. (1999). The treatment of anxiety disorders in children and adolescents. *Biological Psychiatry 46(11),* 1567–1578.
- Mancuso, C.E. Tanzi, M.G. Gabay, M. (2004). Paradoxical reactions to benzodiazepines: Literature review and treatment options. *Pharmacotherapy 24(9)* 1177–1185.
- Nelson, J., Chouinard, G. (1999). Guidelines for the clinical use of benzodiazepines: Pharmacokinetics, dependency, rebound and withdrawal. *Canadian Journal of Clinical Pharmacology 6(2),* 69–83.

HYPNOTICS/SEDATIVES

PRODUCT AVAILABILITY

Chemical Class	Generic Name	Trade Name[A]	Dosage Forms and Strengths	Monograph Statement
Antihistamines Piperazine	Hydroxyzine	Atarax, Vistaril[B]	Capsules: 10 mg, 25 mg, 50 mg, 100 mg(B) Oral syrup: 10 mg/5 ml, 25 mg/5 ml[B] Injection: 25 mg/ml[B], 50 mg/ml	Dosage recommendation provided for children
Ethanolamine	Diphenhydramine	Benadryl	Capsules: 25 mg, 50 mg Chewable tablets: 12.5 mg Oral solution: 6.25 mg/5 ml, 10 mg/5 ml[B], 12.5 mg/5 ml Injection: 10 mg/ml[B], 50 mg/ml	Dosage recommendation provided for children
	Doxylamine[B][D]	Unisom	–	–
Phenothiazines	Promethazine	Phenergan	Tablets: 12.5 mg[B], 25 mg, 50 mg Oral solution: 6.25 mg/5 ml[B], 10 mg/5 ml[C], 25 mg/5 ml[B] Suppositories[B]: 12.5 mg, 25 mg, 50 mg Injection: 25 mg/ml, 50 mg/ml[B], 28.2 mg/ml[C]	Dosage recommendation provided for children over age 2
Barbiturates	Pentobarbital	Nembutal	Capsules: 30 mg[B], 100 mg Injection: 50 mg/ml	Dosage recommendation provided for children
	Phenobarbital	Luminal	Tablets: 15mg, 30 mg, 60 mg, 100 mg Elixir: 4 mg/ml, 5 mg/ml Injection: 30 mg/ml, 120 mg/ml	Dosage recommendation provided for children
	Secobarbital (Quinalbarbitone)	Seconal	Capsules: 50 mg[B], 100 mg	Dosage recommendation provided for children
Benzodiazepines			See pp. 169–183	
Chloral derivative	Chloral hydrate	Noctec	Capsules: 500 mg Oral solution: 500 mg/5 ml	Dosage recommendations provided for children
Acetaldehyde polymer	Paraldehyde	Paral	Injection: 1 mg/ml (100%)	Dosage recommendations provided for children
Amino acid	L-Tryptophan[C][D]	Tryptan	–	–
Cyclopyrrolone	Zopiclone[C] Eszopiclone[B]/[E]	Imovane Lunesta	Tablets: 5 mg, 7.5 mg Tablets: 1 mg, 2 mg, 3 mg	Safety and efficacy not established in children Safety and efficacy not established in children
Imidazopyridine derivative	Zolpidem[B]	Ambien Ambien CR [B]	Tablets: 5 mg, 10 mg Controlled-release tablets[B]: 6.25 mg, 12.5 mg	Safety and efficacy not established in children
Pyrazolopyrimidine	Zaleplon	Sonata[B], Starnoc[C]	Capsules: 5 mg, 10 mg	Safety and efficacy not established in children
Selective melatonin agonist	Remelteon[B][D]	Rozerem	–	–
Antidepressants	Trazodone Mirtazapine		See p. 63 See p. 69	

[A] Generic preparations may be available, [B] Not marketed in Canada, [C] Not marketed in USA, [D] Not generally used in children – not reviewed in this chapter [E] S-isomer of zopiclone

INDICATIONS

Approved in Children and Adolescents

- Anxiety (e.g., hydroxyzine)
- Pruritus (antihistamines)

Approved in Adults

- Nocturnal sedation; short-term management of insomnia
- Preoperative sedation

Other Uses in Children and Adolescents

- Sedative for diagnostic (e.g., EEG, CT scan) or dental procedures
- Hydroxyzine may be helpful in sleep onset problems and nightmares in children with PTSD

GENERAL COMMENTS

- Recommend that stringent sedation guidelines be adhered to (e.g., as formulated by the American Academy of Pediatrics), to ensure patient safety; sedation prior to diagnostic or dental procedures should minimize physical discomfort or pain, as well as negative psychological response to treatment, and maximize amnesia
- Prior to treatment of insomnia, medical and laboratory assessments are recommended as well as identification of any etiological factors and associated syndromes to determine if sleep disturbance is
  - Due to a primary sleep disorder (e.g., sleep apnea, restless legs syndrome, narcolepsy)
  - Due to psychiatric disorder (e.g., depression, mania)
  - Drug-induced (e.g., sympathomimetics, psychostimulants)
  - Due to medical disorder (e.g., thyroid, peptic ulcer, pain)
  - Due to use of excessive caffeine, alcohol
- Treat the primary cause, wherever possible; behavior modification techniques have been found effective, used alone or with drug therapy
- Use of hypnotics is recommended for limited time periods; long-term, continuous treatment is not recommended
- Short-acting benzodiazepines may have a role in brief treatment of insomnia associated with anxiety

PHARMACOLOGY

- Hypnotics suppress the reticular formation of the midbrain to various degrees resulting in sedation, sleep, or anesthesia
- Benzodiazepines bind to the "benzodiazepine"-GABA-chloride receptor complex in the brain; they act non-selectively at 2 central receptor sites (omega 1 & 2), omega-1 receptor modulates sedative activity and omega-2 in responsible for memory and cognitive functioning
- Zolpidem, zopiclon, eszopiclone and zaleplon bind selectively to $GABA_{A1}$ receptors
- Antihistamines antagonize H_1 receptors

DOSING

- See pp. 193–194 for individual agents
- Dosage should be adjusted in patients with hepatic impairment

PHARMACOKINETICS

- See pp. 193–194
- Zaleplon: absorption and peak plasma level decreased with high fat meal (C_{max} and T_{max} decreased by 35%). Japanese patients showed increased C_{max} and AUC by 37% and 64%, respectively
- Zolpidem: CR preparation formulated with immediate-release layer and slow-release layer; C_{max} occurs later and is higher than with regular-release product. Peak plasma level increased (by more than 50%) and half-life increased in cirrhosis
- Eszopiclone: AUC increased 2-fold in moderate to severe liver disease

Hypnotics/ Sedatives

Hypnotics/Sedatives (cont.)

ONSET AND DURATION OF ACTION

- See chart pp. 193–194
- Tolerance to effects of many hypnotics occurs after 2 weeks of continuous use

ADVERSE EFFECTS

- See chart pp. 195–196
- Daytime sedation and impairment dependent on drug dosage, half-life, and patient tolerance
- Anterograde amnesia is dependent on drug potency and dose
- Rebound insomnia is dependent on drug dose, half-life, and duration of use
- High dose can impair respiration and blood pressure

DISCONTINUATION SYNDROME

- See Precautions in chart pp. 195–196 for specific drugs
- Discontinuation of hypnotics can produce:
  - Withdrawal: occurs within 1–2 days (short-acting) to 3–7 days (long-acting) following discontinuation of regular use of most hypnotics (for more than 2 weeks); suggested to occur less frequently with zopiclone and zolpidem. Common symptoms include insomnia, agitation, anxiety, perceptual disturbances (e.g., photophobia), malaise and anorexia. Abrupt withdrawal of high doses may result in seizures and/or psychosis
  - Rebound: occurs hours to days after drug withdrawal; described as worsening of insomnia beyond pretreatment levels. More likely to occur with short-acting agents
  - Relapse: recurrence of the insomnia, to pretreatment levels, when the hypnotic is discontinued
- Can occur with chronic use of all hypnotics

Management

- Withdrawal of a hypnotic (after chronic use) should be tailored to each patient, with gradual tapering of the drug over several weeks
- Typically, tapering regimens suggest reducing dose by 10–25% q 3–7 days –depends on dose, duration of use, and patient sensitivities to withdrawal symptoms
- As no single agent is completely effective or safe, cardiorespiratory monitoring is recommended for children undergoing sedation for diagnostic procedures
- Tolerance and physician dependence can occur after prolonged use of any agent used for sedation or analgesia

PRECAUTIONS

- Abrupt withdrawal may produce anxiety, insomnia, dizziness, nausea, vomiting, twitching, hyperthermia, tremors, convulsions, and death. Taper drug gradually after prolonged use
- Long-term administration of barbiturates has been associated with osteomalacia/rickets in adults, because of altered vitamin D metabolism
- Avoid use in addiction-prone individuals; recreational abuse occurs particularly with benzodiazepines to achieve a "high"
- Abuse may result in clouding of consciousness and visual hallucinations
- Use in individuals with sleep apnea is contraindicated
- CR preparation of zolpidem reported to cause incidents of sleepwalking, driving while "asleep", and food binging while "asleep"

TOXICITY

- See table pp. 195–196

See pp. 195–196 for individual agents. For benzodiazepines, see p. 175

Breast Milk

- The American Academy of Pediatrics considers many hypnotics/sedatives compatible with breastfeeding – see chart pp. 195–196

NURSING IMPLICATIONS

- Counsel patient regarding chronic use of hypnotic and loss of efficacy of drug over time (tolerance)
- Monitor hyperactive children taking antihistamines for paradoxical excitation
- Chloral hydrate solution should be well diluted with water, fruit juice, or ginger ale to minimize gastric irritation
- Moisten suppositories slightly prior to insertion
- Suggest that abrupt withdrawal after chronic use may result in serious side effects and rebound symptoms; drugs should be tapered over time (i.e., decrease dose by 10–25% q 3–7 days)
- Suggest alternative methods of treating insomnia (e.g., do relaxation exercises, avoid daytime naps, avoid caffeine, cognitive therapy)
- Assess personal sleep habits to determine causes or contributing factors to insomnia (e.g., alcohol, caffeine, etc.)

PATIENT INSTRUCTIONS

- Detailed instructions for patients and caregivers are provided in the Information Sheet on p. 324.

DRUG INTERACTION

- Clinically significant interactions are listed below
- For drugs interacting with benzodiazepines see pp. 175–177.

Class of Drug	Example	Interaction Effect
Antibiotic/Antiinfective	Clarithromycin	*Eszopiclone:* increased plasma level of hypnotic due to inhibited metabolism via CYP3A4
	Doxycycline	*Barbiturates* indce the metabolism and reduce the efficacy of doxycycline
	Erythromycin	*Zopiclone, zaleplon,* and *zolpidem* increased plasma level of hypnotic due to decreased clearance
	Linezolid	*Diphenhydramine:* case report of acute delirium
Anticoagulants	Dicumarol, Warfarin	*Choral hydrate* will displace drugs that are protein-bound and temporarily enhance hypoprothrombinemic response; increased or decreased PT ratio or INR response *Barbiturates* will induce metabolism and decrease the efficacy of anticoagulants; on withdrawal, excess bleeding can occur *Paraldehyde:* decreased PT ratio or INO response
Anticonvulsant	Carbamazepine, phenyton	*Zopiclone:* decreased plasma level of zopiclone due to induced metabolism via CYP3A4
	Valproate	*Zolpidem:* case of somnambulism *Barbiturates:* induce the metabolism and decrease the efficacy of valproate
Antidepressant SSRI, RIMA, MAOI	Fluoxetine, moclobemide, phenelzine, tranylcypromine	L-*Tryptophan* combination may produce increased serotonin activity resulting in twitching, agitation ("serotonin syndrome")
SSRI	Fluoxetine, fluvoxamine	Increased sedation and side effects of *chloral hydrate* due to inhibited metabolism
SSRI/NDRI	Sertraline, bupropion	*Zolpidem:* case reports of hallucinations and delirium sertraline, fluoxentine, paroxetine, venlafaxine and bupropion
SNRI	Venlafaxine	*Zolpidem:* case report of hallucinations and delirium *Diphenhydramine*: decreased metabolism of venlafaxine via CYP2D6

Hypnotics/ Sedatives

Hypnotics/Sedatives (cont.)

Class of Drug	Example	Interaction Effect
Tricyclics	Imipramine	*Zolpidem:* in one study 5/8 patients on combination experienced anterograde amnesia
	Desipramine	*Zolpidem:* case rwport of visual hallucinations with combination
	Amitriptyline, clomipramine, desipramine, imipramine	*Diphenhydramine:* increased plasma level of antidepressants metabolized primarily by CYP2D6 due to inhibited metabolism
Antifungal	Ketoconazole, itraconazole	*Eszopiclone:* increase C_{max} and $T_{\frac{1}{2}}$ of eszopiclone (1.4-and 1.3-fold, respectively, with ketoconazole) due to decreased metabolism via CYP3A4 *Zolpidem:* decreased clearance of zolpidem by 41%; half-life increased by 26% with ketoconazole *Zopiclone:* increased AUC and elimination half-life due to decreased metabolism *Zaleplon:* increased plasma level of zaleplon due to decreased metabolism Barbiturates induce the metabolism and reduce the efficacy of griseofulvin *Remelteon:* increased C_{max} and AUC (34% and 84% respectively due to inhibited metabolism by ketoconazole via CYP3A4
	Griseofulvin	*Barbiturates:* induce the metabolism and reduce the efficacy of griseofulvin
Antipsychotics	Chlorpromazine, fluphenazine, perphenazine, thiothixene, risperidone	*Diphenhydramine:* possible increase in plasma level of antipsychotic metabolized via CYP2D6 due to inhibited metabolism Additive CNS depression and psychomotor impairment
Antitubercular Drug	Rifampin	*Zolpidem:* decreased peak plasma level of zolpidem by 60% and increased elimination half-life by 36% *Zaleplon:* decreased AUC of zaleplon by 80% due to induced metabolism *Zopiclone:* decreased AUC of zopiclone by 80% due to induced metabolism *Eszopictone:* decreased AUC of eszopiclone due to induced metabolism *Remelteon:* decreased C_{max} and AUC of remelteon by 40–90% due to induced metabolism
Anxiolytic	Lorazepam	Additive CNS effects *Eszopiclone:* C_{max} of both drugs increased by 22%
β-Blocker	Propranolol	*Barbiturates:* induce metabolism and reduce efficacy of propranolol
	Metoprolol	*Diphenhydramine:* decreased clearance of metoprolol 2-fold due to inhibited metabolism
Ca-channel blocker	Diltiazem	*Diphenhydramine:* initial sharp increase seen in diltiazem concentration secondary to displacement from tissue binding sites, followed by an increase in steady-state plasma levels secondary to inhibited metabolism via CYP2D6
Caffeine	Tea, coffee, colas	May counteract sedation and increase insomnia
Cimetidine		*Zaleplon:* increased peak plasma level and AUC of zaleplon by 85% due to inhibited metabolism via CYP3A4 and aldehyde oxidase *Zopiclone* and *zolpidem:* increased plasma level of hypnotic due to inhibited metabolism *Diphenhydramine:* increased AUC and half-life, and decrease clerence of diphenhydramine
CNS depressants	Alcohol, opiods, antipsychotics	Increased CNS depression and psychomotor impairment; in "high" doses coma and respiratory depression can occur
CNS stimulant	Methylphenidate, dextroamphetamine	May counteract sedation and increase insomnia
Disulfiram		*Paraldehyde:* avoid since it is metabolized to acetaldehyde; an alcohol-like reaction will occur

Class of Drug	Example	Interaction Effect
Flumazenil		*Zolpidem* and *zaleplon*: antagonism of hypnotic effects
Grapefruit juice		*Zaleplon*: increased plasma level of zaleplon due to inhibited metabolism via CYP3A4
Lithium		Increased efficacy and increased plasma level of lithium with L-*tryptophan*
Narcotic	Codeine Methadone	*Diphenhydramine*: inhibited conversion of codeine to its active moiety morphine, via CYP2D6, resulting in decreased analgesic efficacy *Diphenhydramine*: increased plasma levels of methadone possible due to inhibited metabolism via CYP2D6
Oral contraceptive		*Chloral hydrate*: decreased efficacy of the oral contraceptive due to induction of microsomal enzymes *Barbiturates* induce the metabolism and reduce the efficacy of oral contraceptives
Protease inhibitors	Ritonavir Ritonavir, sequinavir	*Zolpidem and eszopiclone*: increased plasma level of zolpidem due to decreased metabolism via CYP3A4 *Barbiturates* induce the metabolism and reduce the efficacy of protease inhibitors
Corticosteroid **Theophylline** **Oxtriphylline** **Phenylbutazone** **Quinidine**	Dexamethasone	*Barbiturates* induce the metabolism and reduce the efficacy of these drugs

Comparison of Hypnotics/Sedatives

Drug	Usual Doses in Children	Onset of Action	Bioavail-ability	Protein Binding	Half-life	CYP-450 Metabo-lizing Enzymes[c]	CYP-450 Effect[d]	Indications
Antihistamines Diphenhydramine (Benadryl, Nytol)	PO/IM/IV: 5 mg/kg/day to a maximum of 50 mg/dose or 300 mg/day	15–60 min	40–60%	80–85%	1–3 h	2D6	2D6 inhibitor	Sedation, insomnia
Hydroxyzine (Atarax)	Sedative – oral: 0.6 mg/kg IM: 1.1 mg/kg	15–30 min	?	?	8–10 h	2D6, 3A4[e]	2D6 inhibitor	Anxiety, pruritis Preoperative or postoperative adjunctivemedication
Promethazine (Phenergan)	Oral or rectal: (0.25–0.5 mg/kg) 12.5–25 mg Preop sedation: 1 mg/kg	2–3 h	25%	?	16–19 h	2D6	2D6 inhibitor	Anxiety, sedation, vomiting Preoperative, postoperative or dental sedation
Barbiturate Pentobarbital	Sedation – oral: 2–6 mg/kg/day Hypnotic – IM: 2–6 mg/kg to a maximum of 100 mg/dose or 50 mg IV (with additional doses if needed at 1 min intervals) Preop sedation: 2–6 mg/kg to a maximum of 100 mg/dose	15 min	61%	35–45%	21–42 h	3A4, 2C19	Inducer of 2A6, 2B6, 2C9, 3A4	Preoperative sedation for diagnostic procedures to minimize anxiety and tension Anesthesia

Hypnotics/ Sedatives

Comparison of Hypnotics/Sedatives (cont.)

Drug	Usual Doses in Children	Onset of Action	Bioavail-ability	Protein Binding	Half-life	CYP-450 Metabo-lizing Enzymes[c]	CYP-450 Effect[d]	Indications
Phenobarbital	Sedative – oral: 2 mg/kg tid Preop sedation: 1–3 mg/kg	Over 60 min	?	?	2–6 days	3A4, 2C9, 2C19, 2E1	Inducer of 1A2, 2A6, 2D6, 2B6, 2C9, 3A4, 2C19	Sedation Preoperative sedation
Secobarbital	Sedative – oral: 2 mg/kg tid Hypnotic – IM: 3–5 mg/kg to a maximum of 100 mg/dose Preop sedation: 2–6 mg/kg to a maximum of 100 mg/dose	15 min	80%	30–45%	2–3 h	3A4, 2C19	Inducer of 2A6, 2B6, 2C9, 3A4	Preoperative sedation for diagnostic or dental procedures, sleep EEG's Acute convulsive disorders
Chloral hydrate (Noctec)	Sedative – oral or rectal: 25 mg/kg/dose Hypnotic – oral or rectal: 50–100 mg/kg/dose	30 min	> 95% (active metabolite trichloro-ethanol)	35–41% (trichloro-acetic acid metabolite = 71–88%)	4–8 h	2B, 2E1	Inducer	Insomnia Dental and pre-operative sedation
Eszopiclone[a] (Lunesta)	No data in children and adolescents	1 h (2 h after high fat meal)	?	52–59%	5–7 h	3A4, 2EI	–	Insomnia
Paraldehyde (Paral)	Sedative – oral: 0.15 ml/kg Rectal: 0.2–0.4 ml of undiluted paraldehyde/kg/dose given q 4–8 h to a maximum of 30 ml (can administer rectally as a 30–50% solution in oil or normal saline)	10 min	?	?	4–8 h	?	?	Preoperative sedation for diagnostic procedures Excited psychiatric states, convulsive control in tetany and poisoning
Zaleplon (Sonata, Starnoc)	5 mg	Rapid Peak level: 0.9–1.5 h (See p. 189)	30%	60%	0.9–1.1 h	3A4, aldehyde-oxi-dase	CYP3A4 inducer	Insomnia Not adequately studied in children
Zolpidem[a] (Ambien)	5–10 mg	30 min Peak level 1.6 h CR:2.5–8 h (See p. 189)	70%	92%	1.5–4.5 h CR: 2.8 h	1A2[w], 3A4, 2C9[w], 2D6	–	Insomnia Not adequately studied in children
Zopiclone[b] (Imovane)	3.75–15 mg	30 min Peak level: 90 min	> 75%	45%	3.8–6.5 h	1A2, 2C9, 3A4	–	Insomnia (increasing the dose above 15 mg may not produce increased efficacy) Not adequately studied in children

[a] Not marketed in Canada, [b] Not marketed in USA, [c] Cytochrome P-450 isoenzymes involved in drug metabolism, [d] Effect of drug on cytochrome enzymes, [e] Pertains to metabolite, [w] Weak activity

	Pregnancy/Lactation	Precautions	Main Side Effects	Toxicity
Antihistamine	In animals, teratogenicity seen in high doses; case reports in humans, but correlation not proven Excreted into human milk; newborn have increased sensitivity to antihistamines	May precipitate seizures in patients with focal lesions Paradoxical excitation can occur Diphenhydramineis a potent inhibitor of CYP2D6 and may interact with various drugs (See Interaction p. 191–193)	Sedation, fatigue, incoordination, GI disturbances; anticholinergic effects (dry mouth, blurred vision) Confusion, delirium, hallucinations	At high doses: paradoxical excitation, insomnia, restlessness, EPS, convulsions; promethazine can cause respiratory depression, apnea and death.
Barbiturate	Barbiturates cross the placenta; an increase in congenital defects and hemorrhagic disease of newborn reported Prolonged elimination of barbiturate reported in fetus Withdrawal symptoms seen in new-born Excreted in breast milk; American Academy of Pediatrics considers secobarbital compatible with breast-feeding	**AVOID** barbiturates in: severe hepatic impairment, porphyria, uncontrolled pain (delirium may result), and pulmonary insufficiency Chronic use has been associated with hyperkinetic states with symptoms such as reduced attention span, and destructive or aggressive reactions; developmental delays reported with mental slowing With low doses, patient may become euphoric, excited, restless, or violent; at high doses, can develop acute confusional state and respiratory depression Risk of unintentional suicide due to low lethal dose Risk of tolerance; high potential for abuse and dependence	CNS: drowsiness, agitation, confusion, hangover, weight gain Skin rash (1–3%), nausea, and vomiting (2–8%) Can cause severe depression (risk of suicide)	Symptoms include excitement, restlessness, delirium and nystagmus; may progress to CNS depression, oliguria, hypotension, tachycardia, circulatory collapse, respiratory depression, and coma Death reported with doses above 2 g Treatment: symptomatic and supportive
Chloral hydrate	Crosses placenta; no reports of congenital defects in newborn Excreted in breast milk; one report of drowsiness in newborn; American Academy of Pediatrics considers drug compatible with breast-feeding	**CAUTION** in hepatic and renal impairment, gastritis, peptic ulcer, and cardiac distress Doses above 1.5 g can impair respiration and decrease blood pressure Tolerance can occur with chronic use; withdrawal reactions reported Will induce hepatic enzymes and affect metabolism of other drugs; will displace other drugs from protein binding	Nausea, vomiting, hangover, hyperactivity (2–5%), skin rash, respiratory depression (9%) Does not accumulate with chronic use	Toxic symptoms reported with doses above 1.5 g. Symptoms can progress to severe hypotension, hypothermia, arrhythmias, edema, and cardiac failure Death reported with doses above 4 g Treatment: symptomatic and supportive
Eszopiclone	Not teratogenic in animals No studies in humans Not known if excreted into breast milk	High doses (> 6 mg) can produce amnesia, euphoria, and hallucinations Caution in respiratory impairment, liver dysfunction, depression, and in combination with CY3A4 inhibitors	Unpleasant taste (> 15%), headache (> 10%), dry mouth; dizziness Withdrawal effects and rebound insomnia have been reported	Symptoms include confusion, sedation, mood changes, restlessness/anxiety. severe lethargy, and ataxia

**Hypnotics/
Sedatives**

Comparison of Hypnotics/Sedatives (cont.)

	Pregnancy/Lactation	Precautions	Main Side Effects	Toxicity
Paraldehyde	Crosses placenta; fetal concentration equals that of maternal blood; respiratory depression seen in neonates	**AVOID** in gastroenteritis, liver damage, bronchopulmonary disease; may produce excitement or delirium in presence of pain Decomposed product should not be used (acetic acid odor). Do not give to persons receiving disulfiram Dissolves plastic; use glass container/syringe; use product immediately after drawing up in syringe Tolerance can occur with chronic use; withdrawal reactions reported	Unpleasant taste, odor imparted into exhaled air; may irritate throat and mucous membranes if administered chronically – dilute liberally Injection can be painful if more than 5 ml injected; give deep IM Toxic hepatitis and nephrosis reported after prolonged use; metabolic acidosis can occur with confusion and agiation	Toxic symptoms reported with doses above 1.5 g. Symptoms can progress to severe hypotension, hypothermia, arrhythmias, edema, and cardiac failure Death reported with doses above 4 g Treatment: symptomatic and supportive
Zaleplon	Safety in pregnancy not established Excreted in breast milk; not recommended for nursing mothers	Due to rapid onset of action, should be taken immediately before bedtime Rebound insomnia reported	Drowsiness, headache, GI upset, asthenia, myalgia, paresthesias, dry mouth, hangover, anterograde amnesia Rarely sleepwalking, confusion, hallucinatious and mania	Symptoms include CNS depression ranging from somnolence, lethargy, confusion to ataxia, hypotonia, and respiratory depression. Coma rare. Treatment: symptomatic and supportive
Zolpidem	Not teratogenic in animal studies Total drug excreted in milk does not exceed 0.02% of administered dose Considered compatible with breastfeeding by the American Academy of Pediatrics	**CAUTION** in liver dysfunction, respiratory impairment Abuse reported Withdrawal reactions reported including GI symptoms, flushing, lightheadedness, panic attacks, nervousness, crying, confusion, disorientation, insomnia, suicidal ideation, tremors and seizures	Drowsiness, dizziness, ataxia, agitation, nightmares, diarrhea, nausea, headache, hangover, anterograde amnesia, sleep walking and sleep talking Dysphoria reported at high doses; rarely delirium and psychosis reported with perceptual distortions and hallucinations (case reports primarily in females) Residual sedation upon awakening reported especially with CR preparation	Symptoms include impairment of consciousness ranging from somnolence to coma. Treatment: symptomatic and supportive
Zopiclone	Not teratogenic in animal studies Crosses placenta; no congenital abnormalities reported in humans. New-borns have significantly lower birth weights and lower gestational Excreted in breast milk; infant receives approx. 1% of administered dose – effect unknown	**CAUTION** in respiratory impairment, liver dysfunction and depression Anticholinergic agents may decrease plasma level Dependence rare and withdrawal effects are mild; rebound insomnia reported	Bitter metallic taste, (up to 30%) dry mouth, GI distress, palpitations, dyspnea, tremor, rash, chills, sweating, agitation, nightmares Severe drowsiness, confusion and incoordination Rarely hallucinations and behavioral disturbances	Symptoms include drowsiness, lethargy, and ataxia; in severe cases somnolence, confusion, reduced or absent refluxes, and coma can occur Treatment: symptomatic and supportive

- Lader, M. (1998).Withdrawal reactions after stopping hypnotics in patients with insomnia. *CNS Drugs 10(6),* 425–440.
- Wagner, J., Wagner, M.L., Hening, W.A. (1998). Beyond benzodiazepines: Alternative pharmacological agents for the treatment of insomnia. *Annals of Pharmacotherapy 32(6),* 680–691.
- Walsh, J.K. (2004). Pharmacologic management of insomnia. *Journal of Clinical Psychiatry 65(Suppl. 16),* 41–45.
- Wang, J.S., DeVane, C.L. (2003). Pharmacokinetics and drug interactions of the sedative hypnotics. *Psychopharmacology Bulletin 37(1),* 10–29.
- Younus, M., Labellarte, M.J. (2002). Insomnia in children: When are hypnotics indicated? *Pediatric Drugs 4(6),* 391–403.

Hypnotics/
Sedatives

MOOD STABILIZERS

GENERAL COMMENTS   • Mood stabilizers can be classified as follows:

Chemical Class	Agent	Page
Lithium	Example: Lithium carbonate	See p. 199
Anticonvulsant	Carbamazepin gabapentin Clonazepam Lamotrigine Oxcarbazepine Topiramate valproate	See p. 208
Second and third-generation antipsychotics	Risperidone, olanzapine Aripiprazole	See p. 115 See p. 127
Antipsychotic/antidepressant combination	Olanzapine/fluoxetine (Symbyex)[B]	Capsules 6/25 mg, 6/50 mg, 12/25 mg, 12/50 mg

[B] Not available in Canada

Levels of Evidence for Efficacy in Pediatric Patients

DRUG	BIPOLAR 1 DISORDER manic or mixed without psychosis	BIPOLAR 1 DISORDER manic or mixed with psychosis	Bipolar Depression
Lithium	A&B	A&B	B&C
Anticonvulsants			
Carbamazepine	B	B	–
Gabapentin	+/– contradictory data as augmenting agent	–	C
Oxcarbazepine	D (+/–)	D (+/–)	–
Valproate	B&C	B&C	C
Lamotrigine	C	C	B&D
Topiramate	C	C	–

DRUG	BIPOLAR 1 DISORDER manic or mixed without psychosis	BIPOLAR 1 DISORDER manic or mixed with psychosis	Bipolar Depression
Antipsychotics			
Risperidone	B&C	B&C	–
Olanzapine	B&C	B&C	B
Quetiapine	B&C	B&C	B
Ziprasidone	B&C	B&C	–
Clozapine	C	C	–
Aripiprazole	B&C	B	–

Adapted from: Kowatch, R.A. et al. *JAACAP* 44(3) 213–235, 2005
A = good research-based evidence (e.g., >1 RCT).
B = at least one randomized placebo-controlled trial
C = non-randomized studies
D = minimal research-based evidence; case reports

Lithium

PRODUCT AVAILABILITY

Chemical Class	Generic Name	Trade Name[A]	Dosage Forms and Strengths	Monograph Statement
Lithium salt	Lithium carbonate	Lithotabs Eskalith, Lithane[C], Carbolith[C] Eskalith CR, Duralith[C], Lithobid SR	Tablets: 300 mg Capsules: 150 mg, 300 mg, 600 mg Extended-release tablets: 300 mg, 450 mg[B]	Not recommended for children under age 12
	Lithium citrate	Cibalith-S	Oral solution: 300 mg/5 ml (8 mmol/5 ml)	Not recommended for children under age 12

[A] Generic preparations may be available, [B] Not marketed in Canada, [C] Not marketed in USA

Lithium (cont.)

INDICATIONS

Approved in Children and Adolescents

- Long-term maintenance or prophylaxis of bipolar disorder (BD) (approved for children > 12 years in the USA)

Approved (for Adults)

- Long-term maintenance or prophylaxis of bipolar disorder (BD) I and II
- Treatment of acute mania and mixed states; open trials in children and adolescents suggest benefit in mania

Other Uses in Children and Adolescents

- Prevention or diminution of the intensity of subsequent episodes of mania, hypomania, and depression
- Double-blind study suggests benefit in adolescents with BD and comorbid substance use disorder
- Augments the action of antidepressants in depression
- Behavioral symptoms of pervasive developmental disorders, treatment of chronic aggression/antisocial behavior/impulsivity; may be useful in patients with an affective component to symptoms; reduces aggression in conduct disorders (moderatate effect)
- Acute psychotic episodes with affective features
- Migraine, cluster headaches
- Case reports of antisuicidal properties

GENERAL COMMENTS

- Adolescent BD is suggested to be less responsive than in adults (though one small study had a 68% response rate and an open study had a 63% response rate on bipolar mania); often combination therapy with two mood stabilizers or an atypical antipsychotic is required, and tends to provide better outcome than lithium used alone.
- "Classic" mania responds best (up to 60%). Other possible predictors of response include: family history of lithium response in a first degree relative and few prior episodes of mania or depression
- Less response noted in patients with dysphoric/psychotic mania or mixed states, rapid-cycling BD, in patients with prepubertal onset of BD, or early onset of ADHD, those with multiple prior episodes, substance abuse, personality disorders, or comorbid medical conditions
- There is a high degree of comorbid disorders in adolescents and children (e.g., ADHD, conduct disorders, substance abuse) which may require concurrent treatment
- May be more effective in preventing manic or mixed episodes than depressive episodes
- Administration of lithium requires 10–14 days before the complete effect is observed, therefore acute mania is often treated with an antipsychotic and/or clonazepam; lithium is subsequently added to the treatment regimen
- As some rapid-cycling may be contributed to by lithium-induced hypothyroidism, it is important to regularly assess thyroid function

PHARMACOLOGY

- Exact mechanism of action unknown; postulated that lithium may stabilize catecholamine receptors, and may alter calcium-mediated intracellular functions and increase GABA activity. Lithium blocks the ability of neurons to restore normal levels of the second messenger system (phosphatidylinositol biphosphate), thereby reducing the responsiveness of neurons to stimuli from muscarinic, cholinergic, and α-adrenergic neurotransmitters

- Research data suggest that chronic lithium use increases N-acetylaspartate levels in the brain, and may exert neuroprotective effects
- May alter cation transport across membranes in nerve and muscle cells

DOSING

- Initiating lithium: A test dose of 300 mg is recommended to assess how well lithium is tolerated (also see Monitoring Recommendations p. 205)
- Increase dose slowly (150–300mg every 2–3 days) to minimize side effects; the following target doses have been suggested; in patients under 25 kg, give 600 mg/day; 25–39 kg, give 900 mg/day; 40–50 km, give 1200 mg/day; if > 50 kg, give 1500 mg/day; the final dose should be guided by the plasma level and clinical response
  - Acute treatment: 0.8–1.2 mmol/l
  - Maintenance: 0.6–1.0 mmol/l
  - In chronic aggressive disorders: 0.8–1.55 mmol/l
- Once patient is stabilized, once-daily dosing is possible (if patient can tolerate)
- Younger subjects have lower brain-to-serum lithium concentrations than adults; children and adolescents may require higher maintenance serum lithium concentrations to ensure that brain lithium concentrations reach therapeutic levels
- Patients sensitive to side effects that are related to high peak plasma levels, e.g., tremor, urinary frequency and GI effects (i.e., nausea), may respond to slow release preparations (e.g., Duralith)
- Discontinuation of lithium within 18 months is associated with high relapse rates; some clinicians recommend continuing lithium therapy throughout adolescence
- Missed doses or drug interactions may reduce lithium levels and precipitate relapse

PHARMACOKINETICS

- Peak plasma level: 0.5–2 h (slow release preparation = 4 h)
- Half-life: 17.9 h (mean) – shorter than in adults due to more efficient clearance; once-daily dosing preferred (improved compliance and decreased urine volume and renal toxicity), half-life increases with duration of therapy (e.g., up to 58 h after 1 year's therapy)
- Patients in an acute manic episode may have an increased tolerance to lithium
- Excreted primarily (95%) by the kidney; therefore, adequate renal function is essential in order to avoid lithium accumulation and intoxication; clearance is faster than in adults, and is significantly correlated with total body weight. Close relationship between level of dehydration and renal clearance
- Monitoring: measure first plasma level 5 days after starting therapy (unless toxicity is suspected). Measure once weekly for the first 2 weeks, thereafter at clinical discretion (at least every 6 months), or whenever a new drug is prescribed or if the dose is increased. Blood levels should be measured at trough, i.e., 9–13 h after last dose
- Lithium is secreted in saliva reaching concentrations 3 times that seen in plasma – saliva composition is altered (see Adverse Effects, GI Effects below)

ADVERSE EFFECTS

- Younger children may experience more side effects than older children

CNS Effects

- General weakness and fatigue common; dysphoria, and restlessness are usually transient and may coincide with peaks in lithium concentration
- Drowsiness, tiredness

Lithium (cont.)

- Cognitive blunting, memory difficulties, decreased speed of information processing, confusion, lack of drive, productivity or creativity [Management: assess lithium plasma level and thyroid function; slow-release preparation or a lower dose may improve cognitive function]
- Slurred speech, ataxia – evaluate for lithium toxicity
- Dizziness and vertigo [Management: administer with food, use slow-release preparation to avoid peak lithium levels, or reduce dosage]
- Neuromuscular: incoordination, muscle weakness, fine tremor/shakiness common; more frequent at higher doses and in combination with antidepressant or antipsychotic, with excessive caffeine use, or alcoholism. Frequency of tremor decreases with time [Management: reduce dose, eliminate dietary caffeine; β-blocker (e.g., propranolol or atenolol) may be of benefit]. A coarse tremor may be a sign of lithium toxicity. Cogwheel rigidity and choreoathetosis reported
- Chronic treatment can affect the peripheral nervous system involving motor and sensory function
- Seizures rare
- Headaches common; rarely, papilledema/elevated intracranial pressure (pseudotumor cerebri) reported
- Cases of somnambulism in adults

| GI Effects |

- Usually coincide with peaks in lithium concentration and are probably due to rapid absorption of lithium; most disappear after a few weeks; if occur late in therapy, evaluate for lithium toxicity
- Nausea – over 50% incidence, abdominal pain [Management: administer with food, or use slow-release preparation]
- Vomiting; higher with increased plasma level [Management: use multiple daily dosing, change to a slow-release preparation, or lower dose]
- Diarrhea, loose stools. Slow release preparation may worsen this side effect in some patients [Management: if on a slow-release product, change to a regular lithium preparation; less problems noted with lithium citrate preparations; if all else fails and cannot decrease the lithium dose, loperamide prn]
- Metallic taste: composition of saliva altered (ions and proteins)
- Excessive thirst, dry mouth, mucosal ulceration (rare), hypersalivation occasionally reported
- Weight gain common; may be related to increased appetite, fluid retention, altered carbohydrate and fat metabolism or to hypothyroidism [Management: reduce caloric intake]. May be dose-related and higher with drug combinations

| Cardiovascular Effects |

- Bradycardia
- ECG changes: benign T-wave changes at therapeutic doses; use lithium cautiously in patients with pre-existing cardiac disease; arrhythmias and sinus node dysfunction occur less frequently (sinus node dysfunction reported with lithium-carbamazepine combination, with high plasma levels of lithium, and in patients taking other drugs that may affect conduction) [assess patient who has syncopal episode]

| Renal Effects |

- Usually seen after chronic use
- Enuresis, polyuria, and polydipsia – over 50% incidence (dose-related); monitor for fluid and electrolyte imbalance – usually reversible if lithium stopped; however, several cases of persistent diabetes insipidus reported up to 57 months after lithium stopped [potassium-sparing

diuretic (amiloride 10 mg/day) or DDAVP (10 µg nasal spray or tablets 0.2 mg) may be useful]; sustained-release preparations may cause less impairment of urine concentrating function
- Changes in distal tubular function including impaired urine concentrating ability in about 50% of patients (not always reversible) and chronic focal interstitial nephritis
- Reduced glomerular filtration rates reported with chronic treatment especially in patients who have had one or more episodes of lithium intoxication
- Histological changes include: a) interstitial fibrosis, tubular atrophy and glomerulosclerosis – primarily those with impaired urine concentrating ability; b) distal tubular dilatation and macrocyst formation
- Rare cases of nephrotic syndrome with proteinuria, glycosuria and oliguria, edema and hypoalbuminemia

Dermatological Effects	

- Dry skin common
- Skin rash, pruritus, "de-novo" or exacerbation of psoriasis
- Acne common
- Dryness and thinning of hair – may be related to hypothyroidism; alopecia reported in patients on chronic therapy
- Case reports of nail pigmentation

Endocrine Effects	

- Reports of irregular or prolonged menstrual cycles
- Long-term effects: clinical hypothyroidism may be more common in regions of high dietary iodine (monitor TSH level – may require levothyroxine therapy). Subclinical hypothyroidism (high TSH and normal free T_4) found in 25% of patients on lithium
- Goiter (not necessarily associated with hypothyroidism) – may be more common in regions of iodine deficiency
- Hyperparathyroidism with hypercalcemia reported; lithium may decrease bone density by altering the concentration of parathyroid hormone. Potential interactions with the developmental maturation of a child (e.g., skeletal growth) has not been studied

Other Adverse Effects	

- Blurred vision may be related to peak plasma levels; reduction in retinal light sensitivity, nystagmus
- Changes in sexual function
- Edema, swelling of extremities – evaluate for sodium retention [use diuretics with caution – see Drug Interactions – spironolactone may be preferred]
- Anemia, leukocytosis, leucopenia, albuminuria; rarely thrombocytopenia

DISCONTINUATION SYNDROME

- Rarely anxiety, instability, and emotional lability reported following abrupt withdrawal
- Rapid discontinuation may increase the risk of relapse
- 50% rate of manic or depressive recurrence within 3 to 5 months among previously stable patients reported with abrupt withdrawal

PRECAUTIONS

- Good kidney function, adequate salt and fluid intake are essential
- Excessive loss of sodium (due to vomiting, diarrhea, use of diuretics, etc.) causes increased lithium retention, possibly leading to toxicity; lower doses of lithium are necessary if the patient is on a salt-restricted diet (which includes most low-calorie diets)
- Heavy sweating can lead to changes in plasma level of lithium
- Avoid severe dehydration

Mood Stabilizers

Lithium (cont.)

- Use cautiously in patients with brain damage or thyroid disease
- Low margin of safety – can be lethal in overdose; assess factors affecting compliance (e.g., chaotic family situation, uncooperative patient) before prescribing

CONTRAINDICATIONS

- Sodium depletion
- Renal disease
- Cardiovascular disease
- Severe debilitation

TOXICITY

Mild Toxicity

- At lithium levels of 1.5–2 mmol/l; occasionally occurs with levels in the range of 1.0–1.2 mmol/l
- Develops gradually over several days
- Side effects such as ataxia, coarse tremor, confusion, diarrhea, drowsiness, fasciculation, and slurred speech may occur

Management

- Stop lithium; check renal function; consider a lower dose of lithium in 1–2 days

Moderate/Severe Toxicity

- At lithium levels in excess of 2 mmol/l
- Severe poisoning may result in coma with hyperreflexia, muscle tremor, hyperextension of the limbs, pulse irregularities, hypertension or hypotension, ECG changes, peripheral circulatory failure, and epileptic seizures; acute tubular necrosis (renal failure) can occur
- Lithium toxicity may manifest as a catatonic stupor
- Deaths have been reported; when serum lithium level exceeds 4 mmol/l the prognosis is poor

Management

- Symptomatic: Reduce absorption, restore fluid and electrolyte balance, correct sodium depletion and remove drug from the body
- Blood lithium concentration may be reduced by forced alkaline diuresis or by prolonged peritoneal dialysis or hemodialysis
- Excretion may be facilitated by IV urea, sodium bicarbonate, acetazolamide, or aminophylline
- Convulsions may be controlled by a short-acting barbiturate (thiopental sodium)

USE IN PREGNANCY

- Avoid in pregnancy (esp. first trimester), overall risk of fetal malformations is 4–12%; cardiovascular malformations can occur (tricuspid valve malformations; 0.05– 0.1% risk of Ebstein's anomaly) – can be detected by fetal echocardiography and high resolution ultrasound at 16–18 weeks gestation. If necessary, use lowest dose possible, in divided doses, to avoid peak concentrations. Monitor lithium levels during pregnancy, weekly in last month, during and immediately after delivery
- Lithium clearance increased by 50–100% in third trimester of pregnancy because of increases in plasma volume and greater glomerular filtration rate; rate returns to pre-pregnancy levels after delivery; dose should be decreased or drug discontinued 2–3 days prior to delivery
- Use of lithium near term may produce severe toxicity in the newborn, which is usually reversible, including nontoxic goiter, nephrogenic diabetes insipidus, floppy baby syndrome; can be minimized by withholding maternal lithium 24 h before delivery; can be minimized by withholding maternal lithium 24 h before delivery
- Do neonatal electrocardiogram if lithium was used in first trimester; observe infant for lithium toxicity for first 10 days of life

Breast Milk

- Present in breast milk at a concentration of 30–50% of mother's serum (infant's serum concentration is approximately equal to or less than that of the milk). Reported symptoms include hypotonia, cyanosis, lethargy, hypothermia, T-wave changes and heart murmur
- Infant has decreased renal clearance; the American Academy of Pediatrics considers lithium contraindicated during breastfeeding. Avoid until infant is at least 5 months old, due to decreased renal clearance
- If breastfeeding is undertaken, the mother should be educated about signs and symptoms of lithium toxicity and risks of infant dehydration; monitor infant lithium levels and consider periodic thyroid evaluation

MONITORING RECOMMENDATIONS

At beginning of treatment and at every admission:
1) Serum electrolytes
2) Hb, Hct, WBC and differential
3) TSH (total T4, T4 uptake if TSH level abnormal)
4) BUN, creatinine
5) Calcium
6) Parathormone
7) ECG

On an out-patient basis, repeat tests (2) + (3) every 6 months; (4) every 6 to 12 months; (5) every 2 years; (6) every 5 years. As some rapid cycling may be due to lithium-induced hypothyroidism, it is important to regularly assess thyroid function
- Plasma level monitoring – see Pharmacokinetics p. 201

NURSING IMPLICATIONS

- Accurate observation and assessment of patient's behavior before and after lithium therapy is initiated is important
- Be alert for, observe, and report any signs of side effects, or symptoms of toxicity; if toxic withhold the dose and call doctor immediately
- Have patient maintain normal salt intake and check fluid intake and output; adjust fluid and salt ingestion to compensate if excessive loss occurs through vomiting or diarrhea
- Expect nausea, thirst, frequent urination, and generalized discomfort during the first few days; therapeutic effects occur gradually and may take up to 3 weeks
- May give lithium with meals to avoid GI disturbances
- Caffeine intake should not be dramatically altered while taking lithium
- Withhold morning dose of lithium until after the blood draw, on mornings when blood is drawn for a lithium level
- The patient and family should be educated regarding the drug's effects and toxicities
- Slow release preparations should not be broken or crushed. They may decrease side effects that occur as a result of high peak plasma levels (i.e., 1–2 h post dose), e.g., tremor
- Because lithium may cause drowsiness, caution patient to avoid activities requiring alertness until response to drug has been determined
- Due to low margin of safety, the importance of compliance should be emphasized

PATIENT INSTRUCTIONS

- Detailed instructions for patients and caregivers are provided in the Information Sheet on p. 325

Lithium (cont.)

DRUG INTERACTIONS   • Clinically significant interactions are listed below

Class of Drug	Example	Interaction Effects
Alcohol		Increased tremor/shakiness with chronic alcohol use
Anesthetic	Ketamine	Increased lithium toxicity due to sodium depletion
Angiotensin-converting enzyme (ACE) inhibitor	Captopril, enalapril, lisinopril	Increased lithium toxicity due to sodium depletion; average increase in lithium level of 36% reported
ACE-2 inhibitor	Cardesartan, losartan, valsartan	Reports of lithium toxicity possibly due to reduced aldosterone levels
Antibiotic/anti-infective	Ampicillin, doxycycline, tetracycline, spectinomycin, levofloxacin, metroni dazole	Case reports of increased lithium effect and toxicity due to decreased renal clearance of lithium. Monitor lithium level if combination used
Anticonvulsant	Carbamazepine, phenytoin, valproate	Increased neurotoxicity of both drugs at therapeutic doses Synergistic mood-stabilizing effect with carbamazepine and valproate Valproate may aggravate action tremor
Antidepressant Cyclic, MAOIs, RIMA	Desipramine, tranylcypromine, moclobemide	Synergistic antidepressant effect in treatment-resistant patients May increase lithium tremor
SSRIs	Fluoxetine, fluvoxamine, sertraline	Elevated lithium serum level, with possible neurotoxicity and increased serotonergic effects (see p. 46)
Antihypertensive	Amiloride, spironolactone, thiazides, triamterene, methyldopa	Increased lithium effects and toxicity due to decreased renal clearance of lithium
	Acetazolamide, mannitol, urea	Increased renal excretion of lithium, decreasing its effect
	β-blockers: propranolol, oxprenolol	Beneficial effect in treatment of lithium tremor; propranolol lowers glomerular filtration rate and has been associated with a 19% reduction in lithium clearance
Antipsychotics	Molindone	Increased plasma level of molindone reported; variable effects on plasma level of neuroleptics as well as lithium seen
	Haloperidol, perphenazine	Increased neurotoxicity possible at therapeutic doses; may increase EPS; cases of NMS reported
	Clozapine	Possible increased risk of agranulocytosis with clozapine; two cases of seizures reported with combination
Antiviral agent	Zidovudine	Reversal of zidovudine-induced neutropenia
Benzodiazepines	Clonazepam	Increased incidence of sexual dysfunction (up to 49%) reported with the combination
Ca-channel blocker	Verapamil, diltiazem	Increased neurotoxicity of both drugs; increased bradycardia and cardiotoxicity with verapamil due to combined calcium blockade
Caffeine		Increased renal excretion of lithium resulting in decreased plasma level May increase lithium tremor

Class of Drug	Example	Interaction Effects
Herbal diuretics	Agrimony, dandelion, juniper, licorice, horsetail, uva ursi	Elevated lithium level possible due to decreased renal clearance
	Cola nut, guarana, maté	Increased excretion and decreased lithium level possible due to high content of caffeine in herbal preparations
Iodide salt	Calcium iodide	May act synergistically to produce hypothyroidism. AVOID
L-Tryptophan		Increased plasma level and increased efficacy and/or toxicity of lithium
Metronidazole		Decreased renal clearance of lithium resulting in elevated plasma levels. Monitor lithium level, creatinine and electrolyte levels and osmolality
NSAID	Ibuprofen, ketorolac, diclofenac, indomethacin, mefenamic acid, naproxen, celecoxib, rofecoxib, sulindac (no interaction with ASA)	Increased lithium level and possible toxicity due to decreased renal clearance of lithium (up to 133% increase reported with celecoxib, up to 448% with rofecoxib, up to 300% with mefenamic acid); serum creatinine increased in several reports. Use caution and monitor lithium level every 4–5 days until stable
Neuromuscular blocker	Succinylcholine, pancuronium	Potentiation of muscle relaxation
Psyllium	Metamucil, Prodiem	Decreased lithium level if drugs taken at the same time. Increased water drawn into the colon by the bulk laxatives would increase the amount of ionized lithium, which would remain unabsorbed
Sodium salt		Increased intake results in decreased lithium plasma level; decreased intake causes increased lithium plasma level
Theophylline	Aminophylline, oxtriphylline, theophylline	Enhanced renal lithium clearance and reduced plasma level (by approx. 20%) May increase lithium tremor
Trimethoprim/Sulfamethoxazole		Case report of lithium toxicity within days of starting antimicrobial
Triptan	Sumatriptan, zolmitriptan	Increased serotonergic effects possible – monitor
Urinary alkalizer	Potassium citrate, sodium bicarbonate	Enhanced renal lithium clearance and reduced plasma level

Mood Stabilizers

Anticonvulsants

PRODUCT AVAILABILITY

Chemical Class	Generic Name	Trade Name[A]	Dosage Forms and Strengths	Monograph Statement
First generation	Clonazepam	Rivotril[C], Klonopin[B]	See p. 179	
Second generation	Carbamazepine	Tegretol[C]	Tablets: 100 mg[B], 200 mg, 300 mg[B], 400 mg[B] Chewable tablets: 100 mg, 200 mg Oral suspension: 100 mg/5 ml	Dosage recommendations available for children
		Tegretol CR[C]	Controlled-release tablets[C]: 200 mg, 400 mg	
		Carbatrol[B], Tegretel XR[B], Equetro[B]	Extended release capsules[B]: 100 mg, 200 mg, 300 mg, 400 mg	
	Divalproex sodium	Epival ECT[C]	Enteric-coated tablets[C]: 125 mg, 250 mg, 500 mg	Dosage recommendations available for children
		Epival ER[C], Depakote ER[B]	Extended release tablets: 250 mg[B], 500 mg	
		Depakote[B]	Delayed-release tablets: 125 mg, 250 mg, 500 mg	
	Valproic acid	Depakene, Valproic acid EC[C]	Enteric-coated capsules[C]: 500 mg Capsules: 250 mg, 500 mg[C] Oral syrup: 250 mg/5 ml	Dosage recommendations available for children
		Epiject IV	Injection[C]: 500 mg/5 ml	
	Valproate Sodium[B]		Injection[B]: 100 mg/ml	
Third generation	Gabapentin	Neurontin	Capsules: 100 mg, 300 mg, 400 mg Tablets: 600 mg, 800 mg Oral solution[B]: 250 mg/5 mg	Dosage recommendations available for children
	Lamotrigine	Lamictal	Tablets: 25 mg, 100 mg, 150 mg, 200 mg[B] Chewable tablets: 2 mg, 5 mg, 25 mg[B]	Dosage recommendations available for children
	Oxcarbazepine[D]	Trileptal	Tablets 150mg, 300mg, 600mg Oral suspension: 300 mg/5ml	Dosage recommendations available for children
	Topiramate	Topamax	Tablets: 25 mg, 100 mg, 200 mg Sprinkle capsules: 15 mg, 25 mg	Dosage recommendations available for children

[A] Generic preparations may be available, [B] Not marketed in Canada, [C] Not marketed in USA, [D] Not reviewed in this chapter

INDICATIONS

	Carbamazepine	Oxcarbazepine [A]	Valproate	Gabapentin[A]	Lamotrigine[A]	Topiramate[A]
Acute mania/hypomania	▲ [A] (+ case reports and open trials in C+A)	+	▲ [A] (+ open trials in C+A)	+/– (Bipolar II) (adjunctive drug – data contradictory)	+/– (data contradictory)	+/– (adjunctive drug – data preliminary in children)

	Carbamazepine	Oxcarbazepine [A]	Valproate	Gabapentin [A]	Lamotrigine [A]	Topiramate [A]
Prophylaxis of BD	▲ [A]	+/−	+/− (data contradictory)	+/− (open trials, adjunctive drug)	+ (Bipolar I depression)	−
Rapid-cycling BD	+/−	−	+	+/− (adjunctive drug – data contradictory)	+ (Bipolar II)	+ (ultrarapid cycling – preliminary data)
Mixed states	▲ [A]	+ (preliminary data, adjunctive drug)	+ (open trials in C+A)	+/− (open trials, adjunctive drug)	+	+/−
Bipolar depression	+ (data contradictory)	+ (preliminary data)	+/− (data adjunctive)	+ (open trials)	+ (Bipolar I) (open trial; adjunctive data in adolescents)	+/− (adjunctive – preliminary data)
Anticonvulsant	▲ Prophylaxis and treatment of complex partial and limbic region seizures	▲ Partial seizures (sole or adjunctive agent)	▲ Absences, simple and complex partial generalized seizures	▲ Adjunctive in refractory epilepsy	▲ Adjunctive or sole therapy in refractory epilepsy	▲ Adjunctive therapy in refractory epilepsy
Paroxysmal pain syndromes	▲	+ (neuropathy – open label)	+	▲ Postherpetic neuralgia + (neuropathic pain)	+ (central pain)	+ (neuropathic pain – preliminary data)
Migraine headaches	−	?	▲ [A]	+ (preliminary data)	+/− (preliminary data-contradictory)	▲ [A] Prophylaxis
Behavior disturbances (in dementia, explosive disorder, mental retardation, brain damage)	+/− (alone or in combination with lithium, antipsychotics, or β-blockers)	+ preliminary	+	+ (preliminary data)	+/− (data contradictory in autism)	+
Panic disorder	+ [A]	+ (case reports)	+ [A]	+ (double-blind trials)	no data	−
Social phobia, generalized anxiety disorder	−	no data	+/− [A] (open trial)	+	no data	+ (preliminary data – open trial)
Posttraumatic stress disorder	+ (open-trials)	Case report	+ [A] (open trials)	+ (adjunctive – preliminary data)	+	+ (open trials)
Obsessive compulsive disorder	+/− (augmenting drug - preliminary data)	+ (case report – adjunctive drug)	−	+ (adjunctive to SSRIs – preliminary data)	+/− (case report – adjunctive drug)	+ (open trial – adjunctive drug)
Movement disorders	Dystonic disorder in children	−	−	Management of tardive dyskinesia in psychotic patients with mood features (preliminary data)	−	Essential tremor (preliminary data)

Mood Stabilizers

Anticonvulsants (cont.)

	Carbamazepine	Oxcarbazepine [(A)]	Valproate	Gabapentin[(A)]	Lamotrigine[(A)]	Topiramate[(A)]
Drug dependence	Aid in alcohol or sedative/hypnotic withdrawal; may play a role in cocaine dependence	–	Aid in alcohol withdrawal (open trials)	May reduce craving for cocaine as well as its usage Aid in alcohol withdrawal (open trials)	Aid in alcohol withdrawal (open trials) May reduce cravings for cocaine	Aid in treatment of alcohol dependence together with behavior modification (comormid trail)
Diabetes Insipidus	+	–	–	–	–	–

▲ Approved indications, for adults **No anticonvulsant is approved for use in mood disorders in either children or adolescents**
[(A)]☐

GENERAL COMMENTS

- No controlled trials have been done with anticonvulsants in children and adolescents with BD; open studies in children and adolescents suggest some efficacy with valproate and carbamazepine
- The younger the age, the less chance of robust response to a mood stabilizer; only about 30% of young adults do well on monotherapy; for optimal response, combination therapy may be required: e.g., with another mood stabilizer, an antipsychotic, antidepressant, or ECT
- Have been found useful to treat aggression in children and adolescents with conduct disorder and organic brain syndromes
- Compliance with antimanic medication suggested to markedly decrease recidivism in juvenile delinquents with BD
- Combined treatment with lithium, a second anticonvulsant or a novel antipsychotic tends to provide better outcomes than use of a single agent
- See chart p. 212 for specific agents

DOSING

- See p. 213 for specific agents
- Plasma level monitoring for carbamazepine and valproate (measured at trough) has been used to guide dosing; however, suggested therapeutic ranges are for the treatment and prophylaxis of seizure disorders, not BD
- Younger children, especially those receiving enzyme-inducing drugs, will require higher maintenance doses of valproate to attain therapeutic total and unbound (free) valproate plasma concentrations
- Reduced dosages recommended in hepatic or renal disorders (see p. 213)
- With topiramate a low starting dose and gradual dose increments minimize cognitive and behavioral side effects

PHARMACOKINETICS

- See p. 214 for specific agents
- Clearance of carbamazepine is higher in children than in adults; children may be at risk for major toxicities at lower serum concentrations due to increased production of toxic metabolite; case reports of behavior disturbances, mania and worsening of tics. Males may have higher/faster clearance of carbamazepine than females of similar age and weight
- Extended release carbamazepine contains immediate release, extended release, and enteric coated beads; should not be chewed or crushed, but can be opened and sprinkled on food
- With valproate, pharmacokinetics show significant variation with changes in body weight. Valproate exhibits concentration-dependent protein binding, therefore at high doses and plasma concentrations a larger proportion may exist in unbound (free) form

- Gabapentin shows dose-dependent bioavailability as a result of a saturable transport mechanism (better bioavailability with more frequent dosing;
- plasma level is proportional to the dose). Children under the age of 5 may require approximately 30% larger dose to achieve desired serum concentration due to enhanced clearance. Elimination is almost entirely by the kidneys, and is reduced in patients with renal dysfunction (see p. 213)
- Lamotrigine: increased metabolism in children results in greater formation of reactive arene oxide metabolite and a higher incidence of rash – use lower starting dose and titrate slowly
- Children have lower topiramate concentrations than adults receiving the same dose per body weight

ADVERSE EFFECTS

- See pp. 214–217 for specific agents
- Common (for all anticonvulsants):
  - GI complaints, e.g., nausea [Management: take with food, change to an enteric-coated preparation, use ranitidine 150 mg/day or famotidine 20 mg/day]
  - Dose-related lethargy, sedation, behavior changes/deterioration, reversible dementia/encephalopathy. Children with pre-existing ADHD, developmental delays or learning disabilities are more likely to experience adverse behavioral effects
  - Dose-related tremor; tends to be rhythmic, rapid, symmetrical and most prominent in upper extremities [reduce dose if possible; responds to pro-pranolol]
  - Ataxia
  - Changes in appetite, weight gain (except lamotrigine and topiramate) –more common in females; may be associated with features of insulin resistance. Weight increases with duration of treatment. Obesity may increase risk of hyperandrogenism in females
  - Menstrual disturbances (except gabapentin), including: prolonged cycles, oligomenorrhea, amenorrhea, polycystic ovaries; elevated testosterone – rates may be higher in females who begin taking valproate before age 20
- Occasional (for all anticonvulsants):
  - Dysarthria, incoordination
  - Diplopia, nystagmus
- Rare – Anticonvulsant hypersensitivity syndrome with fever, rash and internal organ involvement; cross-sensitivity reported between carbamazepine and lamotrigine
- Osteoporosis reported with carbamazepine and valproate; bone loss is related to treatment duration and decreased 25-hydroxy vitamin D levels. Some clinicians recommend baseline bone density in adolescents requiring chronic treatment [optimize vitamin D and calcium intake]

Comparison of Anticonvulsants

	Carbamazepine	Oxcarbazepine	Valproate	Gabapentin	Lamotrigine	Topiramate
General comments	Positive predictors of response include: non-classic or secondary mania, an early age at onset, a negative family history of mood disorder, and patients with neurological abnormalities Less response noted in patients with severe mania, dysphoric mania and rapid cycling disorder May be equivalent to lithium in the treatment of manic symptoms in adolescent bipolar disorder	Pharmacological activity is exerted primarily through the 10-monohydroxy metabolite (MHD) of oxcarbazepine Early data suggest similar pharmacological activity as carbamazepine with a lower potential for serious adverse effects	Positive predictors of response include: pure mania, mixed or dysphoric mania and patients with secondary or rapid cycling disorder Good response in adolescents and in mania with comorbid substance use disorder Retrospective review suggests efficacy in affective instability, depression, and repetitive behaviors of pervasive developmental disorder Less response noted in patients with comorbid personality disorder, severe mania and those previously treated with antidepressants or stimulants May be more effective in treating and preventing manic and mixed episodes than depressive episodes May be used in adolescents more often than lithium because of better tolerability (less weight gain and acne)	May be more effective as an adjunctive medication in both Bipolar I and Bipolar II disorders (evidence limited to open trials), especially in the presence of significant anxiety Not recommended as a primary mood stabilizer in children with Bipolar disorder	More effective in Bipolar I disorder against depression; suggested to have antidepressant properties First-line agent for treatment of bipolar depression in patients with a history of severe refractory manic episodes: does not induce switches to hypomania or mania Prophylaxis of rapid cycling and Bipolar II disorder Risk of serious skin rash, including Stevens Johnson syndrome	Useful as an adjunct to other mood stabilizers in refractory mania and in ultrarapid or ultradician cycling disorder Not often used in children and adolescents due to minimal efficacy data and cognitive side effects
Pharmacology	Anticonvulsant, antikindling, and GABA-ergic activity Blocks voltage-dependent sodium channels	MHD metabolite has anticonvulsant, antikindling, and GABA-ergic activity Blocks voltage-dependent sodium channels and calcium channels	Anticonvulsant, antikindling, and GABA-ergic activity Block Ca channels Indirectly blocks voltage-dependent sodium channels Increases serotonergic function	Anticonvulsant, antikindling, and GABA-ergic activity Blocks voltage-dependent sodium channels Inhibits excitatory amino acids (glutamate)	Anticonvulsant and GABA-ergic activity Blocks voltage-dependent sodium channels Inhibits excitatory amino acids (glutamate)	Anticonvulsant, antikindling, and GABA-ergic activity Inhibits excitatory amino acids (glutamate) Inhibits carbonic anhydrase and blocks voltage-dependent sodium channels

	Carbamazepine	Oxcarbazepine	Valproate	Gabapentin	Lamotrigine	Topiramate
Dosing	Age < 5: begin at 10–20mg/kg/day in divided doses and increase weekly as needed to a maximum of 35 mg/kg/day Ages 6–12: Begin at 100–200 mg daily in divided doses and increase by 100 mg twice weekly, until either side effects limit dose, or reach therapeutic plasma level Dose range: Children: 200–600 mg/day, Adolescents: 300–1200 mg/day in single or divided doses	Age 4–16; begin at 8–10 mg/kg/day or 600 mg per day (whichever lower) in 2 doses and increase every 3 days up to the mainte-nance dose: < 20 kg = 600–900 mg 21–30 kg = 900–1200 mg 31–40 kg = 1200–1500 mg 41–45 kg = 1200–1500 mg 46–55 kg = 1200–1800 mg 56–65 kg = 1200–2100 mg > 66 kg = 1500–2100 mg Children < 8 years old have increased clearance	Children: give a test dose of 125 mg, then begin at 125 mg bid-tid and increase gradually Adolescents: give a test dose of 250 mg, then be-gin at 250 mg bid-tid and increase dose gradually, until either side effects limit dose, or reach thera-peutic plasma level Dose range: Children: 1000–1200 mg/day Adolescents: 1000–2500 mg/day in divided doses	Begin at 10–15 mg/kg/day given tid and increase gradually q 3–5 days; Ages 3–4: usual effective dose 40 mg/kg/day Over age 5: usual effec-tive dose 30 mg/kg/day Maximum dose: 50 mg/kg/day Usual dose range: 900–1800 mg/day Anxiety: up to 2400 mg/day	Begin at 25–50 mg/day in divided doses and increase by 12.5–25 mg every 7 days to a main-tenance dose of 200–400 mg/day Max dose = 700 mg/day *If given with valproate:* use 0.15–0.3 mg/kg/day Maintenance dose: 1–5 mg/kg/day to a maximum of 150 mg/day *If given with an enzyme inducer:* use 0.6–1 mg/kg/day in two divided doses Maintenance dose: 5–10 mg/kg/day to a maximum of 400 mg/day	Children < 12 years old: give 1–3 mg/kg/day (max 25 mg) hs, and increase dose weekly by 1–3 mg/kg/day (given bid) Usual dose: 5–9 mg/kg/day Higher doses may be needed If given with enzyme inducers (up to 22 mg/kg/day) Children > 12 years: give 25–50 mg hs, and increase dose weekly by 25–50 mg (given bid) to a usual dose of 400 mg/day Increased clearance in young children
Renal impairment	?	Decrease dose by 50% if creatinine clearance < 30 ml/min	Free valproate level dou-bles in renal impairment	Decrease dose if creati-nine clearance (CrCl) < 60 ml/min If CrCl 30–59 ml/min, give drug bid to a maximal daily dose of 1400 mg If CrCl 15–29 ml/min, give drug once daily up to 700 mg/day If CrCl 15 ml/min, give up to a maximum of 300 mg once daily; reduce dose proportionally with decreasing CrCl	Reduced clearance	Moderate: clearance reduced by 42% Severe: clearance reduced by 54%
Hepatic impairment	Reduced clearance	Caution–see hepatic ad-verse effects p. 187	No effect	No effect	Reduce initial and main-tenance doses by 50% in mild to moderate impair-ment and 75% in severe impairment	Reduced clearance
Recommended plasma level	17–54 µmol/l (4–12 µg/ml)	15–35 µg/ml (MHD metabnolite)	350–700 µmol/l (50–115 µg/ml)	–	–	–

Mood Stabilizers

Comparison of Anticonvulsants (cont.)

	Carbamazepine	Oxcarbazepine	Valproate	Gabapentin	Lamotrigine	Topiramate
Pharmacokinetics						
Bioavailability	75–85%	> 95%	78%	Approx 60% (dose-dependent; higher with qid dosing)	98%	80%
Peak plasma level (T_{max})	1–6 h	1–3 h (parent) 4–12 h (active MHD metabolite) and 2–4 h at steady state	Oral valproic acid: 1–4 h (may be delayed by food) Divalproex and extended-release: 3–8 h	2–3 h	1–5 h (rate may be reduced by food)	1.4–5 h (delayed by food)
Protein binding	75–90% (alpha, -acid gly-coprotein and albumin)	40%	80–90% (concentration dependent); increased by lowfat diers	Minimal (< 3%)	55% (primarily albumin)	15%
Half-life	25–65 h (acute use); 8–17 h (chronic use) – stimulates own metabolism	Parent: 1–5 h MHD metabolite: 7–20 h	3.5–20 h; mean of 9 h in children aged 2–14 years	5 h	33 h mean (acute use) 26 h mean (chronic use) – stimulates own metabolism	19–23 h in adults; increased clearance in children
CYP-450 metabolizing enzymes	1A3, 3A4[m], 2C8, 2C9	Rapidly metabolized by cytosolic enzymes to active metabolite MHD	2A6, 2C9, 2C19, UGT	Not metabolized – eliminated unchanged by renal excretion	Metabolized primarily by glucuronic acid conjugation, and by UGT	Not metabolized – 70% eliminated unchanged in urine
CYP-450 effect	Inducer of 1A2, 3A4[p], 2C9, 2B6 Induces own metabolism	Moderate inducer of CYP3A4 Inhibitor of CYP2C19 (does not induce own metabolism)	Inhibitor of 2D6[w], 2C9, 2C19, UGT	–	Inhibits UGT	–
Adverse effects						
CNS	Sedation (15%), cognitive blunting, confusion (higher doses)	Sedation common, lethargy	Sedation common, lethargy, asthenia, behavior changes/deterioration, cognitive blunting, confusion, encephalopathy	Sedation, fatigue, abnormal thinking, problems concentrating, amnesia	Sedation, asthenia, cognitive blunting	Sedation, lethargy, fatigue common, psychomotor slowing, confusion. Deficits in word-finding, concentration and memory (dose dependent)
	Agitation, restlessness, irritability, insomnia, delirium Case reports of behavioral disturbances and mania in patients with mental retardation		Hyperactivity, restlessness, irritability, aggression Rare cases of psychosis Case reports of disinhibition	Nervousness, anxiety, restlessness, irritability (5%), hostility (5%), aggression Emotional lability (6%) Rare switches to hypomania/mania Cases of depression Case reports of disinhibition	Agitation, activation, irritability, insomnia Switches to hypomania/mania	Anxiety, agitation, nervousness, irritability, insomnia Increased panic attacks, worsening of depression or psychosis

	Carbamazepine	Oxcarbazepine	Valproate	Gabapentin	Lamotrigine	Topiramate
	Headache Tremors, ataxia, paresthesias, acute dystonic reactions, chronic dyskinesias Reports of worsening of tics	Headache Ataxia, gait disturbances, tremor	Headache common Tremors (15% in children –tend to be rhythmic, rapid, symmetrical and most prominent in the upper extremities), ataxia, dysarthria, incoordination	Fever Tremors, ataxia, incoordination, dysarthria, myalgia	Headache, fever Tremors, ataxia, incoordination, myalgia, arthralgia	Headache Tremors, ataxia; paresthesias
Anticholinergic	Blurred vision, mydriasis, cycloplegia, ophthalmoplegia, dry mouth, slurred speech Constipation, urinary retention	Blurred vision	–	Dry mouth or throat (2%) Constipation	Blurred vision Constipation	Blurred vision, sweating Acute angle closure reported
Gastrointestinal	Nausea and vomiting Diarrhea, abdominal cramps Weight gain (may be associated with polycystic ovaries)	Nausea common, vomiting	Nausea common, vomiting Weight gain; more common in females and with high plasma levels; may be associated with increased leptin and features of insulin resistance Weight loss	Nausea and vomiting Dyspepsia Weight gain (common with higher doses)	Nausea, vomiting, diarrhea Rarely esophagitis No weight gain	Nausea and vomiting Anorexia; weight loss (not conclusively shown in children) Change in taste of carbonated beverages
Cardiovascular	Dizziness Edema Dysrhythmias, heart block Vasculitis	Dizziness, peripheral edema	Rarely dizziness Vasculitis	Dizziness, hypotension Occasionally hypertension Peripheral edema	Breathlessness, dizziness Conduction changes (prolongation of PR interval)	Dizziness common
Dermatological	Rash (10–15%) – severe dermatological reactions may signify impending blood dyscrasias Hair loss (6%) Photosensitivity reactions Rarely: fixed drug eruptions, lichenoid-like reactions, bullous reactions, exfoliative dermatitis, vasculitis Hypersensitivity syndrome Rare; with fever, skin eruptionsAnd internal organ involvement	Rash; 25–30% of patients are cross-sensitive Stevens-Johnson syndrome, toxic epidermal necrolysis in adults and children	Rash Hair loss (higher incidence with higher doses); changes in texture or color of hair Case reports of nail pigmentation Rare cases of Stevens-Johnson syndrome, toxic epidermal necrolysis, lupus, vasculitis, erythema multiforme, or skin pigmentation	Pruritus	Rash; in 2–3% require drug discontinuation – risk of severe rash increased with rapid dose titration, in those < 16 years of age, and in combination with valproate Stevens-Johnson syndrome in1–2% of children and 0.1% of adults (Usually within first 8 weeks) Rarely, erythema multiforme, hypersensitivity syndrome Photosensitivity reactions	Rash

Comparison of Anticonvulsants (cont.)

	Carbamazepine	Oxcarbazepine	Valproate	Gabapentin	Lamotrigine	Topiramate
Hematologic	Transitory leukopenia, persistent leukopenia Rarely, eosinophilia, aplastic Anemia, thrombocytopenia, purpura, and agranulocytosis	Rare	Reversible thrombocytopenia may be related to high plasma levels; prolongation of bleeding times Macrocytic anemia, coagulopathies	Leukopenia (1%), purpura	Neutropenia Rarely, hematemesis, hemolytic anemia, thrombocytopenia pancytopenia, aplastic anemia	Purpura
Hepatic	Transient enzyme elevation evaluate for hepatotoxicity if elevation > 3 times normal Rarely, hepatocellular and cholestatic jaundice, granulomatous hepatitis and severe hepatic necrosis/failure	Rare	Asymptomatic hepatic transaminase elevation Cases of severe liver toxicity primarily in very young children on multiple medications	Case reports of abnormal liver function	Rare	Cases of severe liver damage
Endocrine	Menstrual disturbances in females Decreased libido in males Elevation of total cholesterol (primarily HDL), low-density lipoproteins and ratio of total cholesterol to low-density lipoproteins Can lower thyroxine levels and TSH response to TRH Polycystic ovaries reported in up to 45% of females Osteopenia; can deplete Vit D levels	Hyperthermia	Menstrual disturbances common, including prolonged cycles, oligomenorrhea, amenorrhea, polycystic ovaries (up to 80%), flushing In females: hyperandrogenism (increased testosterone in 33%), android obesity (in up to 53%), hirsutism, hyperinsulinemia Osteopenia; increased bone resorption and decreased bone mineral density (reported in up to 14%) may conduce to osteoporosis; rarely osteomalacia Decreased levels of HDL, low HDL/cholesterol ratio, increased triglyceride levels	Impotence	Menstrual disturbances, dysmenorrhea, vaginitis	Decreased sweating, hyperthermia
Ocular	Diplopia, nystagmus, blurred Vision, visual hallucinations, lens abnormalities	Diplopia, nystagmus	Diplopia, nystagmus, blurred vision, asterixis (spots before the eyes)	Diplopia, nystagmus, amblyopia	Diplopia, nystagmus, amblyopia	Diplopia, nystagmus Cases of acute myopia and secondary angle closure glaucoma

	Carbamazepine	Oxcarbazepine	Valproate	Gabapentin	Lamotrigine	Topiramate
Other	Hyponatremia and water intoxication – more commonwith higher plasma levels Rarely: acute renal failure, osteomalacia, pancreatitis, splenomegaly, lymphadenopathy, systemic lupus erythematosus and serum sickness	Hyponatremia (26% incidence)	Gingival hyperplasia Carnitine deficiency; Hyperammonemia; usually asymptomatic, but may cause increased sedation, confusion, stupor and/or coma Rarely: pancreatitis, and serum sickness	Rhinitis, pharyngitis Back pain, dysarthria	Rhinitis, pharyngitis Rarely, apnea, pancreatitis	Hyponatremia Nephrolithiasis (renal stone formation) in up to 1.5% with chronbic use Epistaxis Decrease in sodium bicarbonate (up to 30% patients) Metabolic acidosis (may increase risk for nephrolithiasis or nephrocalcinosis and may result in osteomalacia and/or osteoporosis)
Chronic or serious conditions	Bone marrow suppression, ocular effects, SIADH (hyponatremia), hypersensitivity syndrome (0.1%), osteopenia	Hyponatremia Stevens-Johnson syndrome, toxic epidermal necrolysis	Endocrine (females), thrombocytopenia, leukopenia, hyperammonemia, hepatic toxicity, Stevens-Johnson syndrome, pancreatitis, osteopenia, osteoporosis	None known	Rash, Stevens-Johnson syndrome, toxic epidermal necrolysis, hypersensitivity syndrome (0.1%); PR prolongation	Untreated metabolic acidosis, Nephrolithiasis, hyperthermia, acute myopia, reduced growth rate
Use in pregnancy	Avoid during first trimester; if necessary, use lowest amount possible in divided doses and monitor drug levels througout pregnancy Caution; 5.7% risk of teratogenic effects, lower birth rates, and developmental delays Risk of spina bifida up to 1% congenital heart defects 9%, craniofacial defects 1%, fingernail hyperplasia 26%, and developmental delays 20% [Vitamin K and folic acid supplementation recommended] Clearance increased 2-fold during pregnancy; dose may need to be increased by 100%	Crosses placenta; teratogenic effects reported in animals; likely to cause teratogenic effects in humans	AVOID; 11.1% risk of malformations – related to dose anddrug plasm level. Fetal serum concentrations are 1.4 times that of the mother; half-life prolonged in infant Risk of spina bifida 1.2%, neural tube defects up to 5%, neurological dysfunction and developmental deficits seen in up to 71%; musculoskeletal, cardiovascular, pulmonary, genital and skin defects also reported [Vitamin K and folic acid supplementation recommended] Total plasma valproate concentration decreased during pregnancy as a result of increased volume of distribution and clearance; plasma protein binding decreased	Fetotoxicity reported in animal studies; risk to humans is currently unknown	Crosses placenta; levels comparable to those in maternal plasma Half-life increased in infant 3.2% risk of malformations; risk increases to 5.4% for total daily dose > 200mg; increased risk of cleft lip and/or cleft palate [Folic acid supplementation recommended] Lamotrigine metabolism appears to be induced during pregnancy and plasma levels increase rapidly after delivery	Fetotoxicity reported in animal studies. Risk to humans is currently unknown Case reports of hypospasiasin male infants [Folic acid supplementation recommended]

Mood Stabilizers

Comparison of Anticonvulsants (cont.)

	Carbamazepine	Oxcarbazepine	Valproate	Gabapentin	Lamotrigine	Topiramate
Breast milk	American Academy of Pediatrics considers carbamazepine compatible with breastfeeding Breast milk contains 7–95% of maternal drug concentration; infant serum level is 6–65% of mother's Educate mother about signs and symptoms of hepatic dysfunction and CNS effects of drug in the infant Monitor liver enzymes and CBC of infant and mother No long-term cognitive or behavioral effects reported in infant	Excreted into breast milk at levels up to 50% of those in maternal plasma Effects on infant unknown	American Academy of Pediatrics considers valproate compatible with breastfeeding Infant plasma level of valproate is up to 40% of that of mother; half-life in infants is significantly longer than in adults Educate mother about the signs and symptoms of hepatic dysfunction and those of hematological abnormalities in the infant Monitor liver enzymes and CBC of infant and mother No long-term cognitive or behavioral effects reported in infant	Amount of gabapentin in breast milk is approximately equivalent to that in maternal serum; effects on infant are unknown No long-term cognitive or behavioral effects reported in infant	Breastfeeding is not recommended Excreted in breast milk; the mild/plasma ratio is about 0.6 Infant serum levels are 25–30% of those of mother Consider risk of life-threatening rash	Breastfeeding not recommended due to possible psychomotor slowing and somnolence in infant

$^{(m)}$ Moderate, $^{(p)}$ Potent activity, $^{(w)}$ Weak activity

DISCONTINUATION SYNDROME

- No evidence of psychological or physical dependence to anticonvulsants (with the exception of benzodiazepines and barbiturates)
- Myoclonic jerks have been reported following the tapering of carbamazepine or valproate
- Abrupt discontinuation (especially in patients with a seizure disorder) may provoke rebound seizures – taper gradually

PRECAUTIONS

- Prior to treatment laboratory investigations should be performed (see p. 221)

Carbamazepine

- Carbamazepine induces its own hepatic metabolism; therefore, bi-weekly determinations of serum carbamazepine should be done for the first 2 months, monthly for 6 months, then at clinical discretion (at least every 6 months) or when there is a change in drug regimen
- Carbamazepine induces the metabolism of drugs metabolized by the cytochrome P-450 system (see Drug Interactions pp. 223–225)
- Because of its anticholinergic effects, give cautiously to patients taking other medications with anticholinergic activity
- Orientals may need lower doses
- Any cutaneous eruption, with fever, should be investigated for internal organ involvement. Check blood (CBC) if patient reports fever, sore throat, petechiae or bruising. Mild degree of blood cell suppression can occur; stop therapy if WBC levels drop below 3,000 white cells/mm^3; erythrocytes less than 4×10^6 mm^3; platelets less than 100,000 mm^3; hemoglobin less than 11 g/dl; reticulocyte count below 3%; or if serum iron rises above 150 mg/dl

- Administer cautiously in patients with a history of cardiac, hepatic, or renal disease
- Discontinue MAOI for at least 2 weeks prior to starting carbamazepine
- Patients who develop cutaneous reactions to carbamazepine should avoid the use of amitriptyline (as carbamazepine has a similar tricyclic structure)
- Do not administer carbamazepine suspension together with any other liquid preparation as formation of an insoluble precipitate can occur
- Higher peak concentrations may occur with liquid preparations
- A hypersensitivity syndrome with fever, skin eruptions and internal organ involvement occurs rarely – cross-sensitivity with other anticonvulsants (e.g., lamotrigine, oxcarbazepine)

Oxcarbazepine

- 25–30% of patients who exhibited hypersensitivity reactions to carbamazepine may also have these reactions with oxcarbazepine
- Monitor sodium levels with chronic use due to risk of hyponatremia
- Cases of Stevens-Johnson syndrome and toxic epidermal necrolysis reported in both adults and children
- A hypersensitivity syndrome with fever, skin eruptions, and internal organ involvement occurs rarely – cross-sensitivity possible with other anticonvulsants (e.g., lamotrigine, carbamazepine)

Valproate

- Children ages 3–10 taking other anticonvulsants are at higher risk for developing fatal hepatotoxicity than adults
- Hepatic toxicity may show no relation to hepatic enzyme levels but is usually preceded by malaise, weakness, lethargy, facial edema, rash, anorexia, and vomiting. Monitor liver function prior to therapy and periodically during the first 6 months. Caution in patients with history of hepatic disease. In high-risk patients, monitor serum fibrinogen and albumin for decreases in concentration, and ammonia for increases. Stop drug if hepatic transaminase 2–3 times the upper limit of normal
- Hyperammonemic encephalopathy should be considered in children and adolescents with unexplained lethargy, vomiting, or changes in mental status [measure serum ammonia – if elevated, discontinue valproate and carnitine may be of benefit]
- In patients with severe abdominal pain, lethargy and weight loss, rule out pancreatitis – serum amylase level should be done
- Platelet counts and bleeding time determinations should be considered prior to therapy and at periodic intervals; withdraw if hemorrhage, bruising, or coagulation disorder is detected
- Diabetic patients on valproic acid may show false-positive ketone results
- In patients with decreased or altered protein binding it may be more useful to monitor unbound (free) valproate concentrations rather than total concentrations
- Valproate will inhibit the metabolism of a number of drugs metabolized by cytochrome P-450 (see Drug Interactions pp. 225–227)
- Use in children and adolescents may result in increased risk of hyperandrogenism and polycystic ovarian syndrome, delayed or prolonged puberty; excessive weight gain, hyperinsulinemia and dyslipidemia. In females, assess for menstrual irregularities and symptoms of polycystic ovarian syndrome. Consider changing to a different mood stabilizer if symptoms of hyperan-drogynism or polycystic ovarian syndrome occur
- Risk of osteoporosis in children and adolescents on chronic therapy

Gabapentin

- Use cautiously in patient with renal dysfunction (see p. 213); use in children < 1 years of age with impaired renal function has not been evaluated

Mood Stabilizers

Comparison of Anticonvulsants (cont.)

Lamotrigine

- Severe, potentially life-threatening rashes have been reported – higher incidence in children (1%) than adults (0.1%), with rapid dosage titration and in combination with valproate. Most occur within first 8 weeks of starting lamotrigine. Patient should be educated to report any rash or systemic symptoms (fever, malaise, pharyngitis, flu-like symptoms), sores or blisters on soles, palms, or mucus membranes to the physician immediately. DO NOT rechallenge with lamotrigine
- Use cautiously in patients with renal dysfunction or moderate to severe hepatic dysfunction as elimination half-life of lamotrigine is increased, see p. 213
- Due to potential of PR prolongation, lamotrigine should be used cautiously in patients with conduction abnormalities

Topiramate

- Use cautiously and decrease dose in patient with poor renal or hepatic function, see p. 213
- Use cautiously in patients with a history of allergy to sulpha preparations
- Risk of renal (Ca phosphate) stone formation – ensure adequate fluid intake and avoid excessive antacid use
- Acute myopia and secondary angle closure glaucoma reported; ophthalmological consult recommended for patients with complaints of acute visual blurring and/or painful/red eyes
- Reports of decreased sweating and hyperthermia in children
- Decrease in sodium bicarbonate; symptoms include fatigue, anorexia, hyperventilation, cardiac arrhythmia, and stupor. Chronic metabolic acidosis may increase risk for nephrolithiasis or nephrocalcinosis and may result in osteomalacia and/or osteoprosis with an increase in risk of fractures [reduce dose or taper and discontinue drug]
- Cognitive side effects are related to dose

CONTRAINDICATIONS

- Patients with a history of hepatic or cardiovascular disease or with a blood dyscrasia
- Hypersensitivity to any tricyclic compound (carbamazepine), and demonstrated hypersensitivity to any of the other agents
- Patients prescribed clozapine due to increased risk of agranulocytosis (carbamazepine)
- Urea cycle disorders (valproate)

TOXICITY

Carbamazepine

- Usually occurs with plasma levels above 50 μmol/l; children may be at risk for toxicity at lower serum concentrations due to increased production of toxic epoxide metabolite. Measurement of epoxide level may be beneficial in patients who develop clinical signs of carbamazepine toxicity at therapeutic concentrations of the parent drug
- The maximum plasma concentration may be delayed for up to 70 h after an overdose; onset of symptoms begin 1–3h after ingestion of extended-release capsules

- Signs:
    - Dizziness, blood pressure changes, sinus tachycardia, ECG changes
    - Drowsiness, stupor, agitation, disorientation, EEG changes, seizures and coma
    - Nausea, vomiting, decreased intestinal motility, urinary retention
    - Tremor, involuntary movements, opisthotonos, abnormal reflexes, myoclonus, ataxia (PROMINENT)
    - Mydriasis, nystagmus
    - Flushing, respiratory depression, cyanosis
- No known antidote, treat symptomatically

Oxcarbazepine

- No deaths reported following overdose of up to 24,000 mg; no known antidote–treat symptomatically

Valproate

- Maximum plasma concentration may not occur for up to 18 h following an overdose, and serum half-life may be prolonged
- Onset of CNS depression may be rapid (within 3 h); enteric-coated preparations may delay onset of symptoms by 8 h or more
- Signs/symptoms: severe dizziness, hypotension, supraventricular tachycardia, bradycardia; severe drowsiness; trembling; irregular, slow or shallow breathing, apnea, respiratory depression and coma; loss of tendon reflexes, generalized myoclonus, seizures; cerebral edema – evident 2 to 3 days after overdose and may last up to 15 days; hematological changes, electrolyte and metabolic abnormalities; optic nerve damage
- Overdose can result in coma and death; naloxone may reverse the CNS depressant effects, and may also reverse anti-epileptic effects
- Supportive treatment

Gabapentin

- Signs and symptoms: double vision, slurred speech, drowsiness, lethargy and diarrhea – all patients recovered
- Gabapentin can be removed by hemodialysis

Lamotrigine

- Overdose can result in ataxia, nystagmus, delirium, seizures, intraventricular conduction delay, and coma
- No known antidote – treat symptomatically

Topiramate

- Emesis and gastric lavage recommended; topiramate can be removed by hemodialysis – treat symptomatically

MONITORING

	Carbamazepine	Oxcarbazepine	Valproate	Gabapentin	Lamotrigine	Topiramate
Biochemical work-up	1) CBC including platelets and differential 2) Serum electrolytes 3) Liver function	Serum electrolytes	1) CBC including platelets and differential 2) Liver function 3) Total and HDL cholesterol and triglycerides 4) In females: body weight/BMI 5) Consider serum testosterone level in young females	BUN and serum creatinine	None required	Baseline body weight, serum bicarbonate BUN and serum creatinine (optional)

Mood Stabilizers

Comparison of Anticonvulsants (cont.)

	Carbamazepine	Oxcarbazepine	Valproate	Gabapentin	Lamotrigine	Topiramate
Follow-up	Repeat CBC after the first month, then 2–3 times a year Serum electrolytes every 6 months	Sodium levels periodically and when patient has symptoms of hyponatremis	Repeat test #1 and #2 monthly for 2 months, then 2–3 times a year Test #3 and #4 annually Test #5 if symptoms of hyperandrogenism or menstrual irregularities occur; also test prolactin, LH, and TSH as well as for insulin resistance syndrome and hypertension Ammonia level in event of lethargy, mental status changes	LH and TSH Renal function if suspect toxicity	None required	Weight at 1 month; then every 3 months Renal function if suspect toxicity Periodic serum bicarbonate (to rule out metabolic acidosis)
Plasma level monitoring	Measure drug level 5 days after start of therapy and 5 days after change in close or addition / deletion of any other drug (see Drug Interactions pp. 223–225)	None required	Measure drug level 5 days after change in dose or addition/deletion of any other drug (see Drug Interactions pp. 225–227 and Precautions p. 219)	None required	None required	None required

NURSING IMPLICATIONS

- Watch out for signs of fever, sore throat, and bruising or jaundice
- Close clinical and laboratory supervision should be maintained (see Adverse Effects and Monitoring) throughout treatment to detect signs of possible blood dyscrasia or liver involvement
- A rash, especially with *carbamazepine* or *lamotrigine*; may signal incipient blood dyscrasia; advise the physician
- Anorexia, nausea, vomiting, edema, rash, malaise and lethargy may signify hepatic toxicity
- A rash with fever may signify multi-organ hypersensitivity reaction (by Stevens-Johnson syndrome)
- Check for constipation with *carbamazepine*; increase fluids to lessen constipation. Avoid grapefruit juice as it can elevate the blood level of carbamazepine
- Liquid *carbamazepine* should not be mixed or taken at the same time as any other liquid medication
- Liquid *valproate* should not be administered with carbonated beverages
- Controlled-release tablets or extended release capsules should not be chewed or crushed. Capsules can be opened and contents sprinkled on food
- Do not administer *gabapentin* within 1 h of an antacid as bioavailability is decreased by 24%
- In females (particularly on *valproate*) obtain baseline body weight/BMI, and measure periodically, monitor for menstrual disturbances, hirsutism, obesity, alopecia and infertility – two or more of these symptoms may be associated with polycystic ovaries
- Monitor patient's height, weight, and body mass index
- Patients on *topiramate* should drink plenty of fluids especially before and during activities such as exercise or exposure to warm temperatures; monitor for decreased sweating and hyperthermia, to minimize risk of renal stone formation. Concurrent use of antacids (e.g., Tums, Malox, Rolaids) should be avoided

- Patients on *topiramate* should report eye pain or continued visual disturbances to the physician
- To treat occasional pain avoid the use of acetylsalicylic acid (ASA or aspirin) as it can affect the blood level of *valproate* – acetaminophen or ibuprofen (and related drugs) are safer alternatives
- Advise patient to store medication away from heat and humidity as the drug may lose potency
- Detailed instructions for patients and caregivers are provided in the Information Sheet on p. 328

- Clinically significant interactions are listed below

DRUGS INTERACTING WITH CARBAMAZEPINE

Class of Drug	Example	Interaction Effects
Acetazolamide		Increased plasma level of carbamazepine due to inhibited metabolism
Anesthetic	Halothane	Enzyme induction may result in hepatocellular damage
	Methoxyflurane, isoflurane, sevoflurane	Enzyme induction may result in renal damage
Antibiotic	Erythromycin, troleandomycin, clarithromycin	Increased plasma levels of carbamazepine due to reduced clearance (by 5–41%)
	Doxycycline (no interaction with other tetracyclines)	Decreased serum level and half-life of doxycycline due to enhanced metabolism (Alternatively, tetracycline can be used or doxycycline can be dosed q 12 h)
	Quinupristin/dalfopristin	Increased plasma level of carbamazepine due to inhibited metabolism via CYP3A4
Anticoagulant	Dicumarol, warfarin	Enhanced metabolism of anticoagulant and impaired hypoprothombinemic response; decreased PT ratio or INR response
Anticonvulsant	Felbamate	Decreased carbamazepine level by 50%, but increased level of epoxide metabolite Decreased felbamate level
	Phenytoin, primidone, Phenobarbital	Decreased carbamazepine level due to increased metabolism via CYP3A4, but ratio of epoxide metabolite increased Altered plasma level of co-prescribed anticonvulsant
	Clonazepam, clobazam, ethosuximide, topiramate, tiagabine, zonisamide, oxcarbazepine	Clearance of the anticonvulsants is increased by carbamazepine, with possible decrease in efficacy (40% decrease in concentration of topiramate and of oxcarbazepine metabolite)
	Valproate, valproic acid	Increased plasma level of epoxide metabolite of carbamazepine; may result in toxicity even at therapeutic carbamazepine concentrations Decreased valproate level due to increased clearance and displacement from protein binding. Effects on carbamazepine levels are variable and inconsistent
	Lamotrigine	Increased plasma level of epoxide metabolite of carbamazepine by 10–45% with resultant increased side effects Increased metabolism of lamotrigine; half-life and plasma level decreased by 30–50%
	Topiramate	Increased plasma level of carbamazepine by 20%
Antidepressant SSRI	Fluoxetine, fluvoxamine	Increased plasma level of carbamazepine and its active metabolite with fluoxetine; increased nausea with fluvoxamine
	Sertraline	Decreased plasma level of sertraline due to enzyme induction via CYP3A4 (case report)
Cyclic (non-selective)	Imipramine, doxepin, amitriptyline	Decreased plasma level of antidepressant by up to 46% due to enzyme induction
SARI	Trazodone	Decreased plasma level of trazodone Increased plasma level of carbamazepine with nefazodone due to decreased metabolism via CYP3A4
MAOI	Phenelzine	Possible decrease in metabolism and increased plasma level of carbamazepine

Comparison of Anticonvulsants (cont.)

Class of Drug	Example	Interaction Effects
Antifungal	Ketoconazole, fluconazole	Increased plasma level of carbamazepine with ketoconazole (by 29%) due to inhibited metabolism via CYP3A4; clearance decreased by 50% with fl uconazole
	Fluconazole, itraconazole, ketoconazole	Decreased plasma levels of antifungals
Antipsychotic	Phenothiazines, haloperidol, risperidone, thiothixene, olanzapine, zuclopenthixol, flupenthixol	Decreased plasma level of antipsychotic (up to 100% with haloperidol, 44% with olanzapine) Increased akathisia
	Clozapine	Avoid combination due to possible potentiation of bone marrow suppression Decreased plasma level of clozapine by up to 63%
	Loxapine, haloperidol	Increased plasma level of carbamazepine and metabolite
	Chlorpromazine liquid, thioridazine liquid	Precipitation of a "rubbery mass" when carbamazepine suspension is combined with neuroleptic liquid preparations
Antitubercular drug	Isoniazid	Increased plasma level of carbamazepine; clearance reduced by up to 45%
	Rifampin	Decreased plasma level of carbamazepine
Benzodiazepine	Alprazolam, clonazepam	Decreased plasma level of alprazolam (> 50%) and clonazepam (19–37%) due to enzyme induction
β-Blocker	Propranolol	Decreased plasma level of β-blocker due to enzyme induction
Calcium-channel blocker	Diltiazem, verapamil (no interaction with nifedipine)	Increased plasma levels of carbamazepine due to decreased metabolism (total carbamazepine increased 46%, free carbamazepine increased 33%)
Cimetidine		Transient increase in carbamazepine levels and possible toxicity due to inhibited metabolism (no interaction with ranitidine, famotidine and nizatidine)
Corticosteroids		Decreased plasma level of corticosteroid due to enzyme induction
Danazol		Plasma levels of carbamazepine increased by 50–100%; half-life is doubled and clearance reduced by half
Desmopressin (DDAVP)		Concurrent use may increase antidiuretic effect, resulting in decreased sodium concentration with resultant seizures
Diclofenac		Increased plasma level of carbamazepine due to decreased metabolism
Disopyramide		Increased metabolism and decreased plasma level of disopyramide
Etretinate		Therapeutic failure with etretinate due to decreased plasma level
Folic acid		Decreased plasma level of folic acid
Grapefruit juice		Decreased metabolism of carbamazepine resulting in increased plasma level by up to 40%
Hormone	Oral contraceptive	Increased metabolism of oral contraceptive and increased binding of progestin and ethinyl estradiol to sex hormone binding globulin, may result in decreased contraceptive efficacy
Immunosuppressant	Cyclosporin	Decreased plasma level and efficacy of cyclosporin due to enzyme induction via CYP3A4
Influenza vaccine		Decreased elimination and increased half-life of carbamazepine

Class of Drug	Example	Interaction Effects
Isotretinoin		Decreased plasma level of carbamazepine and its metabolite
Lithium		Increased neurotoxicity of both drugs; sinus node dysfunction reported with combination
Modafinil		Decreased plasma level of modafinil due to enhanced metabolism
Metronidazole		Increased plasma level of carbamazepine due to inhibited metabolism
Muscle relaxant (non-depolarizing)	Gallamine, pancuronium	Decreased efficacy of muscle relaxant
Narcotic	Methadone	Decreased effect of methadone (up to 60%) due to enhanced metabolism
Propoxyphene		Increased plasma level of carbamazepine due to reduced metabolism
Protease inhibitor	Ritonavir, saquinavir, indinavir, nelfinavir	Increased metabolism and decreased plasma level of ritonavir and saquinavir with possible loss of efficacy Increased plasma level of carbamazepine due to inhibited metabolism via CYP3A4
Quinine		Increased plasma level of carbamazepine (by 37%) and AUC (by 51%) due to inhibited metabolism
Stimulant	Methylphenidate	Decreased plasma level of methylphenidate and its metabolite
Theophylline		Decreased theophylline level due to enzyme induction by carbamazepine; decreased carbamazepine level by up to 50%
Thyroid hormone		Decreased plasma level of thyroid hormone due to enzyme induction

DRUGS INTERACTING WITH OXCARBAZEPINE

Class of Drug	Example	Interaction Effects
Anticonvulsant	Carbamazepine, phenytoin, phenobarbital Valproate	Decreased plasma levels of oxcarbazepine MHD metabolite by 40% Increased level of phenytoin (by 40%) and phenobarbital (by 14%) due to inhibited metabolism via CYP2C19
CNS depressant	Alcohol, hypnotics, narcotics	Increased sedation, disorientation
Hormone	Oral contraceptives	Increased metabolism of ethinyl estradiol through induction of CYP3A4
Verapamil		Reduced oxcarbazepine MHD metabolite plasma level by about 20% – mechanism unknown

DRUGS INTERACTING WITH VALPROATE

Class of Drug	Example	Interaction Effects
Antibiotic	Erythromycin	Increased valproate plasma level due to decreased metabolism
Anticoagulant	Warfarin	Inhibition of secondary phase of platelet aggregation by valproate, thus affecting coagulation; increased PT ratio or INR response Displacement of protein binding of warfarin (free fraction increased by 33%)

Comparison of Anticonvulsants (cont.)

Class of Drug	Example	Interaction Effects
Anticonvulsant	Phenobarbital, primidone	Increased level of anticonvulsant (by 30–50%) due to decreased metabolism caused by valproate
	Carbamazepine	Decreased valproate levels due to increased clearance and displacement for protein binding Effects on carbamazepine levels are variable and inconsistent Synergistic mood-stabilizing effect in treatment-resistant patients
	Phenytoin, mephenytoin	Enhanced anticonvulsant effect due to displacement from protein binding (free fraction increased by 60%) and inhibited clearance (by 25%); toxicity can occur at therapeutic levels Possible decrease in valproate level
	Felbamate	Increased plasma level of valproate (by 31–51%) due to decreased metabolism
	Lamotrigine	Increased lamotrigine plasma level (by up to 200%), half-life (by up to 50%) and decreased clearance (by up to 60%) Both decreases and increases in plasma level of valproate reported. This combination may be dangerous due to high incidence of Stevens-Johnson syndrome and toxic epidermal necrolysis
	Ethosuximide	Increased half-life of ethosuximide (by 25%)
	Topiramate	Case reports of delirium and elevated ammonia levels
Antidepressant Tricyclic	Amitriptyline, nortriptyline	Increased plasma level and adverse effects of antidepressant
SSRI	Fluoxetine	Increased plasma level of valproate (up to 50%)
Antipsychotic	Phenothiazines	Increased neurotoxicity, sedation, and extrapyramidal side effects due to decreased clearance of valproate (by 14%)
	Clozapine	Both increased and decreased clozapine levels reported; changes in clozapine/norclozapine ratio Case report of hepatic encephalopathy
	Haloperidol	Increased plasma level of haloperidol by an average of 32%
	Olanzapine	Combination associated with high incidence of weight gain
Antitubercular drug	Isoniazid	Increased plasma level of valproate due to inhibited metabolism
	Rifampin	Increased clearance of valproate (by 40%)
Antiviral agent	Zidovudine	Increased level of zidovudine (by 38%) due to decreased clearance
	Acyclovir	Decreased level of valproate
Anxiolytic	Clonazepam, chlordiazepoxide, lorazepam	Decreased metabolism and increased pharmacological effects of benzodiazepines resulting in increased sedation, disorientation (lorazepam clearance reduced by 41%)
	Clonazepam	Concomitant use may induce absence status in patients with a history of absence type seizures
	Diazepam	Increased plasma level of diazepam due to displacement from protein binding (free fraction increased by 90%)
Cimetidine		Decreased metabolism and increased half-life of valproate
CNS depressant	Alcohol, hypnotics	Increased sedation, disorientation Valproate displaces alcohol from protein binding and potentiates intoxicating effect

Class of Drug	Example	Interaction Effects
Hypnotic	Zolpidem	Case of somnambulism with combination
Lithium		Synergistic mood-stabilizing effect in treatment-resistant patients Valproate may aggravate action tremor
Salicylate	Acetylsalicylic acid, bismuth subsalicylate	Displacement of valproate from protein binding and decreased clearance, leading to increased level of free drug (4-fold), with possible toxicity
Sulfonylurea	Tolbutamide	Increase in free fraction of tolbutamide from 20% to 50% due to displacement from protein binding
Thiopental		Displacement of thiopental from protein binding resulting in an increased hypnotic/anesthetic Effect

DRUGS INTERACTING WITH GABAPENTIN

Class of Drug	Example	Interaction Effects
Antacid	Al/Mg containing antacids	Co-administration reduces gabapentin bioavailability by up to 24%
CNS depressant	Alcohol, hypnotics	Increased sedation, disorientation
Narcotic	Hydrocodone	Decreased effectiveness of hydrocodone reported
	Morphine	Enhanced analgesic effects

DRUGS INTERACTING WITH LAMOTRIGINE

Class of Drug	Example	Interaction Effects
Anticonvulsant	Carbamazepine, phenytoin, phenobarbital, primidone	Decreased plasma level and half-life of lamotrigine due to increased metabolism (clearance increased by 30–50% with carbamazepine; by 125% with phenytoin) Increased plasma level of epoxide metabolite of carbamazepine by 10–45% with resultant increased side effects
	Valproate	Increased plasma level of lamotrigine (by up to 200%), half-life (by up to 50%) and decreased clearance (by up to 60%); both decreases and increases in valproate levels reported Increased risk of life-threatening rash with combination (Stevens-Johnson syndrome and toxic epidermal necrolysis)
	Topiramate	Decreased plasma level of lamotrigine
Antidepressant	Sertraline	Increased plasma level of lamotrigine (data contradictory)
	Fluoxetine	Decreased plasma level of lamotrigine (mechanism unclear)
Antipsychotic	Olanzapine	AUC of lamotrigine decreased by 24%
CNS depressant	Alcohol, hypnotics	Increased sedation, disorientation
Hormones	Oral contraceptive	Decreased plasma level of lamotrigine by 27–64% Reports of breakthrough bleeding and unexpected pregnancies
Lithium		Decreased plasma level of lamotrigine
Protease inhibitor	Lopinavir/ritonavir	Decreased plasma level of lamotrigine by 50% due to increased metabolism

Comparison of Anticonvulsants (cont.)

DRUGS INTERACTING WITH TOPIRAMATE

Class of Drug	Example	Interaction Effects
Antacid		Excessive use may increase renal stone (calcium phosphate) formation
Anticonvulsant	Carbamazepine, oxcarbazepine, phenytoin, phenobarbital, primidone	Decreased plasma levels of topiramate reported; by 40% with carbamazepine and 48% with phenytoin Increased plasma level of carbamazepine (by 20%) and of phenytoin
	Lamotrigine	Decreased plasma level of lamotrigine
	Valproate	Case reports of delirium and elevated ammonia levels
Carbonic anhydrase inhibitor	Acetazolamide, zonisamide	Excessive use may increase renal stone (calcium phosphate) formation
CNS depressant	Alcohol, hypnotics, narcotics	Increased sedation, disorientation
Digoxin		Decreased levels of digoxin by 12%
Hormone	Oral contraceptive	Possibly decreased metabolism of oral contraceptive

Adverse Reactions to Mood Stabilizers at Therapeutic Doses

Reaction		Lithium	Carbamazepine	Oxcarbazepine	Valproate	Gabapentin	Lamotrigine	Topiramate
CNS	Drowsiness, sedation	>10%	>10%	>10%	>10%	>10%	>10%	>10%[d]
	Headache	> 2%	> 2%	>30%	>10%	> 2%	>10%	>10%
	Cognitive blunting, memory impairment	>10%	> 2%	> 2%	> 2%	< 2%	> 2%	> 2%[d]
	Weakness, fatigue	>30%	>10%	>10%	>10%	>10%	> 2%	>10%
	Insomnia, agitation	< 2%	< 2%	> 2%	> 2%	>2%	> 2%	>10%
Neurological	Incoordination	< 2%[f]	>10%	> 2%	> 2%	< 2%	> 2%	> 2%
	Dizziness	–	>10%	> 2%	>10%	>10%	>30%	>10%[d]
	Ataxia	< 2%[f]	>10%	> 10%	> 2%	>10%	>10%	> 2%[d]
	Tremor	>30%[f]	>30%	> 2%	>10%	> 2%	> 2%	> 2%
	Paresthesias	–	> 2%	> 10%	> 2%	< 2%	< 2%	>10%
	Diplopia	–	>10%	> 2%	>10%	> 2%	>10%	> 2 %
Anticholinergic	Blurred vision	> 2%	> 2%	> 2%	> 2%	< 2%	>10%	> 2%
Cardiovascular	ECG changes[a]	>10%	> 2%	< 2%	> 2%	–	< 2%	–
Gastrointestinal	Nausea, vomiting	>30%	>10%	>10%	>10%	> 2%	>10%	> 2%
	Diarrhea	>10%[f]	> 2%	> 2%	>10%	–	> 2%	> 2%
	Weight gain	>30%	> 2%	> 2%	>30%	>10%[d]	< 2%	–
	Weight loss	< 2%	< 2%	< 2%	> 2%	< 2%	> 2%	>10%[d]
Endocrine	Hair loss, thinning	>10%	> 2%	< 2%	>10%	–	–	< 2%
	Menstrual disturbances	>10%	>30%	< 2%	>30%	–	> 2%	–
	Polycystic ovary syndrome	–	>10%	?	>30%	–	–	–
	Hypothyroidism	>30%	< 2%	?	< 2%	–	< 2%	–
	Polyuria, polydipsia	~>30%	> 2%	< 2%	–	–	–	–
Skin reactions	Rash	>10%[c]	>10%[g]	> 2%	> 2%	< 2%	>10%[g]	< 2%
Sexual dysfunction		> 2%	< 2%	–	> 2%	< 2%	–	–
Blood dyscrasia	Transient leukopenia	< 2%	>10%	< 2%	< 2%	< 2%	< 2%	< 2%
	Leukocytosis	>30%	< 2%	< 2%	< 2%	–	–	–
	Thrombocytopenia	–	> 2%	–	>30%[d]	–	< 2%	–
Hepatic	Transient enzyme elevation[b]	–	>10%	< 2%	>30%[d]	< 2%	< 2%	–

[a] ECG abnormalities usually without cardiac injury, including ST segment depression, flattened T waves, and increased U wave amplitude; [b] Evaluate for hepatotoxicity if elevation >3 times normal; [c] Worsening of psoriasis reported; [d] Greater with higher doses; [f] Higher incidence and more pronounced symptoms with higher serum lithium concentration; may indicate early toxicity – monitor level; [g] May be first sign of impending blood dyscrasia

Anticonvulsants – References and Selected Readings

- AACAP official action. Practice parameters in the assessment and treatment of children and adolescents with bipolar disorder (1997). *Journal of the American Academy of Child and Adolescent Psychiatry 36(1),* 138–157.
- Bowden, C.L. (2005). Atypical antipsychotic augmentation of mood-stabilizer therapy in bipolar disorder. *Journal of Clinical Psychiatry 66 (Suppl. 3),* 12–19.
- Chengappa, K.N.R., Gershon, S., Levine, S. (2001). The evolving role of topiramate among other mood stabilizers in the management of bipolar disorder. *Bipolar Disorder 3,* 215–232.
- Davis, L.L., Ryan, W., Adinoff, B. et al. (2000). Comprehensive review of the psychiatric uses of valproate. *Journal of Clinical Psychopharmacology 20(1)(Suppl. 1),* 1S– 17S.
- Dunner, D.L. (2000). Optimizing lithium treatment. *Journal of Clinical Psychiatry 61(Suppl. 9),* 76–81.
- Ernst, C.L., Goldberg, J.F. (2002). The reproductive safety profile of mood stabilizers, atypical antipsychotic, and broad-spectrum psychotropics. *Journal of Clinical Psychiatry 63(Suppl. 4),* 42–55.
- Hebert, A.A., Ralston, J.P. (2001). Cutaneous reactions to anticonvulsant medications. *Journal of Clinical Psychiatry 62(Suppl. 14),* 22–26.
- James, A.C.D., Javaloyes, A.M. (2002). Practitioner Reviews: The treatment of bipolar disorder in children and adolescents. *Journal of Child Psychology and Psychiatry 42(4),* 439–449.
- Keck, P.E., McElroy, S.L. (2002). Clinical pharmacodynamics and pharmacokinetics of antimanic and mood-stabilizing medications. *Journal of Clinical Psychiatry 63(Suppl. 4),* 3–11.
- Ketter, T.A., Wang, P.W. (2002). Predictors of treatment response in bipolar disorders: Evidence from clinical and brain imaging studies. *Journal of Clinical Psychiatry 63 (Suppl. 3),* 21–25.
- Knowles, S.R. (1999). Adverse effects of antiepileptics. *Canadian Journal of Clinical Pharmacology 6(3),* 137–148.
- Kowatch, R.A., Fristad, M., Birmaher, B. (2005). Treatment guidelines for children and adolescents with bipolar disorder. *Journal of the American Academy of Child and Adolescent Psychiatry 44(3),* 213–235.
- McIntyre, R.S., Mancini, D.A., Parikh, S. et al. (2001). Lithium revisited. *Canadian Journal of Psychiatry 46,* 322–327.
- Mercke, Y., Sheng, H., Khan, T. et al. (2000). Hair loss in psychopharmacology. *Annals of Clinical Psychiatry 12(1),* 35–42.
- Pavuluri, M.N., Naylor, M.W., Janicak, P.G. (2002). Recognition and treatment of pediatric bipolar disorder. *Contemporary Psychiatry 1(1),* 1–9.
- Sachs, G.S. (2003). Decision tree for the treatment of bipolar disorder. *Journal of Clinical Psychiatry 64(Suppl. 8),* 35–40.
- Schapiro, N.A. (2005). Bipolar disorder in children and adolescents. *Journal of Pediatric Health Care* 19(3), 131–141,
- Stahl, S.M. (2004). Psychopharmacology of anticonvulsants: Do all anticonvulsants have the same mechanism of action? *Journal of Clinical Psychiatry 65(2),* 149–150.
- Suppes, T., Dennehy, E.B., Swann, A.C. et al. (2002). Report of the Texas Consensus Conference Panel on medication treatment of bipolar disorder 2000. *Journal of Clinical Psychiatry 63(4),* 288–299.
- Swann, A.C. (2001). Major system toxicities and side effects of anticonvulsants. *Journal of Clinical Psychiatry 62(Suppl. 14),* 16–21.
- Wagner, K.D. (2004). Diagnosis and treatment of bipolar disorder in children and adolescents. *Journal of Clinical Psychiatry 65(Suppl. 15),* 30–35.
- Weller, E. (2004). Pharmacotherapy of adolescents with bipolar disorder. *International Drug Therapy Newsletter 39(11),* 81–87.
- Weller, E. (2004). Pharmacotherapy of children with bipolar disorder. *International Drug Therapy Newsletter 39(10),* 73–80.
- Working Group on Bipolar Disorder (2002). Practice guidelines for the treatment of patients with bipolar disorder. *American Journal of Psychiatry 159(4, Suppl.),* 1–50.
- Wozniak, J. (2005). Recognizing and managing bipolar disorder in children. *Journal of Clinical Psychiatry 66(Suppl. 1),* 18–23.
- Yatham, L.N. Kusumaker, V., Calabrese, J.R. et al. (2002). Third generation anticonvulsants in bipolar disorder: A review of efficacy and summary of clinical recommendations. *Journal of Clinical Psychiatry 63(4),* 275–383.

- This chapter gives a general overview of common drugs of abuse and is not intended to deal in detail with all agents, or be a complete guide to treatment
- Slang names of street drugs change rapidly and vary with country, region, and drug subculture

CLASSIFICATION

- Drugs of abuse can be classified as follows:

Chemical Class	Agents[A]		Page
Stimulant	Examples:	Amphetamine, crystal meth Cocaine Sympathomimetics (incl. caffeine)	See p. 234
Hallucinogen	Examples:	Lysergic acid diethylamide Cannabis Phencyclidine	See p. 239
Alcohol	Alcohol		See p. 243
Opiate/Narcotic	Examples:	Morphine Heroin Pentazocine	See p. 247
Inhalant/Aerosol	Examples:	Glue Paint thinner	See p. 250
Gamma-hydroxy butyrate			See p. 252
Sedative/Hypnotic	Examples:	Flunitrazepam Barbiturates* Benzodiazepines* Hypnotics*	See p. 254 See p. 188 See p. 169 See p. 188
Nicotine*	Examples;	Cigarettes, cigars	

[A] Only includes examples of most commonly used substances
* Not dealt with specifically in this chapter

DEFINITIONS

Drug Abuse

- Acute or chronic intake of any substance that:
    - a) has no recognized medical use,
    - b) is used inappropriately in terms of its medical indications or its dose

Drugs of Abuse (cont.)

Drug Dependence	
A. Psychological	• Craving or desire for continuous administration of a drug to provide a desired effect or to avoid discomfort
B. Physical	• A physiological state of adaptation to a drug which usually results in development of tolerance to drug effects and withdrawal symptoms when the drug is stopped – also called addiction
Tolerance	• Phenomenon where increasing doses of a drug are needed to produce a desired effect

PHARMACOLOGY

• Research data have demonstrated that many drugs of abuse increases dopamine activity in the nucleus accumbens of the brain; the increased dopamine is suggested to be associated with the pleasurable effects produced by the drug

GENERAL COMMENTS

• The effect which any drug of abuse has on an individual depends on a number of variables:
1) dose (amount ingested, injected, sniffed, etc.)
2) potency and purity of drug
3) route of administration
4) past experience of the user (this will predispose to selective behavioral response either on a pharmacologic or conditioning basis)
5) present circumstances, i.e., environment, other people present, whether other drugs are taken concurrently
6) personality and genetic predisposition of user
7) age of user
8) clinical status of user, i.e., type of psychiatric illness, degree of recent stress or loss, occurrence of a vulnerable phase of a circadian or ultradian rhythm, user's expectations, and present feelings
• Some users may have different experiences with the same drug on different occasions. They may encounter both pleasant and unpleasant effects during the same drug experience
• Many street drugs are adulterated with other chemicals, and may differ from what the individual thinks they are; potency and purity of street drugs vary greatly
• It is questionable whether drugs of abuse cause persistent psychiatric disorders in otherwise healthy individuals, or whether they precipitate latent psychiatric illness in predisposed individuals who already have significant premorbid psychopathology. Many abusers tend to be multiple drug users, therefore to say that a specific drug was implicated in a psychiatric disorder is difficult. Overall, in non-treatment community samples, it is estimated over 50% of drug users have at least one other psychiatric disorder
• Substance abuse has been associated with earlier onset of schizophrenia, decreased treatment responsiveness of positive symptoms and poor clinical functioning; similarly decreased treatment responsiveness in bipolar disorder can occur in adolescents abusing substances

ADVERSE EFFECTS

- See pharmacological/psychiatric effects under specific drugs
- Reactions are unpredictable and depend on the potency and purity of drug taken
- Psychiatric reactions secondary to drug abuse may occur more readily in individuals already at risk
- Renal, hepatic, cardiorespiratory, neurological, and gastrointestinal complications as well as encephalopathies can occur with chronic abuse of specific agents
- Intravenous drug users are at risk for infection, including cellulitis, hepatitis and AIDS
- Impurities in street drugs (especially if inhaled or injected) can cause tissue and organ damage (blood vessels, kidney, lungs, and liver)
- Psychological dependence can occur; the drug becomes central to a person's thoughts, emotions, and activities, resulting in craving
- Physical dependence can occur; the body adapts to the presence of the drug and withdrawal symptoms occur when the drug is stopped, resulting in addiction

DETECTION OF DRUGS OF ABUSE

- Factors affecting detection of a drug in urine depend on dose and route of administration, drug metabolism, and characteristics of screening and confirmation assays; for intance:
  - Amphetamines in urine can be positive for up 5 days
  - Marihuana (THC) in urine can be positive 2–4 days after acute use and for up to 1–3 months after chronic use
  - Cocaine in urine can be positive for up to 1.5 days after I.V. use, for up to 1 week with street doses used by different routes, and for up to 3 weeks after use of very high doses
  - Heroin in urine can be positive for up to 1.5 days when administered parenterally or intranasally

TREATMENT

- See specific agents
- The diagnosis of the type of substance abused can be difficult in an Emergency Room when a patient presents as floridly psychotic, intoxicated or delirious. Blood and urine screens take time, therefore diagnosis must include mental status, physical and neurological examination, as well as a drug history, whenever possible; collateral history should be sought
- In severe cases, monitor vitals and fluid intake
- Agitation can be treated conservatively by talking with the patient and providing reassurance until the drug wears off (i.e., "talking down"). When conservative approaches are inadequate or if symptoms persist, pharmacological intervention should be considered
- Avoid low-potency neuroleptics due to anticholinergic effects, hypotension, and tachycardia

DISCONTINUATION SYNDROME

- See specific agents
- Identification of drug(s) abused is important; toxicology may help in identification whenever multiple or combination drug use is suspected
- If 2 or more drugs have been chronically abused, withdraw one drug at a time, starting with the one that potentially represents the greatest problem: e.g., in alcohol/sedative abuse, withdraw the alcohol first

LONG-TERM TREATMENT

- The presence of comorbid psychiatric disorders in substance abusers can adversely influence outcome in treatment of the substance abuse as well as the psychiatric disorder

Stimulants

PHARMACOLOGICAL/ PSYCHIATRIC EFFECTS

- Differ somewhat depending on type of drug taken, dose, and route of administration
- Effects occur rapidly, especially when drug used parenterally
- Acute toxicity reported with doses ranging from 5 to 630 mg of amphetamine; chronic users may ingest extremely high doses
- Following acute toxicity, psychiatric state usually clears within one week of amphetamine discontinuation

Physical

- Elevated BP, tachycardia, increased respiration and temperature, sweating, pallor, tremors, decreased appetite, dilated pupils, reduced fatigue, insomnia, increased sensory awareness, increased sexual arousal/libido combined with a delay in ejaculation

Mental

- Euphoria, exhilaration, alertness, improved task performance, exacerbation of obsessive-compulsive symptoms
- Methamphetamine reported to induce paranoia and hallucinations in non-schizophrenic subjects; flashbacks reported

High Doses

- Anxiety, excitation, panic attacks, grandiosity, delusions, visual, auditory and tactile hallucinations, paranoia, mania, delirium, increased sense of power, violence
- Fever, sweating, headache, flushing, pallor, hyperactivity, stereotypic behavior, cardiac arrhythmias, respiratory failure, loss of coordination, collapse, cerebral hemorrhage, convulsions, and death

Chronic Use

- Decreased appetite and weight, abdominal pain, vomiting, difficulty urinating, skin rash, increased risk for stroke, high blood pressure, irregular heart rate, electrolyte abnormalities (e.g., hyponatremia), impotence, headache, anxiety, delusions of persecution, violence)
- Tolerance to physical effects occurs but vulnerability to psychosis remains
- Chronic high-dose use causes physical dependence; psychological dependence can occur even with regular low-dose use
- Recovery occurs rapidly after amphetamine withdrawal, but psychosis can be chronic

DISCONTINUATION SYNDROME

- Anxiety, distorted sleep, chronic fatigue, irritability, difficulty concentrating, craving, depression, suicidal or homicidal ideation, and paranoid psychosis
- Nausea, diarrhea, anorexia, hunger, myalgia, diaphoresis, convulsions

COMPLICATIONS

- Exacerbation of hypertension or arrhythmias
- Strokes and retinal damage due to intense vasospasm, especially with "crack"

TREATMENT

- Use calming techniques, reassurance, and supportive measures
- Supportive care of excess sympathomemetic stimulation may be required (e.g., temperature, BP); monitor hydration, electrolytes, and for possible serotonin syndrome (see p. 46)
- For severe agitation and to prevent seizures, sedate with benzodiazepine (e.g., diazepam, lorazepam)
- For psychosis, use a high-potency neuroleptic (haloperidol); avoid low-potency neuroleptics
- Antidepressants (e.g., desipramine) can be used to treat depression following withdrawal, and to decrease craving. Preliminary data suggests flupenthixol depot injection may be useful in withdrawal; positive results also reported with buspirone, bromocriptine, and amantadine
- Hypertonic saline/fluid restriction for symptomatic hyponatremia
- Cold I.V. fluids/cooling washes for hyperthermia

Drug of Abuse	Interacting Drugs	Reaction
STIMULANTS (general)	Antipsychotics	Diminished pharmacological effects of stimulants
	Irreversible MAOIs, e.g., phenelzine	Severe palpitations, tachycardia, hypertension, headache, cerebral hemorrhage, agitation, seizures; AVOID
Amphetamines	Antidepressants, general – Tricyclics	Enhanced antidepressant effect Increased plasma level of amphetamine due to inhibited metabolism
	Guanethidine	Reversal of hypotensive effects
	Phenothiazines, e.g., chlorpromazine	Increased plasma level of amphetamine due to inhibited metabolism Phenothiazines can decrease CNS excitation from amphetamines
	Urinary acidifiers, e.g., ammonium chloride	Increased elimination of amphetamine due to decreased renal tubular reabsorption and increased elimination
	Urinary alkalizers, e.g., potassium citrate, sodium bicarbonate	Prolonged pharmacological effects of amphetamine due to decreased urinary elimination of unchanged drug
Cocaine	Alcohol	Ethanol promotes the formation of a highly addicting metabolite, cocoethylene Reports of enhanced hepatotoxicity Increased heart rate; variable effect on blood pressure Increased risk of sudden death with combined use (18-fold) Combined use reported to result in more impulsive decision making and poorer performance on tests of learning and memory
	Antidepressants (Cyclic, SSRI) Tricyclics: e.g., desipramine	Decreased craving Decreased seizure threshold Elevated heart rate and diastolic pressure by 20–30%; increased risk of arrhythmia
	Barbiturates	Reports of enhanced hepatotoxicity
	β-blockers	May increase the magnitude of cocaine-induced myocardial ischemia
	Carbamazepine	Augmentation of cocaine-induced increase in heart rate and diastolic BP
	Catecholamines, e.g., norepinephrine	Potentiation of vasoconstriction and cardiac stimulation
	Disulfiram	Increased plasma level (3-fold) and half-life (60%) of cocaine with possible increased risk of cardiovascular effects
	Flupenthixol	Decreased craving
	Marihuana (cannabis)	Increased heart rate; blood pressure increased only with high doses of both drugs Increased plasma level of cocaine and increased subjective reports of euphoria
	Mazindol	May decrease craving for cocaine Increased lethality and convulsant activity reported
	Narcotics, e.g., heroin, morphine	May potentiate cocaine euphoria
	Yohimbine	Enhanced effect of cocaine on blood pressure
MDA/MDMA	MAOIs, e.g., phenelzine	**AVOID**; serotonin syndrome (see p. 46)
	SSRIs, e.g., fluoxetine	Diminished pharmacological effects of MDA
	Protease inhibitor, ritonavir	Case reports of increased plasma level of MDMA due to inhibited metabolism via CYP2D6; death reported

Stimulants (cont.)

DRUG	COMMENTS
STIMULANT AGENTS	
AMPHETAMINE, DEXTROAMPHETAMINE (Dexedrine, Dexampex, Biphetamine, Adderall) Taken orally as tablet, capsule, sniffed, Injected *Slang:* bennies, hearts, pep-pills, dex, beans, benn, truck-drivers, ice, jolly beans, black beauties, crank, pink football, dexies, crosses, hearts, LA turnaround	– Cause the release of amines (NE, 5-HT, DA) from central and peripheral neurons and inhibit their breakdown – Onset of action: 30 min after oral ingestion – Active drug use usually terminated by a psychotic reaction, or by exhaustion with excessive sleeping – Psychosis can last up to 10 days – Tolerance and psychic dependence occurs with chronic use – Excessive doses can lead to heart failure, delirium, psychosis (can last up to 10 days), coma, convulsions, and death – Pregnancy: increase in premature births; withdrawal symptoms and behavioral effects (hyperexcitability) noted in offspring
METHAMPHETAMINE (Desoxyephedrine) (Des-oxyn, Methampex) Powder: taken as tablets, capsules, liquid, injected, snorted, inhaled (smoked) *Slang:* speed, crystal meth, uppers, shit, moth, crank, crosses, ice, methlies quick, jib, fire, chalk, glass, go fast, shabu, krystal, tweak Crystal (ice) is methamphetamine washed in a solvent to remove impurities – smoked in a glass pipe, "chased" on aluminium foil	– Can be manufactured using ephedrine or pseuodoephedrine; (>300 ways to manufactures) – Synthetic drug related chemically to amphetamines and ephedrine – Enhances release and blocks uptake of catecholamines. Also can block metabolism of aminos (unlike cocaine) – Very rapid onset of action; can last 10–12 h – Can be highly addicitive – A "run" refers to the use of the drug several times a day over a period of several days – Physical effects: tachycardia, tachypnea, diaphoresis, hyperthermia, mydriasis, hypertension; appetite, thirst, and sleep suppression – CNS effects: anxiety, agitation, euphoria, alertness, delirium, psychosis, paranoia, violence – Chronic use has been associated with neuronal damage and malnutrition – Toxic effects: dysrhythmias, hypertension, heart failure, hyperthermia, seizures, encephalopathy, rhabdomyolysis – After abrupt discontinuation withdrawal effects peak in 2–3 days and include GI distress, headache, depression, irritability
COCAINE Extract from leaves of coca plant Leaves chewed, applied to mucous membranes, powder Taken orally, snorted, smoked, injected can last for weeks or months *Slang:* coke, snow, flake, lady, toot, blow, big C, candy, crack, joy dust, star-dust, rock, nose, boulders, bump, charlie, coca, blanca, perico, nieve, soda **"Crack"** Free base cocaine; more potent Volatilized and inhaled	– Inhibits dopamine and serotonin reuptake – stimulates brain's reward pathway; >47% of receptors need to be blocked to feel cocaine's effect – Onset of action and plasma half-life varies depending on route of use (e.g., IV: peaks in 30 s, half-life 54 min; snorting: peaks in 15–30 min, half-life 75 min); metabolized via CYP3A4 – Often adulterated with amphetamine, ephedrine, procaine, ylocaine, or lidocaine – Used with heroin ("dynamite," "speedballs"), morphine ("whizbang"), or marihuana ("cocoa puffs") for increased intensity – Used with flunitrazepam to moderate stimulatory effect – CNS effects: rapid euphoria, anxiety, agitation, delusion, hallucinations – Physical effects: nausea, vomiting, tachycardia, hypertension, pyrexia, diaphoresis, mydriasis, ataxia; tactile hallucinations ("coke bugs") occur – Tolerance develops to some effects (appetite), but increased sensitivity (reverse tolerance) develops to others (convulsions, psychosis) – Powerful psychological dependence occurs; physical dependence seen in crack users; withdrawal symptoms can last for weeks or months – Depression commonly occurs after drug use; dysphoria promotes repetitive use – Chronic users can develop panic disorder, paranoia; with repetitive administration or use of high doses, euphoria may be replaced by dysphoria, irritability, assaultive behavior, paranoia and delirium – Snorting can cause stuffy, runny nose, eczema around nostrils, atrophy of nasal mucosa, bleeding and perforated septum – Smokers are susceptible to respiratory symptoms and pulmonary complications – Sexual dysfunction is common – Chronic users of "crack" can develop "crack keratitis": abrasions on eye due to excessive rubbing, microvascular changes in the eyes, lungs and brain; respiratory symptoms include asthma and pulmonary hemorrhage and edema – Dehydration can occur due to effect on temperature regulation, with possible hyperpyrexia – Toxic effects: hyperthermia, hypertension, paroxysmal atrial tachycardia, hyper-reflexia, irregular respiration, seizures, unconsciousness, death; fatalities more common with IV use, or when cocaine-filled condoms are swallowed (by smugglers) then burst – Pregnancy: associated with spontaneous labor and abortion; increase in premature births; infants have lower weight, length, and head circumference, jitteriness, irritability, poor feeding, EEG abnormalities

DRUG	COMMENTS
KHAT (*Catha edulis*) Leaves chewed	– Grows as a bush in Africa and the Middle East; used by certain communities to attain religious euphoria – Cathinone is principal psychoactive agent – Symptoms occur within 3 h and last about 90 min – Acute symptoms include: euphoria, excitation, grandiosity, increased blood pressure, flushing – Chronic use can cause: anxiety, agitation, confusion, dysphoria, aggression, visual hallucinations, paranoia
METHYLPHENIDATE Tablets crushed and snorted, swallowed, injected *Slang:* Vitamin R, R-ball, skippy, the smart drug, JIF, MPH	See p. 19 – Large doses can cause psychosis, seizures, stroke, and heart failure
SYMPATHOMIMETICS Ephedrine, phenylpropanolamine, caffeine Taken as capsules, tablets *Slang:* look alikes, Herbal Bliss, Cloud 9, Herbal X	– Known as Herbal Ecstasy and sold as "natural" alternative to Ecstasy – Misrepresented as amphetamines and sold in capsules or tablets that resemble amphetamines – Doses of ingredients vary widely – Reports of hypertension and seizures; death due to stroke can occur after massive doses
DRUGS WITH STIMULANT AND HALLUCINOGENIC PROPERTIES	
NUTMEG (Active ingredient related to trimethoxyamphetamine and to mescaline) Seeds eaten whole, ground, powdered; sniffed	– Effects occur slowly and last several hours (duration of hallucinogenic effects is dose related) – Hallucinations are usually preceded by nausea, vomiting, diarrhea, and headache – Lightheadedness, drowsiness, thirst, and hangover can occur
3, 4-methylene-dioxymethamphetamine (MDMA) Powder, usually in tablets or capsules; may also be snorted or smoked "bumped" or coated on lollypops or pacifiers *Slang:* ecstasy; MDMA, "Adam," XTC, X, E, EVE, love drug, business man's special, clarity, lover's speed, hugs, beans	– Causes a calcium-dependent increase in serotonin release into the synaptic cleft and inhibits serotonin reuptake; increases levels of serotonin, norepinephrine and, to a smaller extent, dopamine – May decrease serotonin's intracellular synthesis if used long term – Many MDMA products are contaminated with other compounds including dextromethorphan, caffeine, phenylpropanolamine, MDA, ephedra, paramethoxyamphetamine (PMA), ketamine, methylsalicylate – Typical dose varies from 50–150 mg, but amount of drug per tablet can be from 0 to 100 mg – Onset of effects 30–60 min; duration of action 3–6 h; metabolized primarily by CYP2D6 and may inhibit CYP2D6; slow metabolizers of CYP2D6 may develop toxicity at moderate doses due to drug accumulation – CNS effects: Produces wakefulness, increases energy, endurance and sexual arousal and decreases fatigue and sleepiness; creates feelings of euphoria and well-being together with derealization, depersonalization, impaired memory and learning, and heightened tactile sensations (action believed to be mediated through release of serotonin); commonly used at "raves" – Common physical effects include increased blood pressure and heart rate, increased salivation, urinary retention; mydriasis, bruxism, trismus, increased tension, headache, restless legs, blurred vision, dry mouth, nausea, and suppressed appetite, thirst, and sleep – Severe physical reactions include hypertension, tachycardia, dysrhythmia, hyperthermia, followed by hypotension, ischemic stroke, fatal brain hemorrhage, seizures; coma; death can occur from excessive physical activity ("raves") that may result in disseminated intravascular coagulation, rhabdomyolysis, hyponatremia, acute renal and hepatic failure, and multiple organ failure – High doses can precipitate panic disorder, hallucinations, paranoid psychosis, aggression, and flashbacks – After-effects include: drowsiness, muscle aches, generalized fatigue, anorexia, irritability, anxiety, and depression (last 1–2 days due to half-life of drug of about 8 h) – Tolerance to euphoric effects with chronic use – Chronic regular use may result in mood swings, depression, impulsivity and lack of self-control, memory loss, and parkinsonism; can lead to psychological dependence – Suggested that chronic use can produce changes in serotonin function in the CNS and the development of progressive neurodegeneration. May also stress the immune system and increase susceptibility to infections disease

Stimulants (cont.)

DRUG	COMMENTS
3, 4-methylene-dioxyamphetamine (MDA) Chemically related to both mescaline and amphetamine (synthetic drug) Used orally as a liquid, powder, tablet; injection *Slang:* love drug	– Typical doses: 60–120 mg – Effects occur after 30–60 min (orally), or sooner if injected, and last about 8 h – Hallucinations and perceptual distortions rare; feeling of peace and tranquility occurs – High doses: hyperreactivity to stimuli, agitation, hallucinations, violent and irrational behavior, delirium, convulsions and coma
N-ethyl-3, 4-methylene-dioxyamphetamine (MDE) Chemically related to MDMA (synthetic drug) *Slang:* Eve	– Effects as for MDMA (above) – Onset of eff ects within 30 min; duration of action 3–4 h
Paramethoxyamphetamine (PMA) Synthetic drug Used as powder, capsules	– Often sold as MDMA but has more pronounced hallucinogenic and stimulant effects – Causes major increase in BP and pulse, hyperthermia, increased and labored breathing – Highly toxic; convulsions, coma, and death reported – Metabolized by CYP2D6
2, 5-dimethoxy-4-methylamphetamine (STP/DOM) Chemically related to both mescaline and amphetamine Used orally *Slang:* serenity, tranquility, peace	– Effects last 16–24 h – More potent than mescaline, but less potent than LSD – "Bad trips" occur frequently; prolonged psychotic reactions reported in people with psychiatric history – Tolerance reported; no evidence of dependence – Anticholinergic effects, exhaustion, convulsions, excitement, and delirium reported
Trimethoxyamphetamine (TMA) Synthetic drug related to mescaline Used orally, as powder, injection	– Effects occur after 2 h – Often misrepresented as MDA – More potent than mescaline – More toxic if injected or higher doses used – Can cause unprovoked anger and aggression

Hallucinogens

PHARMACOLOGICAL/ PSYCHIATRIC EFFECTS

- Differ somewhat depending on type of drug taken and route of administration (see specific agents below)
- Effects occur rapidly and last from 30 min (e.g., DMT) to several days (e.g., PCP)

Physical

- Increased BP, tachycardia, dilated pupils, nausea, sweating, flushing, chills, hyperventilation, incoordination, muscle weakness, trembling, numbness

Mental

- Alteration of perception and body awareness, impaired attention and short-term memory, disturbed sense of time, depersonalization, euphoria, mystical or religious experiences, grandiosity, anxiety, panic, visual distortions, hallucinations (primarily visual), erratic behavior, aggression

High Doses

- Confusion, restlessness, excitement, anxiety, emotional lability, panic, mania, paranoia, "bad trip"
- Cardiac depression and respiratory depression (mescaline), hypotension, convulsions and coma (PCP)

Chronic Use

- Anxiety, depression, personality changes
- Tolerance (tachyphylaxis) can occur with regular use (except with DMT); reverse tolerance (supersensitivity) has been described
- "Woolly" thinking, delusions and hallucinations reported; may persist for months after drug discontinuation
- Flashbacks – recurrent psychotic symptoms, may occur years after discontinuation
- Regular (weekly) marihuana use has been associated with increased risk of tardive dyskinesia in schizophrenic patients on antipsychotics
- Cohort studies suggest that chronic use of cannabis by teenagers is associated with a greater than 5-fold increase in risk of later-life depression and anxiety, as well as an increased risk (by 30%) of schizophrenia. Prolonged exposure to cannabis may cause an initial increase in synaptic dopamine and then lead to more prolonged changes in the endogenous cannabinoid system – may be more profound in adolescents

TREATMENT

- Supportive care of excess CNS stimulation may be required; monitor hydration, electrolytes, and for possible serotonin syndrome (see p. 46)
- Provide reassurance and reduction of threatening external stimuli
- In severe cases, the "trip" should be aborted chemically as rapidly as possible. This reduces the likelihood of flashbacks or recurrences in the future; in mild cases "talking down" may be more appropriate
- Avoid low-potency neuroleptics with anticholinergic and α-adrenergic properties (e.g., chlorpromazine) to minimize hypotension, tachycardia, disorientation, and seizures
- Use high-potency neuroleptic (e.g., haloperidol) for psychotic symptoms
- Use benzodiazepines (diazepam, lorazepam) to control seizures or agitation and to sedate, if needed
- Propranolol, ammonium chloride, or ascorbic acid (+ diuretic) may minimize effects of PCP and aid in its excretion
- Nitroprusside for hypertensive crisis

Drugs of Abuse

Hallucinogens (cont.)

• Clinically significant interactions are listed below

Drug of Abuse	Interacting Drugs	Reaction
Cannabis/Marihuana	Antidepressant: – Tricyclic, e.g., desipramine	Case reports of tachycardia, light-headedness, mood lability and delirium with combination Cardiac complications reported in children and adolescents
	– MAOI: tranylcypromine	Caution: Cannabis increases serotonin levels and may result in a serotonin syndrome (see p. 46)
	Antipsychotic, e.g., chlorpromazine, thioridazine	Drugs with anticholinergic and α-adrenergic properties can cause marked hypotension and increased disorientation
	Barbiturate	Additive effect causing anxiety and hallucinations
	Cocaine	Increased heart rate; blood pressure increased with high doses of both drugs; increased plasma level of cocaine and euphoria
	Disulfiram	Synergistic CNS stimulation reported, hypomania
	Lithium	Clearance of lithium may be decreased
	Morphine	THC blocks excitation produced by morphine
	Protease inhibitor: indinavir, nelfinavir	Inhaled marihuana reported to reduce indinavir AUC by 17% C_{max} of nelfinavir by 21%; no effect on viral load
LSD	SSRI antidepressant, e.g., fluoxetine	Tonic clonic seizures reported Recurrence or worsening of flashbacks reported with fluoxetine, sertraline, paroxetine
	Protease inhibitor: ritonavir	Elevated levels of LSD possible due to inhibited metabolism
PCP	Acidifying agents: cranberry juice, ammonium chloride	Increased excretion of PCP
	Protease inhibitor: ritonavir	Elevated levels PCP possible due to inhibited metabolism.

DRUG	COMMENTS
HALLUCINOGENIC AGENTS	
CANNABIS	
Marihuana – crushed leaves, stems, and flowers of female hemp plant, *Cannabis sativa* Smoked (cigarettes or water pipe), swallowed *Slang*: grass, pot, joint, hemp, weed, reefer, smoke, Mary Jane, Indian hay, ace, ganja, gold, J, locoweed, shit, herb, Mexican, ragweed, bhang, sticks, blunt, dope, sinsemilla, skunk, Hydro (hydroponic marihuana), blunts, mota, yerba, grifa **Hashish** – resin from flowers and leaves; more potent than marihuana Smoked or cooked and swallowed *Slang*: hash, hash oil, weed oil, weed juice, honey oil, hash brownies, tea, black, solids, grease, smoke, boom, chronic, gangster, hemp	– Tetrahydrocannabinol (THC) is the active ingredient: 5–11% in marihuana and up to 28% in hashish – THC undergoes first pass metabolism to form the psychoactive metabolite 11-OH-THC. Initial $T_{1/2}$ is 1–2 h and elimination $T_{1/2}$ is 24–36 h. Metabolized by 2D6, 2C9, and 2C19. Weak inhibitor of CYP 1A2, 3A4, 2C9, and 2C19. – Effects occur rapidly and last up to several hours; accumulates in fat tissue for up to four weeks before being released back into the bloodstream – effects may persist. – Early data suggest THC may have some benefit in the treatment of tics in Tourette's syndrome and for chronic neuropathic pain – Tolerance and psychic dependence may occur; reverse tolerance (supersensitivity) described – Combined with other drugs including PCP ("killer weed"), opium ("o.j."), heroin ("A-bomb") or flunitrazepam to enhance effect – Most users experience euphoria with feelings of self-confidence and relaxation; some become dysphoric, anxious, agitated and suspicious. Can cause psychotic symptoms with confusion, hallucinations, emotional lability (very prolonged or heavy use can cause serious and potentially irreversible psychosis) – Increased craving for sweets, decreased concentration, "amotivational syndrome" – Chronic use: bronchitis, weight gain, bloodshot eyes, loss of energy, apathy, "fuzzy" thinking, impaired judgment, decreased testosterone in males; increased risk of depression, anxiety and schizophrenia – Cannabis cigarettes have a higher tar content than ordinary cigarettes and are potentially carcinogenic – Pregnancy: can retard fetal growth, and cause withdrawal reactions in the infant – Breast-feeding: can reach high levels in milk, especially with heavy use

DRUG	COMMENTS
KETAMINE (Ketalar) General anesthetic in day surgery Taken orally as capsules, tablets, powder, crystals, and solution; injected, snorted, smoked *Slang*: K, special K, vitamin K, ket, green, jet, kit-kat, cat valiums, Ketalar SV	−NMDA receptor antagonist; prevents glutamate activation; inhibits reuptake of catacholamines (5-HT, NE, DA) −Used as a club drug at raves −Related to PCP and involved in "date rapes" −Doses of 60–100 mg injected; consciousness maintained at this dose, but get disorientation and analgesia −Physical effects: increased heart rate and blood pressure, nausea, vomiting, increased tone, nystagmus, stereotypic movements, numbness −Effects start within 60 sec. (IV) and 10–20 min (PO) −CNS effects: dream-like state, confusion, hostility, delirium, hallucinations, amnesia, depersonalization − Highly addictive −Toxic effects: delirium, respiratory depression, loss of consciousness, catatonia; 1 gm can cause death
LYSERGIC ACID DIETHYLAMIDE (LSD) Semi-synthetic drug derived from ergot (grain fungus) White powder: used as tablet, capsule, liquid, snorted, smoked, inhaled, injected *Slang*: acid, cubes, purple haze, Raggedy Ann, sunshine, LBJ, peace pill, big D, blotters, domes, hits, tabs, doses, window-pane, microdot, boomers	−5-HT2 receptor agonist −Used as a club drug at raves −Effects occur in less than 1 h and last 2–18 h −CNS effects with 25 microgram dose −Combined with cocaine, mescaline, or amphetamine to prolong effects −Physical effects: mydriasis, nausea, muscle tension, decreased appetite, hyperthermia, hypertension, numbness, weakness, tremors −Can cause agitation, visual hallucinations, suicidal, homicidal, and irrational behavior and dysphoria; panic, psychotic reactions can last several days; sedation reported −Flashbacks occur without drug being taken −Tolerance develops rapidly; psychological dependence occurs −Pregnancy: increased risk of spontaneous abortions; congenital abnormalities have been reported
MESCALINE From peyote cactus buttons; pure product rarely available Cactus buttons are dried, then sliced, chopped, or ground; used as powder, capsule, tablet, inhaled or injected *Slang*: mesc, peyote, buttons, cactus	−Effects occur slowly and last 10–18 h −Less potent than LSD, but cross-tolerance reported −High doses: anxiety, disorientation, impaired reality testing, headache, dry skin, numbness, tremors, increased temperature and heart rate, hypertension or hypotension, cardiac and respiratory depression −Chronic mental disorders and flashbacks reported −Dependence not reported but tolerance to effects occurs quickly
MORNING GLORY SEEDS Active ingredient is lysergic acid amide; 1/10th as potent as LSD Seeds eaten whole, or ground, mushed, soaked, and solution injected *Slang*: flying saucers, licorice drops, heavenly blue, pearly gates	−Effects occur after 30–90 min when seeds ingested and immediately when solution injected −Commercial seeds are treated with insecticides, fungicides, and other chemicals and can be poisonous
PEYOTE From cactus *Lophaphora williamsii* Dried, chewed, and swallowed, used as capsules, solution	−Used for centuries by native people of North and South America −Effects occur 1–2 h after ingestion −Geometric brilliant colors, weightlessness, time distortion, anxiety, panic, dizziness, severe nausea

Hallucinogens (cont.)

DRUG	COMMENTS
PHENCYCLIDINE General anesthetic used in veterinary medicine; often misrepresented as other drugs Powder, chunks, crystals; used as tablets, capsules, liquid, inhaled (dipped onto cigarettes or joints), snorted, injected (IM or IV) *Slang*: PCP, angel dust, hog, horse tranquilizer, animal tranquilizer, peace pill, killer, weed, supergrass, crystal, "CJ," dust, rocket fuel, boat, loveboat	–Blocks reuptake of satacholamines (5-HT, NE, and DA) –Glutamate agonist at NMDA receptor –Effects occur in a few minutes and can last several days to weeks (half-life 18 h) –Frequently sold on street as other drugs (easily synthesized); mis-synthesis yields a product that can Cause abdominal cramps, vomiting, coma, and death –Intermittent vomiting, drooling, diaphoresis, miosis, nystagmus, hypertension and ataxia can occur –Can cause apathy, estrangement, feelings of isolation, indifference to pain, delirium, disorientation with amnesia, depression, psychosis, and violence (often self-directed); can feel intermittently anxious, fearful, euphoric, disinhibited –Toxic effects: hypoglycemia, muscle rigidity, rhabdomyolysis, respiratory depression, coma; deaths have occurred secondary to uncontrollable seizures, or to hypertension resulting in intracranial hemorrhage, hyperthermia –Flashbacks occur –Psychological dependence occurs –Pregnancy: signs of toxicity have been reported in newborns –Breast-feeding: drug concentrates in milk and detectable for weeks after heavy use
PSILOCYBIN From *Psilocybe mexicana* mushroom Used as dried mushroom, white crystal, powder, capsule, injection; eaten raw, cooked or steeped as tea *Slang*: magic mushrooms, sacred mushrooms, mushroom, shroom, purple passion	–Chemically related to LSD and DMT –Increased release of catacholamines (5-HT, DA, and NE) –Effects occur within 30 min and last several hours –Pure drug rarely available; injection dangerous as foreign particles present –Mental effects: altered perceptions, nervousness, paranoia, flashbacks; chronic mental disorders –Physical effects: nausea and vomiting after ingestion –Tolerance develops rapidly; cross-tolerance occurs with LSD –Physical or psychological dependence not reported –Mistaken identity with "death-cap" (Amanita) mushroom can result in accidental poisoning
SALVIA DIVINORUM Member of the mint family Leaves chewed, or crushed and the juice ingested as tea, smoked *Slang*: diviner's sage, magic mint, Maria Pastora	–Main active ingredient is Salvinorin A; a potent kappa opioid agonist –Used in traditional spiritual practices by native people of Mexico –Effects, when taken orally, depend on the absorption of Salvinorin A through the oral mucosa as it is inactivated by the GI tract –Can cause dramatic, and sometimes frightening, hallucinogenic experiences
TRYPTAMINES Soaked in parsley, dried and snorted or smoked, used as liquid (tea), injected *Slang*: lunch-hour drug, businessman's lunch, FOXY(=MeO-DIPT)	DIMETHYLTRYPTAMINE (DMT), ALPHA-METHYLTRYPTAMINE (AMT), 5-METHYL-DI-ISOPROPYL-TRYPTAMINE(5-MeO-DIPT) –Appear in nature in several plants in South America; easily synthesized –Monoamine oxidase inhibitors; interact with a variety of drugs and foods –Effects vary widely depending on amount ingested; occur almost immediately with DMT and last 30–60 min –Readily destroyed by stomach acids –Often mixed with marihuana –Produce intense visual hallucinations, loss of awareness of surroundings –Anxiety and panic frequent due to quick onset of effects

Alcohol

SLANG

- Booze, hooch, juice, brew

PHARMACOLOGICAL/ PSYCHIATRIC EFFECTS

- Signs and symptoms are associated with blood alcohol level of approximately 34 mmol/l (higher in chronic users; 60–70 mmol/l)
- Effects of a single drink occur within 15 min and last approximately 60 min, depending on amount taken; renal elimination is about 10 g alcohol per hour (about 30 ml (1 oz) whiskey or 1 bottle of regular beer). Blood alcohol level declines by 4–7 mmol/l per hour.

Acute

- Disinhibition, relaxation, euphoria, agitation, drowsiness, impaired cognition, judgment, and memory, perceptual and motor dysfunction
- ☞ **Acute alcohol intake decreases hepatic metabolism of co-administered drugs by competition for microsomal enzymes**

Chronic

- Chronic use results in an increased capacity to metabolize alcohol and a concurrent CNS tolerance; psychological as well as physical dependence may occur; hepatic metabolism decreases with liver cirrhosis
- ☞ **Chronic alcohol use increases hepatic metabolism of co-administered drugs**

Physical

- Hand tremor, dyspepsia, diarrhea, morning nausea and vomiting, polyuria, impotence, pancreatitis, headache, hepatomegaly, peripheral neuropathy

Mental

- Memory blackouts, nightmares, insomnia, hallucinations, paranoia, intellectual impairment, dementia, Wernicke-Korsakoff syndrome, and other organic mental disorders
- Chronic alcohol use by patients with schizophrenia suggested to be associated with more florid symptoms, more re-hospitalizations, poorer long-term outcome and increased risk of tardive dyskinesia

RELATED PROBLEMS

- Up to 50% of alcoholics meet the criteria for lifetime diagnosis of major depression
- Withdrawal symptoms, physical violence, loss of control when drinking, surreptitious drinking, change in tolerance to alcohol, deteriorating job performance, change in social interactions, increased risk for stroke, and death from motor vehicle accidents

TOXICITY

- Hazardous alcohol consumption: greater than 80 g ethanol per day (approx. 6 bottles of regular beer, 270 ml (9 oz) spirits, or 720 ml (24 oz) wine)
- Risk increases when combined with drugs with CNS depressant activity
- Symptoms include: CNS depression, decreased or absent tendon reflexes, cardiac dysfunction, flushed skin progressing to cyanosis, hypoglycemia, hypothermia, peripheral vasodilation, respiratory depression, shock, coma

Alcohol (cont.)

DISCONTINUATION SYNDROME

- Occurs after chronic use (i.e., drinking for more than 3 days, more than 500 ml of spirits or equivalent per day)
- Most effects seen within 5 days after stopping

Mild Withdrawal

- Insomnia, irritability, headache
- Usually transient and self-limiting

Severe Reactions

- Phase I: begins within hours of cessation and lasts 3–5 days. Symptoms: tremor, tachycardia, diaphoresis, labile BP, nausea, vomiting, anxiety
- Phase II: perceptual disturbances (usually visual or auditory)
- Phase III: 10–15% untreated alcohol withdrawal patients reach this phase; seizures (usually tonicclonic) last 0.5–4 min and can progress to status epilepticus
- Phase IV: Delirium tremens (DTs) usually occurs after 72 h; includes autonomic hyperactivity and severe hyperthermia; mortality rate of patients who reach phase IV is 20%
- Wernicke's encephalopathy can occur in patients with thiamine deficiency

Protracted Abstinence Syndrome

- Patients may experience subtle withdrawal symptoms that can last from weeks to months – include sleep dysregulation, anxiety, irritability and mood instability
- Cognitive impairment from chronic alcohol use will persist for several weeks after abstinence achieved
- Individuals are at high risk for relapse during this period

TREATMENT

- In acute intoxication minimize stimulation; effects will diminish as blood alcohol level declines (rate of 4–7 mmol/l per hour)
- Withdrawal reactions following chronic alcohol use may require
  a) vitamin supplementation (thiamine 50 mg orally or IM)
  b) benzodiazepine for symptomatic relief and to prevent seizures (chlordiazepoxide, lorazepam, or oxazepam); caution in transferring dependence from alcohol to benzodiazepines
  c) hydration and electrolyte correction
  d) high potency antipsychotic (e.g., haloperidol, zuclopenthixol) to treat behavior disturbances and hallucinations
  e) paraldehyde, or haloperidol and lorazepam, to prevent or treat delirium tremens
- SSRIs (e.g., fluoxetine) and buspirone have shown some efficacy in decreasing alcohol consumption by 9–17%, as well as decreasing interest in and craving for alcohol
- Naltrexone and acamprosete reported to be effective adjuncts to treatment for relapse prevention following alcohol detoxification
- See p. 257 for use of disulfiram in treatment

PRECAUTIONS

- Increased risk of drug toxicity possible in patients with alcohol-induced liver impairment or cirrhosis
- Risk as well as type of drug-drug interaction varies with acute versus chronic alcohol consumption

- Infants born with fetal alcohol syndrome with mental deficiency, irritability, and facial abnormalities
- Withdrawal reactions reported

Breast Milk
- Milk levels attain 90–95% of blood levels; prolonged intake can be detrimental

DRUG INTERACTIONS
- Clinically significant interactions are listed below

Class of Drug	Example	Reaction
Analgesic	Acetaminophen	Chronic excessive alcohol use increases susceptibility to acetaminophen-induced hepatotoxicity
	Salicylates	Increased gastric bleeding with ASA; reduced peak plasma concentration of ASA reported ASA may increase blood alcohol concentration by reducing ethanol oxidation by gastric alcohol dehydrogenase
Antibiotic	Cephalosporins	Disulfiram-like reaction with nausea, hypotension, flushing, headache, tachycardia
	Doxycycline	Chronic alcohol use induces metabolism and decreases plasma level of doxycycline
Anticoagulants	Warfarin	Chronic alcohol use induces warfarin metabolism and decreases hypoprothrombinemic effect. Acute alcohol use can impair warfarin metabolism
Anticonvulsant	Barbiturates, phenytoin	Additive CNS effects Decreased plasma level of ethanol Acute intoxication inhibits phenobarbital metabolism; chronic intoxication enhances metabolism
	Valproic acid, divalproex	Displaces alcohol from protein binding and potentiates intoxicating effect
Antidepressant	Tricyclic	Additive CNS effects Short-term or acute use reduces first-pass metabolism of the antidepressant and increases its plasma level Imipramine and desipramine clearance is increased in chronic alcoholics and during the first month after detoxification; delay in ethanol absorption with antidepressant use
	SSRI	Rate of fluvoxamine absorption increased by ethanol
	NaSSA	Additive CNS effects
Antifungal	Metronidazole, ketoconazole, furazolidone	Disulfiram-like reaction
Antipsychotics		Additive CNS effects Extrapyramidal side effects may be worsened by alcohol
Antitubercular Drug	Isoniazid	Increased risk of hepatotoxicity Tyramine-containing alcoholic beverages may cause a hypertensive reaction (MAOI)
Antiviral	Abacavir	Increased AUC of abacavir by 41%
Ascorbic acid		Increased ethanol clearance
Benzodiazepine	General	Potentiation of CNS effects
	Alprazolam	Alprazolam reported to increase aggression in moderate alcohol drinkers
	Triazolam, estazolam, diazepam	Brain concentrations of various benzodiazepines altered by ethanol: triazolam, and estazolam concentrations decreased, diazepam concentration increased, no change with chlordiazepoxide
Ca-channel blocker	Verapamil	Increased concentration of ethanol due to inhibited metabolism

Alcohol (cont.)

Class of Drug	Example	Reaction
Chloral hydrate		Additive CNS effects Increased plasma level of metabolite of chloral hydrate (trichloroethanol), and of blood ethanol
CNS depresant	Hypnotics, benzodiazepines, narcotics, etc.	Potentiation of CNS effects
Disulfiram		Flushing, sweating, palpitations, headache due to formation of acetaldehyde (see p. 257)
H₂ blocker	Cimetidine, ranitidine	Peak blood alcohol level increased by 92% with cimetidine and 34% with ranitidine – data contradictory (no effect with famotidine)
Narcotic: slow-release opioids	Morphine: sustained-release (Kadian)	Alcohol can speed the release of opioids into the blood stream by dissolving the slow-release system (not all products affected; no problems noted with Codeine Contin, Hydromorph Contin, MS Contin and OxyContin). Use caution with other slow-release products.
Sulfonylurea	Chlorpropamide, tolbutamide	Flushing, sweating, palpitations, headache due to formation of acetaldehyde
Milk		Decreased ethanol absorption by delaying gastric emptying
Stimulant	Cocaine	Ethanol promotes the formation of a highly addicting etabolite, cocoethylene Reports of enhanced hepatotoxicity Increased heart rate; variable effect on blood pressure Increased risk of sudden death with combined use (18-fold) Combined use reported to result in more impulsive decision making and poorer performance on tests of learning and memory
Tianeptine		Rate of tianeptine absorption decreased; plasma level decreased by 30%

Opiates/Narcotics

GENERAL COMMENTS	• High rate of psychopathology, specifically depression, alcoholism, and antisocial personality disorder, have been demonstrated in opiate abusers (often not clear if these are cause or effect) • Polydrug use and co-dependence on benzodiazepines appears particularly common among individuals injecting opioids
PHARMACOLOGICAL/ PSYCHIATRIC EFFECTS	• Differ somewhat depending on type of drug taken, the dose, the route of administration, and whether combined with other drugs • Elderly more sensitive to effects and side effects of opiates
Physical	• Analgesia, "rush" sensation followed by relaxation, decreased tension, slow pulse and respiration, increased body temperature, dry mouth, constricted pupils, decreased GI motility, hypotension, nausea, insensitivity to pain, cough suppression
Mental	• Euphoria, state of gratification, sedation, "deadening of emotions"
High Doses	• Respiratory depression, cardiovascular complications, coma, and death
Chronic Use	• General loss of energy, ambition, and drive, motor retardation, attention impairment, sedation, slurred speech • Tolerance and physical dependence; withdrawal • Cross-tolerance occurs with other narcotics
WITHDRAWAL	• Symptoms include: yawning, runny nose, sneezing, lacrimation, dilated pupils, vasodilation, tachycardia, elevated BP, vomiting and diarrhea, restlessness, tremor, chills, piloerection, bone pain, abdominal pain and cramps, anorexia, anxiety, irritability, insomnia • Acute symptoms can last 10–14 days (longer with methadone)

TREATMENT	• Opioid withdrawal states are generally not life-threatening; "cold turkey" is acceptable to some addicts
	• Non-narcotic alternatives (e.g., benzodiazepines, antipsychotics) usually do not work
	• Drugs are prescribed for the following reasons:
	  a) to reverse effects of toxicity using narcotic antagonists (e.g., naloxone, redundant naltrexone – can precipitate withdrawal)
	  b) to treat the immediate withdrawal reaction (e.g., clonidine, methadone)
	  c) to aid in detoxification, or for maintenance therapy in a supervised treatment program (e.g., methadone, buprenorphine)

DRUG INTERACTIONS	• Clinically significant interactions are listed below

Drug of Abuse	Interacting Drugs	Reaction
Opiates (general)	CNS drugs, e.g., alcohol, benzodiazepines	Additive CNS effects; can lead to respiratory depression
	Cocaine	May potentiate cocaine euphoria
	Narcotic antagonist, e.g., naloxone	Will precipitate withdrawal reaction
Codeine, oxycodone, hydrocodone	Antidepressants, SSRI: e.g., fluoxetine, paroxetine	Loss of analgesic efficacy; inhibited biotransformation of narcotic to active moiety via CYP2D6 (e.g., conversion of codeine to morphine, etc.)
	Protease inhibitor: ritonavir	Moderate decrease in clearance of hydrocodone and oxycodone

Drugs of Abuse

Opiates/Narcotics (cont.)

Drug of Abuse	Interacting Drugs	Reaction
Fentanyl, alfentanyl	Antibiotic: erythromycin, clarithromycin Antifungal: ketoconazole	Increased plasma concentration of fentanyl due to inhibited metabolism via CYP3A4, resulting in prolonged analgesia and increased adverse effects
	Protease inhibitor: ritonavir	Large decrease in clearance of fentanyl and alfentanyl
Heroin	Antidepressant: doxepin	Case reports of delirium when used for heroin withdrawal
	Protease inhibitor: ritonavir, nelfinavir	Increased level of heroin possible due to inhibited metabolism
Meperidine	Antidepressant: MAOIs – irreversible, RIMA	Increased excitation, sweating and hypotension reported; may lead to development of encephalopathy, convulsions, coma, respiratory depression and "serotonin syndrome" (see p. 46)
	Antipsychotic: Phenothiazines, e.g., chlorpromazine	Additive analgesic, CNS and cardiovascular effects
	Anticonvulant: phenytoin, barbiturates	Decreased plasma level of meperidine due to increased metabolism
	H_2 Antagonist: cimetidine	22% decrease in clearance of meperidine
	Protease inhibitor: ritonavir	Large increase in plasma level of meperidine due to inhibited metabolism
Methadone		See pp. 268–269
Opium	Antihistamines: tripelennamine, cyclizine	"Opiate high" reported with combination, euphoria
	H_2 Antagonist: cimetidine	Enhanced effect of narcotic and increased adverse effects due to decreased metabolism
Pentazocine	Antidepressant: SSRIs, e.g., fluoxetine	Excitatory toxicity reported (serotonergic)
Propoxyphene	Protease inhibitor: ritonavir	Large decrease in clearance of propoxyphene

DRUG	COMMENTS
NARCOTIC AGENTS	
HEROIN Diacetylmorphine – synthetic derivative of morphine Injected (IV – "mainlining", or SC – "skin popping"), smoked, inhaled, taken orally *Slang*: "H", horse, junk, snow, stuff, lady, dope, shill, poppy, smack, scag, black tar, Lady Jane, white stuff, brown sugar, skunk, white horse	–Effects almost immediate following IV injection and last several hours; effects occur in 15–60 min after oral dosing –Risk of accidental overdose as street preparations contain various concentrations of heroin –Physical dependence and tolerance occur within 2 weeks; withdrawal occurs within 8–12 h after last dose and peaks in 48–72 h –Combined with flunitrazepam to enhance effects and to ameliorate heroin withdrawal –Toxicity: sinus bradycardia or tachycardia, unstable blood pressure, palpitations, syncope, respiratory depression, coma and death –Pregnancy: high rate of spontaneous abortions, premature labor and stillbirths – babies are often small and have an increased mortality risk; withdrawal symptoms in newborn reported
MORPHINE Principal active component of opium poppy Taken as powder, capsule, tablet, liquid, injected *Slang*: "M", dreamer, sweet Jesus, junk, morph, Miss Emma, monkey, white stuff	–Effects as for heroin, but slower onset and longer-acting –Effects occur in 15–60 min after oral dosing and last 1–8 h –Physical effects: pain relief, nausea, constipation; with high doses can get respiratory depression, unconsciousness, and coma –Mental effects: drowsiness, confusion, euphoria –Dependence liability high (second to heroin) due to powerful euphoric and analgesic effects

DRUG	COMMENTS
METHADONE (Dolophine, Roxane, Metadol) Used as tablets, liquid, injected *Slang*: the kick pill, dolly, meth	– Drug used in withdrawal and detoxification from opiates, but subject to abuse – Effects occur 30–60 min after oral dosing, and last 7–48 h – Chronic use causes constipation, blurred vision, sweating, decreased libido, menstrual irregularities, joint and bone pain, sleep disturbances – Physical dependence and tolerance occur; withdrawal effects peak in 72–96h and can last up to 14 days – Pregnancy: dosing needs should be reassessed (decreased between weeks 14 and 32 and increased prior to term); withdrawal effects reported in neonates – Breastfeeding: small amounts of methadone enter milk; nurse prior to taking dose or 2–6 h after
OPIUM Resinous preparation from unripe seed pods of opium poppy; available as dark brown chunks or as Powder Soaked, taken as solution, smoked *Slang*: big O, black stuff, block, gum, hop	– Contains a number of alkaloids including morphine (6–12 %) and codeine (0.5–1.5 %) – Physical effects: nausea common, constipation; with high doses can get respiratory depression, unconsciousness, and coma – Mental effects: drowsiness, confusion, euphoria
OTHER FREQUENTLY ABUSED PRESCRIPTION NARCOTICS AND RELATED DRUGS	
CODEINE Methylmorphine Used orally, liquid, injected *Slang*: schoolboy, 3s, 4s, Captain Cody, Cody	– Naturally occurring alkaloid from opium poppy – Common ingredient of both prescription and over-the-counter analgesics and antitussives (e.g., Fiorinal-C, Tylenol #1, etc.) – Mixed with glutethimide (called loads, pacs, doors and fours, pancakes, and syrup) – Tolerance develops gradually; physical dependence is infrequent; withdrawal will occur with chronic high-dose use
DEXTROMETHORPHAN (Robitussin DM) Used orally *Slang:* robo, poor man's PCP	– Higher doses can cause euphoria, altered perceptions, ataxia, nystagmus, visual disturbances, and disorientation; may progress to panic attacks, delusions, psychotic/manic behavior, hallucinations, paranoia, and seizures
FENTANYL (Duragesic, Sublimaze) *Slang*: tango, cash, Apache, China girl, China white, dance fever, friend, goodfella, jackpot, murders, TNT	– Effects almost immediate following IV injection and last 30–60 min; with IM use, onset slower and duration of action is up to 120 min – Exposing application site of fentanyl patch to external heat source (e.g., heating pad) can increase drug absorption and result in increased drug effect – Euphoria occurs quickly – Side effects: primarily sedation, confusion, dizziness, dry mouth, constipation, and GI distress – High doses can produce muscle rigidity (including respiratory muscles) respiratory depression, unconsciousness, and coma
HYDROCODONE (e.g., Novahistex DH)	– Related to codeine, but more potent – An ingredient in prescription antitussive preparations; sought by abuser due to easy availability and purity of product – Physical, CNS and toxic effects as for codeine – Tolerance develops rapidly – Lethal dose: 0.5–1.0 g
HYDROMORPHONE (Dilaudid) Used orally *Slang*: juice, dillies	– Semisynthetic narcotic – At low doses side effects less common than with other narcotics; high doses more toxic due to strong respiratory depressant effect
LEVORPHANOL (Levo Dromoran)	– Synthetic narcotic analgesic with effects similar to morphine – High doses can produce cardiac arrhythmias, hypotension, respiratory depression, and coma
MEPERIDINE/PETHIDINE (Demerol) Synthetic opioid derivative Used orally, injected *Slang*: demmies, painkiller	– Metabolite (normeperidine) is highly toxic; may accumulate with chronic use and cause convulsions – High doses produce disorientation, hallucinations, respiratory depression, stupor, and coma

Opiates/Narcotics (cont.)

DRUG	COMMENTS
OXYCODONE (Percodan, Percocet) Semisynthetic derivative Used orally; tablets chewed, crushed and snorted, powder boiled for injection *Slang*: percs, OC, OXY, oxycotton, killers	– An ingredient in combination analgesic products – Very high abuse potential – Physical effects: nausea, constipation; with high doses can get respiratory depression and coma – Mental effects: drowsiness, disorientation, euphoria
PENTAZOCINE (Talwin) Used orally, injected *Slang*: T's, big T, Tee, Tea	– Has both agonist and antagonist properties at opioid receptors – Repeated injections can result in tissue damage at injection site – Mixed with tripelennamine (called T's and blues)
PROPOXYPHENE (Darvon) Used orally, injected *Slang*: yellow football	– Synthetic narcotic analgesic – Abuse results in a state of euphoria – Repeated injections can cause damage to veins and local tissue – Tolerance to analgesic and euphoric effects develops gradually; chronic use results in physical dependence

SUBSTANCES ABUSED

- Volatile gases: butane, propane, aerosol propellants
- Solvents: airplane glue, gasoline, toluene, printing fluid, cleaning solvents, benzene, acetone, amyl nitrite ("poppers"), etc.
- Aerosols: deodorants, hair spray, freon
- Anesthetic gases: nitrous oxide (laughing gas), chloroform, ether

SLANG

- Glue, gassing, sniffing, chemo, snappers
- Amyl and butyl nitrates: pearls, poppers, rush, locker room
- Nitrous oxides: laughing gas, balloons, whippets

GENERAL COMMENTS

- High rate of psychopathology, specifically alcoholism, depression, and antisocial personality disorder, have been demonstrated in individuals with a history of solvent use
- Considered "poor man's" drug of abuse; used by children, and in third world countries to lessen hunger pain
- Fourth most commonly abused substance among teens in Canada; high use in Aboriginal populations
- Amyl nitrite used to promote sexual excitement and orgasm

METHODS OF USE

- "Bagging" – pouring liquid or discharging gas into plastic bag or balloon
- "Sniffing" – holding mouth over container as gas is discharged
- "Huffing" – holding a soaked rag over mouth or nose
- "Torching" – inhaling fumes discharged from a cigarette lighter, then igniting the exhaled air

PHARMACOLOGICAL/ PSYCHIATRIC EFFECTS

- Differ somewhat depending on type of drug taken
- Fumes sniffed, inhaled; use of plastic bag can lead to suffocation
- Rapid CNS penetration – effects occur quickly and last a short time

Physical

- Drowsiness, dizziness, slurred speech, impaired motor function, muscle weakness, cramps, headaches, light sensitivity, nausea or vomiting, salivation, sneezing, coughing, wheezing, decreased breathing and heart rate, hypotension (reflex tachycardia)
- Fatalities can arise from cardiac arrest or inhalation of vomit while unconscious
- Amyl nitrite vasodilates coronary vasculature and decreases after load

Mental

- Changing levels of awareness, impaired judgment and memory, loss of inhibitions, hallucinations, euphoria, excitation, vivid fantasies, feeling of invincibility, delirium

High Doses

- Loss of consciousness, convulsions, cardiac arrhythmia, seizures, death

Inhalants/Aerosols (cont.)

| Chronic Use |

- Fatigue, encephalopathy, hearing loss, visual impairment, sinusitis, rhinitis, laryngitis, weight loss, kidney and liver damage, bone marrow damage, cardiac arrhythmias, chronic lung disease
- Inability to think clearly, memory disturbances, depression, irritability, hostility, paranoia
- Tolerance develops to desired effect; psychological dependence is frequent

TREATMENT

- Effects are usually short-lasting; use calming techniques, reassurance

TOXICITY

- CNS: acute and chronic effects reported, e.g., ataxia, peripheral neuropathy
- Cardiac: an MI can occur, primarily with use of halogenated solvents
- Renal: acidosis, hypokalemia
- Hepatic: hepatitis, hepatic necrosis
- Hematologic: bone marrow suppression primarily with benzene and nitrous oxide use

DRUG INTERACTIONS

- Clinically significant interactions are listed below

Class of Drug	Example	Reaction
CNS depressants	Alcohol, benzodiazepines, hypnotics, narcotics, etc.	Increased impairment of judgment, distortion of reality

Gamma-hydroxybutyrate (GHB)

INDICATIONS

▲ Approved (as Xyrem) for oral treatment of cataplexy and excessive daytime sleepiness in patients with narcolepsy

SLANG

- Liquid ecstasy, liquid X, liquid F, goop, GBH = Grievous Bodily Harm, Easy lay, Ghost Breath, G, Somatomax, Gamma-G, Growth Hormone Booster, Georgia home boy, nature's Quaalude, G-riffick, Soap, Salty Water, Women's viagra

GENERAL COMMENTS

- Prescribing and dispensing restrictions apply for use of Xyrem in patients with narcolepsy
- Used for its hallucinogenic and euphoric effects at raves (or dance parties)
- Marketed as Xyrem in the USA for treatment of cataplexy in patients with narcolepsy – distributed as a "controlled drug" with generic name of sodium oxybate; improves nighttime sleep and reduces daytime sleep attacks and cataplexy at doses of 6–9 g/night
- Has been used in Europe to treat alcohol dependency at a dose of 50 mg/kg/day – reported to reduce alcohol cravings and increase abstinence; also used for sedation and to treat opiate withdrawal
- Originally researched as an anesthetic; shown to have limited analgesic effects and increased seizure risk
- Promoted illegally as a health food product, an aphrodisiac and for muscle building
- Has been used in "date rapes" because it acts rapidly, produces disinhibition and relaxation of voluntary muscles and causes anterograde amnesia for events that occur under the influence of the drug
- Chronic use may result in tolerance and/or psychological dependence
- Products converted to GHB in the body include: gammabutyrolactone (GBL – also called Blue Nitro Vitality, GH Revitalizer, GHR, Remforce, Renewtrient and Gamma G – is sold in health food stores) and the industrial solvent butanediol (BD – also called tetramethylene glycol or Sucol B, and sold as Zen, NRG-3, Soma Solutions, Enliven, and Serenity)

METHODS OF USE

- Xyrem available as an oral solution containing 500 mg/ml
- Abused as a powder mixed in a liquid; usually sold in vials and taken orally; has salty or soapy taste

PHARMACOLOGY

- Produced naturally in the body and is a metabolite of gamma aminobutyric acid (GABA); acts on $GABA_B$ receptor to potentiate gabaergic effects
- Reduces cataplexy
- Shown to increase dopamine levels in the basal ganglia
- Stimulates slow-wave sleep (stages 3 and 4) and decreases stage 1 sleep; with continued use decreases REM sleep
- Some effects of GHB are blocked by opioid receptor antagonists

PHARMACOLOGICAL/ PSYCHIATRIC EFFECTS

- Deep sleep reported with doses of 2.0 g
- At 10 mg/kg produces anxiolytic effect, muscle relaxation, and amnesia
- At 20–30 mg/kg increases REM and slow-wave sleep
- At doses > 60 mg/kg can result in anesthesia, respiratory depression, and coma

PHARMACOKINETICS

- Quickly absorbed orally; onset of action occurs within 30 min; peak plasma concentration reached in 20–60 min
- Elimination half-life approx. 20–30 min; no longer detected in blood after 2–8 h and in urine after 8–12 h

Drugs of Abuse

Gamma-hydroxybutyrate (GHB) (cont.)

ADVERSE REACTIONS

Physical

- With high doses: high frequency of drop attacks – "victim" suddenly loses all muscular control and drops to the floor, unable to resist the "attacker"
- Drowsiness, dizziness, nausea, vomiting, headache, hypotension, bradycardia, ataxia, nystagmus, hypotonia, hypothermia, tremor, muscle spasms, seizures, decreased respiration; symptoms usually resolve within 7 h, but dizziness can persist up to 2 weeks
- Use of sodium oxydate in narcolepsy has been associated with headache, nausea, dizziness, sleepwalking, confusion and urinary incontinence; worsening of sleep apnea
- Use of high doses may lead to unconsciousness and coma – called "G-hold" (particularly dangerous in combination with alcohol)

Mental

- Feeling of well-being, lowered inhibitions, sedation, poor concentration, confusion, amnesia, euphoria, and hallucinations; can cause agitation and aggression

WITHDRAWAL

- Symptoms occur 1–6 h after abrupt cessation and can last for 5–15 days after chronic use
- Initial symptoms include nausea, vomiting, insomnia, anxiety, confusion, and/or tremor; after chronic use, symptoms can include mild tachycardia and hypertension, and can progress to delirium with auditory and visual hallucinations

TOXICITY

- Low therapeutic index; dangerous in combination with alcohol
- Overdoses can occur due to unknown purity and concentration of ingested product
- Symptoms: bradycardia, seizures, apnea, sudden (reversible) coma with abrupt awakening and violence
- Coma reported in doses > 60 mg/kg (4 g)
- Several deaths reported secondary to respiratory failure

Management

- No known antidote

USE IN PREGNANCY

- Schedule B drug

Breast Milk

- Unknown

DRUG INTERACTIONS

- Clinically significant interactions are listed below

Class of Drug	Example	Interaction Effects
Benzodiazepine	Diazepam	Has been used to treat GHB withdrawal effects; theoretically, may worsen respiratory depression
Cannabis		Increased pharmacological effects
CNS depressant	Alcohol	Synergistic CNS depressant effects can occur, especially with high doses of GHB leading to respiratory depression
Protease inhibitors	Ritonavir-saquinavir combination	GHB toxicity – may cause bradycardia, respiratory depression, and seizures
Stimulant	Amphetamines	Increased pharmacological effects

Flunitrazepam (Rohypnol)

SLANG

- Roofies, R-2s, Roches Dos, forget-me pill, Mexican Valium, roofinol, rope, rophies

GENERAL COMMENTS

- Used as a sedative/tranquilizer in some European countries
- Commonly used as a date-rape drug because it acts rapidly, produces dis-inhibition and relaxation of voluntary muscles, and causes anterograde amnesia for events that occur under the influence of the drug
- Alcohol potentiates the drug's effects

METHODS OF USE

- Ingested, snorted or injected
- Purchased in doses of 1 and 2 mg (legal manufacturers have added blue or green dye to formulation to color beverages and make them murky); illegal manufacturing is common
- Added to alcoholic beverages of unsuspecting victim

PHARMACOLOGY

- Fast-acting benzodiazepine (not marketed in Canada or US) structurally related to clonazepam
- Structurally related to clonazepam
- See p. 172

PHARMACOKINETICS

- Effects begin in 30 min; peak within 2 h; last up to 8 h

ADVERSE REACTIONS

- See p. 173
- These reactions are reported following restoration of consciousness

Physical

- Dizziness, impaired motor skills, "rubbery legs," weakness, unsteadiness, visual disturbances, blood shot eyes, slurred speech and urinary retention
- Decreased blood pressure and pulse, slowed breathing; may lead to respiratory depression and arrest

Mental

- Rapid loss of consciousness and amnesia; residual symptoms include drowsiness, fatigue, confusion, impaired memory and judgment, reduced inhibition
- If some memory of the event remains, the "victim" may describe a disassociation of body and mind – a sensation of being paralyzed, powerless, unable to resist

TOXICITY

- See Benzodiazepines p. 174

DRUG INTERACTIONS

- See Benzodiazepines pp. 175–177

Drugs of Abuse – References and Selected Readings

- Anton, R.F. (2001). Pharmacologic approaches to the management of alcoholism. *Journal of Clinical Psychiatry 62(Suppl. 20),* 11–17.
- Buck, M.L. (2000). Managing iatrogenic opioid dependence with methadone. *Pediatric Pharmacotherapy 6(7),* 1–7.
- Chabane, N., Leboyer, M., Mouren-Simeoni, M.C. (2000). Opiate antagonists in children and adolescents. *European Child and Adolescent Psychiatry 9(Suppl. 1),* 144–150.
- Kalant, H. (2001). The pharmacology and toxicology of "ecstasy" (MDMA) and related drugs. *Canadian Medical Association Journal 165(7),* 917–928.
- Kenna, G.A., McGeary, J.E., Swift, R.M. (2004). Pharmacotherapy, pharmacogenomics, and the future of alcohol dependence treatment, Part 2. *American Journal of Health-System Pharmacy 61(22),* 2380–2388.
- McRae, A. (2004). Pharmacotherapy of substance use disorders. *International Drug Therapy Newsletter 39(4),* 25–30.
- Myrick, H., Brody, K.T., Malcolm, R. (2001). New developments in the pharmacotherapy of alcohol dependence. *American Journal of Addictions 10(Suppl.),* 3–15.
- Niederhofer, H., Staffen, W. (2003). Acamprosate and its efficacy in treating alcohol dependent adolescents. *European Child and Adolescent Psychiatry 12(3),* 144–148.
- Schwartz, R.H., Milteer, R. (2000). Drug-facilitated sexual assault ("date rape"). *Southern Medical Journal 93(6),* 558–561.
- Srisurapanant, M., Jarusuraisin, N. (2002). Opioid antagonists for alcohol dependence. *Cochrane Database System Review (2),* CD001867.
- Swift, R.M. (2001). Can medication successfully treat substance addiction? *Psychopharmacology Update 12(1),* 4–5.
- Teter, C.J. (2003). Club Drugs Part I and II. *International Drug Therapy Newsletter 38 (7/8),* 49–56, 57–64.

CLASSIFICATION

- Drugs available for treatment of substance use disorders may be classified as follows:

Primary Indication	Generic Name	Page
Alcohol dependence	▲Disulfiram[B] ▲Acamprosate[B]	See p. 257 See p. 260
Alcohol/opioid dependence	▲Naltrexone	See p. 262
Opioid dependence	▲Methadone ▲Buprenorphine (Subutex)[C] ▲Buprenorphine / Naloxone (Suboxone)[B)(C]	See p. 265
Nicotine dependence	Bupropion (Zyban)	See p. 58
Heroin and nicotine withdrawal	Clonidine	See p. 33

▲ Approved indication in adults, [B] Not marketed in Canada, [C] Not used in children and adolescents and not reviewed in this chapter

Disulfiram

PRODUCT AVAILABILITY

Chemical Class	Generic Name	Trade Name[A]	Dosage Forms and Strengths	Monograph Statement
	Disulfiram[B]	Antabuse	Tablets: 250 mg, 500 mg	No data

[A] Generic preparations may be available, [B] Not marketed in Canada

INDICATIONS

No approved indications in children and adolescents

Approved (for Adults)

- Deterrent to alcohol use/abuse

Other Uses

- Double-blind and open studies suggest benefit in decreasing cocaine use and increasing abstinence in patients with comorbid alcohol abuse (caution – see Drug Interactions p. 259)

GENERAL COMMENTS

- Anti-alcohol drugs are not recommended in children or adolescents; behavioral treatment approaches should be used
- Case reports suggest judicious use of this drug for serious alcohol use disorder in adolescents, following a thorough medical and psychiatric evaluation, careful assessment for comorbid diagnoses, family involvement, education and obtaining signed informed consent

Disulfiram (cont.)

PHARMACOLOGY
- Inhibits alcohol metabolism at the acetaldehyde level; the accumulating acetaldehyde produces an unpleasant reaction consisting of flushing, choking, nausea, vomiting, tachycardia, and hypotension; response is proportional to the dose and amount of alcohol ingested; can occur 10–20 min after alcohol ingestion and may last up to 2 h

DOSING
- 125–500 mg daily (h.s.)

PHARMACOKINETICS
- Onset of action: 3–12 h
- Duration of action: up to 14 days

ADVERSE EFFECTS
- Drowsiness and lethargy frequent, depression, disorientation, headache, restlessness, excitation, optic neuritis and peripheral neuropathy, skin eruptions (up to 5% risk), impotence, garlic-like taste, blood dyscrasias, psychosis
- Transient elevated liver function tests reported in up to 30% of individuals; hepatitis is rare

CONTRAINDICATIONS
- Cardiac and pulmonary disorders, liver disease, renal disorders, epilepsy, diabetes mellitus; psychotic conditions including depression
- Use of alcohol-containing products

PRECAUTIONS
- Do not give to intoxicated individuals or within 36 h of alcohol consumption
- Do not administer without patient's knowledge
- If alcohol reaction occurs, general supportive measures should be used; in severe hypotension, vasopressor agents may be required

TOXICITY
- Alcohol reaction is proportional to dose of drug and alcohol ingested; severe reactions may result in respiratory depression, cardiovascular collapse, arrhythmias, convulsions, and death; supportive measures may involve oxygen, vitamin C, antihistamines or ephedrine

USE IN PREGNANCY
- Possible teratogenicity: report of limb reduction anomalies

Breast milk
- Unknown

NURSING IMPLICATIONS
- Patient should be made aware of purpose of medication and educated about the consequences of drinking; informed consent to treatment is recommended
- Reactions can occur up to 6 days after a dose
- Daily uninterrupted therapy must be continued until the patient has established a basis for self-control
- Drug should not be used alone, without proper motivation and supportive therapy; will not cure alcoholics, but acts as a motivational aid

DRUG INTERACTIONS   • Clinically significant interactions are listed below

Class of Drug	Example	Interactions
Anticoagulant	Warfarin, coumarins	Increased PT ratio or INR response due to reduced metabolism
Anticonvulsant	Phenytoin	Increased anticonvulsant blood levels and toxicity due to reduced metabolism

Antidepressant
  Cyclic
 	
  Irreversible MAOIs
	
	Amitriptyline, desipramine
	
	Tranylcypromine
		
		Increased plasma level of antidepressant due to reduced metabolism; neurotoxicity reported with combination
		Report of delirium, psychosis with combination

Antipsychotic	Clozapine	Inhibited metabolism and increased plasma level of clozapine
Antitubercular Drug	Isoniazid	Unsteady gait, incoordination, behavioral changes reported due to reduced metabolism of isoniazid
Benzodiazepine	Diazepam, alprazolam chlordiazepoxide, triazolam	Increased activity of benzodiazepine due to decreased clearance (oxazepam, temazepam, and lorazepam not affected)
Caffeine		Reduced clearance of caffeine by 24–30%
Metronidazole		Acute psychosis, ataxia, and confusional states reported
Narcotic	Methadone	Decreased clearance of methadone
Paraldehyde		Alcohol-like reaction can occur as paraldehyde is metabolized to acetaldehyde
Protease inhibitor	Ritonavir	Alcohol-like reaction reported (as formulation contains alcohol)
Stimulant	Cocaine	Increased plasma level (3- to 6-fold) and half-life (by 60%) of cocaine; increased risk of cardiovascular effects
St. John's Wort		Alcohol-like reactions reported
Theophylline	Oxtriphylline, theophylline	Increased plasma level of theophyllines due to reduced metabolism

**Treatment of Substance
Use Disorders**

Acamprosate

PRODUCT AVAILABILITY

Chemical Class	Generic Name	Trade Name	Dosage Forms and Strengths	Monograph statement
Calcium acetyl-homotaurine	Acamprosate calcium [(B)]	Campral	Delayed-release enteric-coated tablets: 333 mg (equiv. to 300 mg acamprosate)	Safety and efficacy not established in children

[(B)] Not available in Canada

INDICATIONS

No approved indications in children and adolescents

Approved (for Adults)

* Maintenance of abstinence from alcohol; used in adolescents to reduce alcohol cravings and prevent relapse as an adjunct to psychosocial treatment programs

GENERAL COMMENTS

* May not be effective in patients who are actively drinking at the start of treatment or in patients who abuse other substances; it is not effective for acute withdrawal and does not treat delirium tremens. Initiate treatment as soon as possible after alcohol withdrawal
* Acamprosate treatment should be part of a comprehensive alcohol management program that includes psychosocial support
* Combination with naltrexone increases efficacy and success of abstinence (see Interactions p. 256); acamprosate appears more useful in achieving abstinence, while naltrexone controls alcohol comsumption
* Has been used in combination with disulfiram to increase abstinence

PHARMACOLOGY

* Mechanism of action is not fully understood, but is suggested to affect glutamatergic neurotransmission (restores glutamate tone through action on calcium channels and modulates neuronal hyperxcitability during withdrawal from alcohol)

DOSING

* Adults > 60 kg: 666 mg tid, taken with meals; < 60 kg: 666 mg bid, taken with meals
* Hepatic disorders: no dosage adjustment needed
* Renal dysfunction: give 333 mg tid if creatinine clearance (CrCl) is 30–35 ml/min; avoid in patients with CrCl < 30ml/min

PHARMACOKINETICS

* Food increases absorption of acamprosate; C_{max} decreased by 42% and AUC by 23%
* Bioavailability = 11%; peak plasma level = 3–8 h
* Has low protein binding
* Half-life = 20–33 h
* Is not degraded by the liver and is primarily excreted as unchanged drug by the kidneys – not involved in CYP-450 interactions

ADVERSE EFFECTS

- Common: flatulence and diarrhea (dose-related), headache, nausea, asthenia,
- Depression, anxiety, insomnia, rarely suicidal ideation
- Less common: vomiting, dizziness, fluctuaions in libido, pruritus, maculopapular rash
- Acute renal failure reported

PRECAUTIONS

- Use of acamprosate does not diminish withdrawal symptoms

CONTRAINDICATIONS

- Avoid in severe renal insufficiency (CrCl < 30 ml/min)

TOXICITY

- Diarrhea reported after overdose of 56 g
- Provide supportive treatment

USE IN PREGNANCY

Breast Milk

- Category C; teratogenic effects seen in animal studies - not recommended in humans
- Not known if excreted in human milk

NURSING IMPLICATIONS

- Acamprosate treatment should be part of a comprehensive alcohol management program that includes psychosocial support
- Monitor patients for symptoms of depression or suicidal thinking
- Diarrhea occurs commonly during therapy, is does-generally transient

PATIENT INSTRUCTIONS

- For detailed patient instruction on acamprosate, see the patient information sheet on p. 333

DRUG INTERACTIONS

- Clinically significant interactions are listed below

Class of Drug	Example	Interaction Effects
Naltrexone		Rate and extent of absorption of acamprosate increased; C_{max} increased by 33% and AUC by 25%

Treatment of Substance
Use Disorders

Naltrexone

PRODUCT AVAILABILITY

Chemical Class	Generic Name	Trade Name[A]	Dosage Forms and Strengths	Monograph Statement
	Naltrexone	Revia, Trexan Vivitrol [B][C]	Tablets: 25 mg[B], 50 mg, 100 mg[B] Extended-release injection: 380 mg	Safety and efficacy not established in children < 18 yrs

[A] Generic preparations may be available, [B] Not available in Canada, [C] Not used in children and adolescents and not reviewed in this chapter

INDICATIONS*

No approved indications in children and adolescents

Approved (for adults)

▲ • Adjunct in the treatment of alcohol dependence; preliminary results support efficacy on abstinence in adolescents when combined with supportive psychotherapy
▲ • Adjunct in the treatment of opiate addiction

Other uses in Children and Adolescents

• Has been studied in children for aggression, hyperactivity, stereotypic and ritualistic behavior, self-injurious behavior, autism and mental retardation (dose: 0.5–2 mg/kg/day); effects noted within first hour of administration
• Controlled studies have shown a decrease in hyperactivity, stereotypies, ritualistic behavior in patients with autism; however, worsening of hyperactivity and stereotypies in children with autism also reported
• Has been studied in children for self-injurious behavior in autism and mental retardation (data contradictory as increases in self-injurious behavior have been reported in some patients)
• Open trial suggests benefit in treating adolescent sexual offenders with doses of 100–200 mg/day
• Early data suggest a role in impulse-control disorders and obsessive-compulsive disorders, e.g., binge-eating behavior in females with bulimia, trichotillomania, pathological gambling, alcohol dependence

GENERAL COMMENTS

• Blocks the "craving" mechanism in the brain producing less of a high from alcohol; stops the reinforcing effect of alcohol by blocking the opioid system - promotes abstinence and reduces risk for relapse. Recommended to be used together with psychosocial interventions (double-blind study suggests that it may not have long-term benefits in men with chronic severe alcohol dependence)
• Combination with acamprosate increases efficacy and success of abstinence (see Interaction p. 263); naltrexone controls alcohol consumption while acamprosate is more useful in achieving abstinence
• Does not attenuate craving for opioids or suppress withdrawal symptoms; patients must undergo detoxification before starting the drug
• Does not produce euphoria

PHARMACOLOGY

• Synthetic long-action antagonist at various opiate receptor sites in the CNS; highest affinity for the (sigma) receptor

* ▲ Approved indications

DOSING	• For antisocial behavior/aggression: 0.5–2 mg (kg/day)

PHARMACOKINETICS

- Rapidly and completely absorbed from the GI tract
- Undergoes extensive first-pass metabolism; only about 20% of drug reaches the systemic circulation
- Widely distributed; 21–28% is protein bound
- Onset of effect occurs in 15–30 minutes in chronic morphine users
- Duration of effect is dose-dependent; blockade of opioid receptors lasts 24–72 h
- Metabolized in liver (not via CYP-450); major metabolite, 6-β naltrexone is active as an opiate antagonist
- Elimination half-life is 96 h; excreted primarily by the kidneys

ADVERSE EFFECTS

- GI effects – abdominal pain, cramps, nausea and vomiting (approx 10%) and weight loss; women are more sensitive to GI side effects
- Headache (6.6%), insomnia, anxiety, dysphoria, depression, confusion, nervousness, fatigue
- Joint and muscle pain
- Dose-related elevated enzymes and hepatocellular injury reported; increased ALT and AST associated with concurrent use of NSAIDs, ASA or acetaminophen; liver function tests recommended at start of treatment and monthly for the first 6 months
- Case reports of naltrexone-induced panic attacks

DISCONTINUATION SYNDROME

- No data available

PRECAUTIONS

- Since naltrexone is an opiate antagonist, do not give to patients who have used narcotics in the previous 10 days – may result in symptoms of opiate withdrawal
- Do not use in patients with liver disorders; baseline liver function tests recommended; repeat monthly for 6 months. Liver toxicity has been reported in very obese individuals on high doses and in combination with NSAIDs, ASA and acetaminophen
- Attempts to overcome blockade of naltrexone with high doses of opioid agonists (e.g., morphine) may lead to respiratory depression and death

CONTRAINDICATIONS

- Patients receiving opioids, or those in acute opioid withdrawal
- Acute hepatitis or liver failure

TOXICITY

- No experience in humans; 800 mg dose for 1 week showed no evidence of toxicity

USE IN PREGNANCY

- No adequate well-controlled studies done

Breast Milk

- Unknown whether naltrexone is excreted into breast milk

Treatment of Substance Use Disorders

NURSING IMPLICATIONS

- Naltrexone should be used in conjunction with established psychotherapy or self-help programs
- As naltrexone does not attenuate craving for opioids or suppress withdrawal symptoms, compliance problems may occur; individuals must undergo detoxification prior to starting drug
- Advise patients not to self-medicate with excessive doses of NSAIDs, acetaminophen or ASA

PATIENT INSTRUCTIONS

- For detailed patient instructions on naltrexone, see the Patient Information Sheet on p. 335

DRUG INTERACTIONS

- Clinically significant interactions are listed below

Class of Drug	Example	Interaction Effects
Acamprosate		Rate and extent of absorption of acamprosate increased; C_{max} increased by 33% and AUC by 25%
Antipsychotic	Chlorpromazine	Lethargy, somnolence with combination
Narcotic	Codeine, morphine	Decreased efficacy of narcotic

Methadone

PRODUCT AVAILABILITY

Chemical Class	Generic Name	Trade Name[A]	Dosage Forms and Strengths	Monograph Statement
Narcotic	Methadone		Bulk powder	Government regulations govern the use of methadone in children and adolescents
		Roxane[B], Metadol[C]	Oral liquid: 1 mg/ml[C], 5 mg/5 ml[B], 10 mg/5 ml[B], 10 mg/ml	
		Dolophine[B], Metadol[C]	Tablets: 1 mg[C], 5 mg, 10 mg, 25 mg[C], 40 mg (dispersible)[B] Injection[B]: 10 mg/ml	

[A] Generic preparations may be available, [B] Not marketed in Canada, [C] Not marketed in USA

INDICATIONS

No approved indications in children and adolescents

Approved (for Adults)

- A substitute drug in narcotic analgesic dependence therapy
- Treatment of severe pain; Has been used for postoperative pain in children at doses of 0.2 mg/kg; has a longer duration of action than morphine

GENERAL COMMENTS

- Useful drug in opiate-dependent patients who desire maintenance opiate therapy and who relapse with alternative interventions, because:
  - Effective orally and can be administered once daily, due to its long half-life
  - Suppresses withdrawal symptoms of other narcotic analgesics
  - Suppresses chronic craving for narcotics without developing tolerance
  - Does not produce euphoria in users already tolerant to euphoric effects of narcotic analgesics
- Patients receiving methadone remain in treatment longer, demonstrate a decreased use of illicit opiates, show decreased antisocial behavior and maintain social stability
- Methadone is a narcotic and its prescribing, dispensing and usage is governed by Federal regulations (regulations vary in different countries). It is prepared as a liquid, mixed with orange juice. Most patients receive their methadone, on a daily basis, from the pharmacy and are required to drink the contents of the bottle in the presence of the pharmacist. Some patients (who are stable on their medication) are permitted to carry several days' supply of methadone
- Signed informed consent should be obtained from a parent, or legal guardian prior to use in children
- Effects of prolonged methadone use on physiologic and psychological development of children is not known

Treatment of Substance
Use Disorders

Methadone (cont.)

PHARMACOLOGY

- A synthetic opiate acting on the μ-opiate receptor; blocks reinforcing euphorigenic effects of other administered opiates
- Analgesic and sedative properties – similar in degree to morphine, but with a longer duration of action

DOSING

- Initially 30–40 mg/day, given once daily; increase by 10 mg every 2–3 days to a stable maintenance dose (up to 200 mg/day)
- Oral methadone doses are approximately twice the intravenous dose (due to decreased bioavailability)
- Patients vary in dosage requirements; dosage is adjusted to control abstinence symptoms without causing marked sedation or respiratory depression
- Doses below 60 mg/day are considered to be inadequate in preventing relapse
- In rare cases patients who are rapid metabolizers of methadone may require a divided (split) dose rather than one single daily dose; the situation should be carefully evaluated by the physician

PHARMACOKINETICS

- Bioavailability: 70–80%
- Half-life: 13–55 h (average: 25 h); half-life increases with repeated dosing and drug can accumulate if dosed too frequently
- Peak plasma level: 2–3 h
- 70–85% protein bound
- Metabolized by the liver primarily via CYP3A4 and 2D6 (see Interactions p. 268–269)
- Plasma level measurements are not considered useful, except in specific circumstances where stabilization has posed difficulties (threshold range suggested to be 150–220 ng/ml)
- Urine testing may be done to detect illicit drug use and/or compliance with methadone

ONSET AND DURATION OF ACTION

- Onset of effect: 30–60 minutes
- Duration of action increases with chronic use

ADVERSE EFFECTS

CNS Effects

- Drowsiness, insomnia, euphoria, dysphoria, confusion, cognitive impairment, depression and weakness; tolerance develops to sedating and analgesic effects
- With chronic use: sleep disturbances
- Headache

Anticholinergic Effects

- Sweating, flushing
- Chronic constipation

Cardiovascular Effects

- Dizziness, lightheadedness
- Cases of QT prolongation and torsades de pointes; increased risk with higher doses, drug accumulation, or in combination with drugs that decrease the metabolism of methadone (see Interactions p. 268)

| GI Effects | • Nausea, vomiting, decreased appetite |
| | • Weight changes |

| Sexual Side Effects | • Impotence, ejaculatory problems |

| Other Adverse Effects | • Rarely, pulmonary edema and respiratory depression |
| | • With chronic use: menstrual irregularities, pain in joints and bones |

DISCONTINUATION SYNDROME

- Drug must be tapered (by 5–10% every 1–2 days) if used for longer than 5–7 days; the patient must be continually assessed for withdrawal symptoms
- Rapid withdrawal can result in opiate withdrawal syndrome, which includes CNS effects: restlessness, agitation, insomnia, headache; Autonomic effects: increased blood pressure, heart rate, body temperature and respiration, lacrimation, perspiration, congestion, itching, "gooseflesh"; Neurological effects: muscle twitching, cramps, tremors, seizures; GI effects: nausea, vomiting, diarrhea, anorexia
- Symptoms may begin 24–48 h after the last dose, peak in 72 h, and may last for 6–7 weeks

Management

- Reinstitute dose to previous level; restabilize patient and monitor while tapering dose at a slower rate
- Clonidine may ameliorate withdrawal symptoms

PRECAUTIONS

- Effects of prolonged methadone use on physiological and psychological development of children is not known
- Methadone has a high physical and psychological dependence liability, therefore withdrawal symptoms will occur on abrupt discontinuation – decrease the dose slowly
- Methadone can build up in the body if dosed too frequently, with high doses, or in combination with drugs that decrease its metabolism. Peak respiratory depressant effects occur later, and persist longer, than peak analgesic effects

TOXICITY

- With excessive doses can get marked shallow breathing, pinpoint pupils, flaccidity of skeletal muscles, low blood pressure, slowed heart rate, cold and clammy skin; can progress to cyanosis, coma, severe respiratory depression, circulatory collapse and cardiac arrest

USE IN PREGNANCY

- Dosing needs should be assessed during pregnancy: decreased between weeks 14 and 32 and increased prior to term
- Short-term withdrawal effects reported in infants (not dose-related); no long-term effects demonstrated

Breast Milk

- A small amount of methadone enters breast milk; nurse prior to a dose of methadone, or 2–6 h after dose

NURSING IMPLICATIONS

- Methadone must be prescribed in sufficient doses, on a maintenance basis, to prevent relapse; long-term treatment may be required. Premature withdrawal may lead to relapse
- Methadone is a narcotic and must be prescribed according to Federal regulations. It is prepared as a liquid mixed in orange juice. Many patients pick up their methadone, from the pharmacy, on a daily basis, and drink the medication in the presence of the pharmacist. Some patients (who are stable on their medication) are permitted to carry several days' supply of methadone

Methadone (cont.)

- Each time the patient is to be medicated, he/she should be assessed for impairment (i.e., drowsiness, slurred speech, forgetfulness, lack of concentration, disorientation and ataxia); patients should not be medicated if they appear impaired or smell of alcohol – the physician should be contacted as to management of the patient

PATIENT INSTRUCTIONS

- Detailed instructions for patients and caregivers are provided in the Information Sheet on p. 337

DRUG INTERACTIONS

- Clinically significant interactions are listed below

Class of Drug	Example	Interaction Effects
Alcohol		Acute alcohol use can decrease methadone metabolism and increase the plasma level Chronic alcohol use can induce methadone metabolism and decrease the plasma level
Antacid	Al/Mg antacids	Decreased absorption of methadone
Antiarrhythmic	Quinidine	Possible risk of QT prolongation
Anticonvulsant	Phenytoin, carbamazepine, barbiturates	Decreased plasma level of methadone due to enhanced metabolism (by 50% with phenytoin)
Antidepressant		
Cyclic	Desipramine, amitriptyline	Increased plasma level of desipramine (by about 108%) Increased giddiness, euphoria; suspected potentiation of methadone's "euphoric" effects – abuse with amitriptyline reported
SSRI	Fluvoxamine	Increased plasma level of methadone by 20–100% with fluvoxamine, due to decreased clearance
Antifungal	Fluconazole	Increase in methadone peak and trough plasma levels by 27% and 48%, respectively; clearance decreased by 24%
Antipsychotic	Risperidone	Case reports of precipitation of narcotic withdrawal symptoms (mechanism unclear)
Antitubercular drug	Isoniazid	Decreased clearance and increased plasma level of methadone
	Rifampin	Decreased plasma level of methadone (by up to 50%) due to enhanced metabolism
Antiviral	Efavirenz, nevirapine	Increased clearance of methadone and decreased total concentration (AUC) (by up to 60% with efavirenz and nevirapine) via enzyme induction – withdrawal symptoms reported within 7–10 days
	Didanosine, stavudine	Decreased bioavailability of antiretrovirals due to increased degradation in GI tract by methadone (C_{max} and AUC decreased by 66% and 63%, respectively, for didanosine, and by 44% and 25% for stavudine)
	Zidovudine (AZT)	Inhibited metabolism of AZT by methadone (AUC increased by 43%)
	Abacavir	Abacavir levels decreased ba 34%, however clearance remained the same Methadone plasma level increased by 23% – may result in withdrawal
	Delavirdine	Likely to increase methadone levels via inhibition of metabolizing enzymes

Class of Drug	Example	Interaction Effects
Benzodiazepine	Diazepam, clonazepam Diazepam	Enhanced risk of respiratory depression "Opiate high" reported with combined use
H$_2$ antagonist	Cimetidine	Decreased clearance of methadone
Disulfiram		Decreased clearance of methadone
Narcotic	Pentazocine, nalbuphine, butorphanol Morphine	Occurrence of withdrawal symptoms due to partial antagonist effects of these narcotics Efficacy of narcotic analgesic reduced; dosage may need to be increased
Protease inhibitor	Ritonavir	Variable effects on clearance of methadone reported
	Amprenavir	AUC, C_{max}, and C_{min} of amprenavir decreased by 30%, 27%, and 25%, respectively Methadone levels decreased an average of 35% with amprenavir/abacavir combination
	Indinavir	Variable effects reported on C_{max} of indinavir
	Nelfinavir	Reduced AUC of methadone by 40% AUC of nelfanavir metabolite decreased by 53% – significance unknown
	Lopinavir/ritonavir	Methadone AUC decreased by 36% due to increased clearance (attributed to lopinavir) – may result in withdrawal
	Ritonavir/saquinavir	Displacement from protein binding of methadone and decrease in AUC of both R-methadone and S-methadone
St. John's Wort		Decreased plasma level of methadone; symptoms of withdrawal reported
Urine acidifier	Ascorbic acid	Increased elimination of methadone
Urine alkalizer	Sodium bicarbonate	Decreased elimination of methadone

**Treatment of Substance
Use Disorders**

Treatment of Substance Use Disorder – References and Selected Readings

- Anton, R.F. (2001). Pharmacologic approaches to the management of alcoholism. *Journal of Clinical Psychiatry 62(Suppl. 20),* 11–17.
- Buck, M.L. (2000). Managing iatrogenic opioid dependence with methadone. *Pediatric Pharmacotherapy 6(7),* 1–7.
- Chabane, N., Leboyer, M., Mouren-Simeoni, M.C. (2000). Opiate antagonists in children and adolescents. *European Child and Adolescent Psychiatry 9(Suppl.1),* 144–150.
- Kalant, H. (2001). The pharmacology and toxicology of "ecstasy" (MDMA) and related drugs. *Canadian Medical Association Journal 165(7),* 917–928.
- Kenna, G.A., McGeary, J.E., Swift, R.M. (2004). Pharmacotherapy, pharmacogenomics, and the future of alcohol dependence treatment, Part 2. *American Journal of Health-System Pharmacy 61(22),* 2380–2388.
- McRae, A. (2004). Pharmacotherapy of substance use disorders. *International Drug Therapy Newsletter 39(4),* 25–30.
- Myrick, H., Brody, K.T., Malcolm, R. (2001). New developments in the pharmacotherapy of alcohol dependence. *American Journal of Addictions 10(Suppl.),* 3–15.
- Niederhofer, H., Staffen, W. (2003). Acamprosate and its efficacy in treating alcohol dependent adolescents. *European Child and Adolescent Psychiatry 12(3),* 144–148.
- Schwartz, R.H., Milteer, R. (2000). Drug-facilitated sexual assault ("date rape"). *Southern Medical Journal 93(6),* 558–561.
- Srisurapanant, M., Jarusuraisin, N. (2002). Opioid antagonists for alcohol dependence. *Cochrane Database System Review (2),* CD001867.
- Swift, R.M. (2001). Can medication successfully treat substance addiction? *Psychopharmacology Update 12(1),* 4–5.
- Teter, C.J. (2003). Club Drugs Part I and II. *International Drug Therapy Newsletter 38 (7/8),* 49–56, 57–64.

OTHER TREATMENTS OF PSYCHIATRIC DISORDERS

Biochemical theories on the etiology of specific psychiatric disorders have initiated investigations of various drugs/chemicals that may influence brain neurotransmitters and thereby play a role in the treatment of psychiatric disorders. Several drugs traditionally used to treat medical conditions have been found to be of benefit in ameliorating or preventing symptoms of certain psychiatric disorders in children and adolescents. This section presents a summary of some of these drugs and their uses. **As a rule, these treatments should be reserved for patients highly resistant to conventional therapies. Clinicians should be cognizant of medicolegal issues when prescribing drugs for non-approved indications, as most medications used in children and adolescent psychiatric conditions have not been adequately studied**.

	Anxiety Disorders	Schizophrenia	Antisocial Behavior/ Aggression	ADHD	Drug Dependence Treatment	Pervasive Developmental Disorders	Tourette's Syndrome
β-Blockers, e.g., propranolol, atenolol, pindolol (p. 271)	+		+			Pr	
Cholinesterase Inhibitors (p. 272)				PR			
Modafinil (p. 273)				PR			
Selegiline (p. 273)				+			

C = contradictory results, P = partial improvement, + = positive, S = synergistic effect, PR = preliminary data

Adrenergic Agents

Have membrane-stabilizing effect and GABA-mimetic activity; 5-HT antagonist properties (See p. 161 for treatment of EPS)

Antisocial Behavior/ Aggression

- Propranolol dose: 0.5–1.0 mg/kg/day given q 6–8 h. Slowly increase to a maximum dose of 5 mg/kg/day or 120 mg/day
- Response may take up to 8 weeks
- Useful in controlling rage, violence, irritability, and aggression due to a number of causes (e.g., autism, ADHD, PTSD)
- May be effective in controlling aggressive behavior in children and adolescents with organic brain dysfunction
- Potential side effects include hypotension, bradycardia and worsening of asthmatic symptoms; monitor BP and EKG
- Rebound rage reactions on drug withdrawal reported; taper dose gradually

(Simeon, J.G. (1997). *Child and Adolescent Psychopharmacology News 2(3)*, 11–12; Silver, J.M. et al. (1999). *Journal of Neuropsychiatry and Clinical Neurosciences 1(3)*, 328–335)

Herbal and "Natural" Products

Adrenergic Agents (cont.)

| Anxiety Disorders |

- Propranolol dose: up to 160 mg/day
- Beneficial for somatic or autonomically mediated symptoms of anxiety (e.g., tremor, palpitations) as seen in social phobia and acute panic
- Efficacy reported in children with posttraumatic stress disorder; short-term post-trauma use may reduce severity of symptoms

(Le Melledo, J.M. et al. (1998). *Biological Psychiatry 1:44(5),* 364–366; Pitman, R.K. et al. (2002). *Biological Psychiatry 51,* 189–192)

Cholinergic Agents

CHOLINESTERASE INHIBITORS

Increase the activity of acetylcholine in the brain

| PDD |

- Open trial and case reports suggest donepezil, galantamine and rivastigmine may benefit dysfunctional behaviors, hyperactivity and expressive speech in patients with PDD.

(Hardan, A.Y. et al. (2002). *Journal of Child and Adolescent Psychopharmacology 12,* 237–241; Chez, M.G. et al. (2004). *Journal of Child Neurology, 19,*165–169; Hertzman, M. et al. (2003). *International Journal of Psychiatry in Medicine* 33, 395–398)

| ADHD |

- Dose donepezil: up to 10 g/day
- Open trials suggest that augmentation with donepezil may improve organization, mental efficiency and attention in treatment-refractory children and adolescents with ADHD
- Most adverse effects are due to cholinomimetic activity: nausea, vomiting, diarrhea, constipation and anorexia

(Wilens, T.E. et al. (2000). *Journal of Child and Adolescent Psychopharmacology 10(3),* 217–222)

Dopaminergic Agents

MODAFINIL

Psychostimulant which exhibits weak affinity for dopamine uptake carrier sites; may work by reducing GABA release and increasing the release of glutamate

ADHD

- Dose: 100–400 mg/day in divided doses or 170–425 mg film-coated tablet formulation given once daily
- Beneficial results reported on inattention, hyperactivity and impulsivity in open and double-blind trials of children
- Good response reported in double-blind placebo-controlled study of modafinil (mean dose 206.8 mg/day) with dextroamphetamine, in adults
- Most commonly reported adverse effects in children include: insommia (28%), headache (20%) and decreased appetite (16%); case report of mania in a boy given modafinil for narcolepsy.

(Rugino, T.A. et al. (2001). *Journal of the American Academy of Child and Adolescent Psychiatry 40(2),* 230–235; Taylor, F.B. et al. (2000). *Journal of Child and Adolescent Psychopharmacology 10(4),* 311–320; Rugino, T.A. et al. (2003). *Pediatric Neurology 29(2),* 136–142; Biederman, S. et al. (2005). *Pediatrics 116(6),* e777–784; Vorspan, F. et al. (2005). *American Journal of Psychiatry 162(4),* 813–814)

Miscellaneous

SELEGILINE

Inhibitor of MAO-B, possibly nonselective at higher doses; stimulates nitric oxide production

ADHD

- Dose: 5–10 mg
- Positive effects on ADHD and tic symptoms reported in double-blind placebo controlled crossover studies and in open trials; may have a preferential effect on symptoms of inattention
- Small ($n = 40$) randomized, double blind trial comparing selegiline to methylphenidate found no major differences between treatments after 60 days.

(Popper, C.W. (1997). *Journal of Clinical Psychiatry 58(Suppl. 14),* 14–29; Findling, R.L. (2001). *International Drug Therapy Newsletter 36(12),* 89–93; Akhondzadeh, S. et al. (2003). *Progress in Neuropsychopharmacology and Biological Psychiatry 5,* 841–845; Mohammadi M.R. et al. (2004). *Journal of Child and Adolescent Psychopharmacology 14(3),* 418–25; Rubenstein, S. et al. (2006). *Journal of Child and Adolescent Psychopharmacology 16(4),* 404–415)

Herbal and "Natural" Products

HERBAL AND "NATURAL" PRODUCTS

PRODUCT AVAILABILITY

Drug	Anxiety	Depression	Sleep Disorders	ADHD
Ginkgo Biloba (p. 237)		PR		PR/S
Inositol (p. 238)	PR			
Melatonin (p. 238)			C	
Omega 3 Fatty Acids (p. 239)				PR/C
St. John's Wort (p. 239)		+*		
Valerian (p. 240)			+	

C = contradictory results, P = partial improvement, + = positive, PR = preliminary data, S = synergistic effect. *Mild to moderate depression only

Herbal (natural) products have been traditionally used by many cultures to treat a variety of psychiatric conditions. Very few of these products, however, have been subjected to scientific scrutiny through standardized research methods. Clinicians should always be cognizant of medicolegal issues when recommending herbal products for non-approved indications in children and adolescents.

CAUTION: Quality control of herbal/natural products is variable, depending on the preparation used. As these products are not standardized in North America, the amount of active constituents can vary between preparations, and some products may be adulterated with other herbs, chemicals and drugs.

GINKGO BILOBA

Active ginkgolides obtained from the nuts and leaves of the oldest deciduous tree in the world (ginkgo – also called Maidenhair tree or kew tree) Standardized products contain flavone glycosides (24%) and terpenoids (6%)

Increases vasodilation and peripheral blood flow in capillary vessels and end arteries; may have antioxidant action (free radical scavenger); may increase cholinergic transmission by inhibiting acetylcholinesterase; may have anticonvulsant activity through elevation of GABA levels.

ADHD

- Dose: 50 mg
- Open-label study suggests benefit of ginkgo biloba in combination with panax quinquefolium (American ginseng extract) 200 mg, in children aged 3–17; improvement noted in hyperactivity, impulsiveness, and social problems
- (Lyon, M.R. et al. (2001). *Journal of Psychiatry and Neuroscience 26(3),* 221–228)

INOSITOL

Simple isomer of glucose and a precursor of a "second messenger" system (the phosphotidyl-inositol cycle) used by various receptors including α and 5-HT$_2$

Anxiety Disorders

- 6–18 g/day
- Preliminary data suggest efficacy in treating panic, phobic disorders, obsessive-compulsive disorder and trichotillomania
- May aggravate symptoms of ADHD in children

(Fux, M. et al. (1997). American Journal of Psychiatry 153(9), 1219–1221; Levine, J. (1997). European Neuropsychopharmacology 7, 147–155; Seedat, S. et al. (2001). Journal of Clinical Psychiatry 62(1), 60–61)

MELATONIN

Hormone produced by the pineal gland involved in regulation of circadian rhythms
- Dietary supplement in the USA, not regulated by FDA with regard to purity, efficacy or safety; currently available in Canada only through Special Assess Program

Sleep Disorders

- Dose: 2.5–6 mg/day (0.3 mg = physiological dose – children with neurological disorders may require higher doses; the administration of exogenous melatonin does not appear to affect endogenous production or secretion)
- Peak plasma concentration achieved within 60 min; metabolized by the liver; elimination life = 20–50 h
- Double blind study showed benefit in children with chronic idiopathic insomnia; promoted sleep onset without producing drowsiness and minimized nighttime awakenings, not associated with rebound insomnia or withdrawal effects
- Useful in circadian-based sleep disorders (e.g., jet lag) – can shift circadian rhythms at a rate of 1–2 h/day with taken when physiological plasma levels of melatonin are low (i.e., noon to bedtime)
- Hypnotic effect not fully established, as studies show inconsistent results (due to different populations and variable doses used in trials); shown to decrease sleep latency and increase total sleep time in some studies; may be more effective given 2 h before bedtime, or may exert hypnotic effect only when endogenous concentrations of melatonin are low
- Double-blind studies in children suggest benefit in advancing sleep onset and increasing sleep duration; no benefit seen in wake-up time or sustained attention time
- May facilitate sleep in children with ADHD on psychostimulants (contradictory results)
- Reported to improve sleep quality in patients with diabetes with high HbA1C concentrations
- Early data suggest it may be beneficial in multidisabled and blind children (with neurological or behavioral disorders) with severe insomnia reduces time to sleep onset in doses of 2–10 mg
- Case report of improving insomnia, aborting mania, and stabilizing bipolar disorder in a 10-year-old boy
- Shown to improve sleep efficiency in patients with schizophrenia, in double-blind study
- Adverse effects are rare: abdominal cramps with high doses, fatigue, headache, dizziness and increased irritability; very high doses can exacerbate depression
- Not recommended in patients with autoimmune disorders since melatonin may play a role in immune function
- Cases of worsening of seizures in children with seizure disorders

(Hung, J.C. et al. (1998). Journal of Pediatric Pharmacy Practice 3, 250–256; Shamir, E. et al. (2000). Journal of Clinical Psychiatry 61, 373–377; Andrade, C. et al. (2001). Journal of Clinical Psychiatry 62(1), 41–45; Garfinkel, D. (2001). 17th Congress of the International

Herbal and "Natural" Products

Herbal and "Natural" Products (cont.)

Association of Gerontology, July 6, Vancouver, BC; Robertson, J.M. et al. (1997). Journal of the American Academy of Child and Adolescent Psychiatry 36(6), 822–825; Smits, M.G. et al. (2001). Journal of Child Neurology 16(2), 86–92; Jan, J.E. et al. (1996). Journal of Pineal Research 21, 193–199; Paavonen, E. et al. (2003). Journal of Child and Adolescent Psychopharmacology 3(1), 83–95; Buck, H.L. (2003). Pediatric Pharmacology 9(11), 1–5; Smits, M.G. et al. (2003). Journal of the American Academy of Child and Adolescent Psychiatry 42(11), 1286–1293, Weiss M.D. et al. (2006). Journal of the American Academy of Child and Adolescent Psychiatry 45(5), 512–519)

OMEGA POLYUNSATURATED FATTY ACIDS

Contained in fish oil (e.g., mackerel, halibut, salmon), green leafy vegetables, nuts, flaxseed oil and canola oil; may affect cell membrane composition at neuron synapses and interfere with signal transduction; may also affect monoamine oxidase

ADHD

- Administered as Efamol (evening prempose oil) or decosehaxaenoic acid (DHA)
- Dosage ranges from 500 mg to 4 g/day depending on age and weight
- Suggested that relative deficiencies in highly unsaturated fatty acids may be implicated in some of the behavioral and learning problems associated with ADHD; has been suggested that Efamol may improve or compensate for zinc deficiency
- Contradictory results reported in double-blind studies in combination with psychostimulants (d-amphetamine) in children with ADHD; augmentation studies also inconclusive

(Richardson, A.J. et al. (2002). *Progress in Neuropsychopharmacology and Biological Psychiatry 26(2)*, 233–239; Voigt, R.C. et al. (2001). *Journal of Pediatrics 139(2)*, 189–196; Arnold, L.E. et al. (2000). *Journal of Child and Adolescent Psychopharmacology 10(2)*, 111–117; Hirayama et al. (2004). *European Journal of Clinical Nutrition 58(3)*, 467–473)

ST. JOHN'S WORT

Active ingredients thought to be the naphthodianthrone, hypericum, hyperforin, and other flavonoids; standardized products contain 0.3% hypericin (approximately equivalent to 2–4 g of dried herb); mechanism of action still unclear, but affects number of systems, including NE, 5-HT$_{1A}$, DA, GABA, and MAO enzymes; suggested to inhibit 5-HT reuptake

Depression

- Dose: 300–1800 mg/day in divided doses
- Meta-analysis of clinical trials suggests efficacy in adults with mild to moderate depression; lack of data regarding long-term use
- Open label study of children aged 6–16 with major depressive disorder, showed good response in 25 out of 33, after 8 weeks at doses up to 900 mg per day
- Postmarketing surveillance reports efficacy and good tolerability in 101 children under age 12 with mild to moderate depression
- Adverse effects are rare: GI problems, dry mouth, sedation, fatigue, headache, restlessness, constipation, hair loss, photosensitivity and hypersensitivity reactions; cases of mania and hypomania in bipolar patients, including irritability, disinhibition, agitation, anger, decreased concentration, and disrupted sleep
- Contraindicated in pregnancy, lactation, cardiovascular disease and pheochromocytoma
- Due to possible MAOI activity, use caution with foods containing tyramine and with sympathomimetic or serotonergic drugs

- Interactions
  - Potent inducer of CYP3A4; IA2 and/or the p-glycoprotein transporter; reported to decrease plasma level of cyclosporin, resulting in rejection of transplanted organ; also reported to decrease plasma level of indinavir (57% decrease in AUC), digoxin (up to 25% decrease in AUC), theophylline, irinotican, amiodarone, warfarin, methadone, alprazolam, and amitriptyline; breakthrough bleeding and cases of pregnancy reported in patients on oral contraceptives; may interact with other drugs metabolized by these enzymes
  - May increase levels of serotonin in the CNS; several cases of serotonin syndrome reported in combination with serotonergic drugs

(Wong, A.H. et al. (1998). *Archives of General Psychiatry 55(11),* 1033–1044; Linde, K. et al. (1996). *British Medical Journal 313,* 253–258; Singer A. et al. (1999). *Journal of Pharmacology and Experimental Therapeutics 290(3),* 1363–1368; Gelenberg, A.J. (ed.) (2000). *Biological Therapy in Psychiatry, 23(6),* 22–24; Woelk, H. (2000). *British Medical Journal 321,* 536–539; Shelton, R.C. et al. (2001). *Journal of the American Medical Association 285,* 1978–1986; Hubner, W.D. et al. (2001). *Phytotherapy Research 15(4),* 367–370; Scott, G.N. et al. (2002). *American Journal of Health-System Pharmacy 59(4),* 339–347; Hypericum Depression Study Group (2002). *Journal of the American Medical Association 287(14),* 1807–1814; Findling, R.L. et al. (2003). *Journal of the American Academy of Child and Adolescent Psychiatry 42(8),* 908–914)

VALERIAN

From the plant Valeriana officinalis; active ingredients associated with sedative properties thought to be valepotriates, mono- and sesquiterpenes (e.g., valerenic acid) and pyridine alkaloids; the composition and relative proportions of these compounds vary between species. Interacts with central GABA$_A$ receptors; causes CNS depression and muscle relaxation

Sleep Disorders

- Dose: 200–800 mg/day
- Double-blind placebo-controlled trial in 8 children with various intellectual deficits (and hyperactivity) demonstrated a decrease in sleep latency and nocturnal wake time, increased total sleep time and improved quality of sleep
- Adverse effects rare: include nausea, excitability, blurred vision, headache, vivid dreams, and morning hangover with higher doses
- Will potentiate the effects of other CNS depressants
- Liver dysfunction reported; use with caution in patients with a history of liver disease – periodic liver function tests recommended
- Four cases of hepatotoxicity reported when valerian combined with herbal product, skullcap
- Withdrawal symptoms, including delirium, reported after abrupt discontinuation of chronic use

(Wagner, J. et al. (1998). *Annals of Pharmacotherapy 32(6),* 680–691)

VITAMINS/MINERALS

ADHD

- Zinc supplementation at 55 mg/day, together with methylphenidate produced a marked improvement over methylphenidate alone in 44 children in a double-blind study
- Serum ferritin levels reported to be low in a high proportion of children with ADHD, and correlated with greater cognitive deficits; iron supplementation recommended

(Akhondzadeh, S. et al. (2004). *BMC Psychiatry 4,* 9; Arnold, L.E. et al. (2005). *Journal of Child and Adolescent Psychopharmacology 15(4),* 619–627; Konofal, E. et al. (2004). *Archives of Pediatrics and Adolescent Medicine 158,* 1113–1115, Konofal E. et al. (2005). *Pediatrics 116(5),* e732–734)

Herbal and "Natural" Products

Herbal and Natural Products – References and Selected Readings

- Buck, H.L. (2003). The use of melatonin in children with sleep disturbances. *Pedatric Pharmacology 9(11),* Medscape #464854.
- Facts and Comparisons. The Review of Natural Products (updated loose-leaf binder). St. Louis, MO: Facts and Comparisons Publ.
- Knuppel, L., Linde, K. (2004). Adverse effects of St. John's Worth: A systematic review. *Journal of Clinical Psychiatry 65(11),* 1470–1479.
- Manber, R., Allen, J.J.B., Morris, M.M. (2002). Alternative treatments for depression: Empirical support and relevance to women. *Journal of Clinical Psychiatry 63(7),* 628–640.
- Pies, R. (2000). Adverse neuropsychiatric reactions to herbal and over-the-counter "antidepressants." *Journal of Clinical Psychiatry 61(11),* 815–820.
- Scott, G.N., Elmer, G.W. (2002). Update on natural product-drug interactions. *American Journal of Health-System Pharmacy 59(4),* 339–347.
- Wong, A.H., Smith, M., Boon, M.S. (1998). Herbal remedies in psychiatric practice. *Archives of General Psychiatry 55(11),* 1033–1044.

Miscellaneous References and Selected Readings

- Connor, D.F., Carlson, G.A., Chang, K.D. et al. (2006). Juvenila maladaptive aggression. A review of prevention, treatment, and service configuration and a proposed research agenda. *Journal of Clinical Psychiatry* 67(5), 808–820.
- Pres, R.W. (2002). Pharmacological approaches to psychotropic-induced weight gain. *International Drug Therapy Newsletter 37(7),* 49–53.
- Ramshaw, L., Roberge, J. (eds.) (2001). *Psychiatric Medications, A Practical Guide to Psychotropics.* Toronto: Linacre.
- Riddle, M.A., Kastelic, E.A., Frosch, E. (2001). Pediatric psychopharmacology. *Journal of Child Psychology Psychiatry 42(1),* 73–90.
- Scahill, L., Chappell, P.B., King, R. et al. (2000). Pharmacologic treatment of tic disorders. *Child and Adolescent Psychiatric Clinics of North America 9(1),* 99–117.
- Spiqset, O., Hagg, S. (1998). Excretion of psychotropic drugs into breast-milk: Pharmacokinetic overview and therapeutic implications. *CNS Drugs 9(2),* 111–134.

GLOSSARY

ADHD	Attention deficit hyperactivity disorder		**Ballismus**	Jerking, twisting
Agranulocytosis	Reduction of neutrophil white blood cells to very low levels		**Bioavailability**	Amount of drug available to acton receptors (depends on amount absorbed, first-pass metabolism, distribution, protein-binding, and clearance)
Akathisia	Inability to relax, compulsion to change position, motor restlessness			
Akinesia	Absence of voluntary muscle movement		**Bipolar I Disorder**	Cyclical mood disorder with depression alternating with mania or mixed mania
Alopecia	Hair loss			
Amenorrhea	Absence of menstruation		**Bipolar II Disorder**	Cyclical mood disorder with depression alternating with hypomania
Anorexia	Lack of appetite for food			
Anterocollis	Forward spasm of the neck		**Blepharospasm**	Forceful sustained eye closure
Anticholinergic	Block effects of acetylcholine		**BMI** (body mass index)	Weight (in kg) divided by height (in m^2)
Antiemetic	Helps prevent nausea and vomiting			
Arrhythmia	Any variation of the normal rhythm (usually of the heart beat)		**Bradycardia**	Abnormally slow heart beat
			Bruxism	Teech clenching, grinding
Arteriosclerosis	Hardening and degeneration of the arteries due to fibrous tissue formation		**Cataplexy**	Loss of muscletone and collapse
			Category C Drug	May have fetal risk based on animal studies; no data of harm to humans
Arthralgia	Pain in the joints			
Asterixis	Spots before the eyes		**Category D Drug**	Evidence suggests there may be a risk to human fetus
Asthenia	Weakness, fatigue		**Choreiform**	Purposeless, uncontrolled sinuous movements
Ataxia	Incoordination, especially the inability to coordinate voluntary muscular action		**Choreoathetosis**	Slow, repeated, involuntary sinuous movements or twitching of muscles
Atherosclerosis	Degeneration of the walls of the arteries due to fatty deposits		**Chronic brain syndrome**	Irreversible damage to brain cells = dementia
Atypical depression	As per DSM IV-TR, patient has mood reactivity and at least 2 of the following symptoms: increased appetite or weight, hypersomnia, leaden paralysis and a longstanding pattern of extreme sensitivity to perceived interpersonal rejection		**Clearance**	Rate at which drug is removed from a unit of blood plasma (depends on rate of metabolism by liver and eliminiation from body)
AUC	Area under the concentration vs time curve (on graph depicting drug in the plasma after a single dose) – represents the extent of systemic exposure of the body to the drug		**CNS**	Central nervous system
			CNS depression	Drowsiness, ataxia, incoordination, slowing of respiration which in severe cases may lead to coma and death
Autonomic	The part of the nervous system that is functionally independent of thought control (involuntary)		**Cortex**	The external layer (superficial gray matter) of the brain
BD	Bipolar disorder (manic-depressive illness)		**Coryza**	"Head cold," acute catarrhal inflammation of nasal mucosa

Glossary (cont.)

Cycloplegia	Paralysis of accommodation of the eye
CYP	Cytochrome P–450 enzymes, involved in drug metabolism
DA	Dopamine
DDAVP	Desmopressin acetate
Dermatitis	Inflammation of the skin
Diaphoresis	Perspiration
Diplopia	Double vision
Dysarthria	Impaired, difficult speech
Dysgeusia	Unpleasant taste
Dyspepsia	Pain or discomfort in upper abdomen or chest (gas, feeling of fullness, or burning pain)
Dysphagia	Difficulty in swallowing
Dyskinesia	Abnormal movements, i.e., twitching, grimacing, spasm
Dystonia	Disordered muscle tone leading to spasms or postural change
ECG	Electrocardiogram (tracing of electrical activity of the heart muscle)
ECT	Electroconvulsive therapy, "shock therapy"
Edema	Swelling of body tissues due to accumulation of fluid
EEG	Electroencephalogram (tracing of electrical activity of the brain)
Elimination	Excretion or removal of drug (and/or metabolites) from the body, usually by the kidneys
Emesis	Vomiting
Endocrine	A gland that secretes internally, a ductless gland
Endogenous depression	Depression from within; in DSM-IV, called major depression
Enzyme	Organic compound that acts upon specific fluids, tissues, or chemicals in the body to facilitate chemical action
Enuresis	Involuntary discharge of urine
Eosinophilia myalgia syndrome (EMS)	Connective tissue disease with eosinophilia and myalgia (Eosinophils are blood cells that are usually in low quantities)
Epigastric	Referring to the upper middle region of the abdomen
Epistaxis	Nose bleed
Exacerbation	Increase in severity of symptoms or disease
Extrapyramidal	Refers to certain nuclei of the brain close to the pyramidal tract
Extrapyramidal syndrome	Parkinsonian-like effects of drugs
Fasciculation	Twitching of muscles
Fibrosis	Formation of fibrous or scar tissue
First-pass effect	Drugs absorbed from the intestine first pass through the liver; a portion of the drug is metabolized before it can act on receptors
FSH	Follicle stimulating hormone
GABA	Gamma-amino butyric acid; an inhibitory neurotransmitter
Galactorrhea	Excretion of milk from breasts
GI	Gastrointestinal
Glaucoma	Increased pressure within the eye
Glomerular	Pertaining to small blood vessels of the kidney that serve as filtering structures in the excretion of urine
Gynecomastia	Increase in breast size in males
Half-life	Time required to decrease the plasma concentration of a drug by 50% (depends on drug clearance and volume of distribution)
Histological	Pertaining to microscopic tissue anatomy
Hypercalcemia	An excessive amount of calcium in the blood

Hyperkinetic	Abnormal increase in activity
Hyperpara-thyroidism	Increased secretion of the parathyroid
Hyperreflexia	Increased action of the reflexes
Hypertension	High blood pressure
Hyperthyroid	Excessive activity of the thyroid gland
Hypertrophy	Enlargement
Hypnotic	Inducing sleep
Hypospadias	Developmental abnormality in males in which the urethra opens on the under surface of the penis or in the perineum
Hypotension	Low blood pressure
Hypothyroid	Insufficiency of thyroid secretion
Induration	Area of hardened tissue
INR	International Normalization Ratio; measures coagulation of blood
Jaundice	Yellow skin caused by excess of bile pigment
Kindling	Epileptogenesis caused by adaptive changes in neurons repeated electrical discharges
LDH	Lactic dehydrogenase (an enzyme)
LH	Luteinizing hormone
Libido	Drive or energy usually associated with sexual interest
Limbic system	A system of brain structures common to the brains of all mammals (deals with emotions)
Leukocytosis	Increase in the white blood cells in the blood
Leukopenia	Decrease in the white blood cells in the blood
Macrosomia	Birth weight of infant > 4 kg
MAOI	Monoamine oxidase (an enzyme) inhibitor
Manic depressive psychosis	Conspicuous mood swings ranging from normal to elation or depression, or alternating of the two; in DSM-IV, called bipolar affective disorder
MDD	Major depressive disorder

Metabolism	Process by which liver converts a fat-soluble drug into one that is water-soluble and can be excreted by the kidneys. Most psychotropic drugs are metabolized by cytochrome P450 enzymes
Metabolites	By-products of metabolism by liver cytochrome enzymes to create more water-soluble agents. Some metabolites are pharmacologically active
Micrographia	Decrease in size of handwriting; may be a form of akinesia
Miosis	Constricted pupils
Myalgia	Tenderness or pain in muscles
Mydriasis	Dilated pupils
Narcolepsy	Condition marked by an uncontrollable desire to sleep
Nephritis	Inflammation of the kidneys
Nephrolithiasis	Renal stone formation
Nystagmus	Involuntary movement of the eyeball or abnormal movement on testing
OCD	Obsessive compulsive disorder
Oculogyric crisis	Rolling up of the eyes and the inability to focus
Occipital	In the back part of the head
Ophthalmoplegia	Paralysis of the extraocular eye muscles
Opisthotonus	Arching (spasm) of the body due to contraction of back muscles
Orthostatic hypotension	Faintness caused by suddenly standing erect (leading to a drop in blood pressure)
Osteomalacia	Rickets
PANSS	Positive and negative syndrome scale used in the diagnosis and monitoring of symptoms of schizophrenia
Palinopsia	Visual perseveration, "tracking" or shimmering
Papilledema	Edema of the optic disc
Paresthesia	Feeling of "pins and needles," tingling or stiffness in distal extremities

Glossary (cont.)

Parkinsonism	A condition marked by mask-like facial appearance, tremor, change in gait and posture (resembles Parkinson's disease)
Perioral	Around the mouth
Peripheral neuropathy	Pathological changes in the peripheral nervous system
Petechiae	Small purplish hemorrhagic spots on skin
Photophobia	Sensitivity of the eyes to light
Photosensitivity	light sensitive
Piloerection	"Goose-bumps" or hair standing up
Pisa syndrome	A condition where an individual leans to one side
PMS	Premenstrual syndrome
Polydipsia	Excessive drinking
Polyuria	Excessive urination
Postural hypotension	Lowered blood pressure caused by a change in position
Priapism	Abnormal, continued erection of the penis
Prostatic hypertrophy	Enlargement of the prostate gland
Pruritis	Itching
Psychosis	A major mental disorder of organic or emotional origin in which there is a departure from normal patterns of thinking, feeling and acting; commonly characterized by loss of contact with reality
Psychomotor excitement	Physical and emotional overactivity
Psychomotor retardation	Slowing of physical and psychological reactions
Pyloric	Referring to the lower opening of the stomach
Rabbit syndrome	Tremor of the lower lip
Retardation	Slowing
Retrocollis	Spasm of neck muscles causing the head to twist up and back
Schizophrenia	A severe disorder of psychotic depth characterized by a retreat from reality with delusions and hallucinations
SDAT	Senile dementia Alzheimer's type
Sedative	Producing calming of activity or excitement
Serotonin syndrome	Hypermetabolic syndrome resulting from serotonergic excess. Symptoms include: disorientation, confusion, agitation, tremor, myoclonus, hyperreflexia, twitching, shivering, ataxia, hyperactivity
SIADH	Syndrome of inappropriate secretion of antidiuretic hormone
Sialorrhea	Excessive flow of saliva
Somnambulism	Sleep-walking
Stereotypic	Rhythmic and repetitive
Syncope	A sudden loss of strength or fainting
Tachycardia	Abnormally rapid heart rate
Tachyphylaxis	Tolerance to effects
Tardive dyskinesia	Persistent dyskinetic movements that appear late in neuroleptic therapy
Tardive dystonia	Persistent abnormal muscle tone that appears late in neuroleptic therapy
Therapeutic index	Ratio of median lethal dose of a drug to its median effective dose: i.e., therapeutic index = median lethal dose/median effective dose
Tinnitus	A noise in the ears (ringing, buzzing, or roaring)
Torticollis	Spasm on one side of the neck causing the head to twist
Tortipelvis	Twisting of pelvis due to muscle spasm
Tracking	A reaction in which the medication leaves the original injection site and moves to another

TRH	Thyrotropin-releasing hormone, releases TSH and prolactin	**Ulceration**	An open lesion on the skin or mucous membrane
Trismus	Severe spasm of the muscles of the jaw resembling tetanus (lock jaw); jaw clenching	**Vasoconstrictor**	Causes narrowing of the blood vessels
TSH	Thyroid-stimulating hormone	**Volume of distribution (Vd)**	The extent to which a drug is distributed throughout the body (influenced by drug properties and the patient)
UGT	Uridine diphosphate glucuronosyltransferase enzyme, involved in drug metabolism	**Wernicke-Korsakoff syndrome**	Syndrome characterized by confusion, ataxia, ophthalmoplegia, recent memory impairment and confabulation

PATIENT AND CAREGIVER INFORMATION SHEETS

This section in the *Clinical Handbook of Psychotropic Drugs for Children and Adolescent* contains information that may be passed on to patients and caregivers about some of the most frequently used psychotropic medications. The sheets reproduced on the following pages, designed to be easily understood by patients and carers, give details on such matters as the uses of the drug, how quickly it starts working, how long it should be taken, side effects and what to do if they occur, what to do if a dose is forgotten, drug interactions, and precautions. Information sheets such as these of course cannot replace a proper consultation with and advice from the physician or other medical professional, but can serve as a useful tool to enhance compliance, improve efficacy, and enhance safety. The authors and the publisher would welcome feedback and suggestions from readers (for contact addresses, see the front of the book). Information sheets are included here on the drugs and classes of drug shown at the right.

Contents

PATIENT AND CAREGIVER INFORMATION on PSYCHOSTIMULANTS

The name of your medication is _____.

Use

Psychostimulants are primarily used in the treatment of Attention Deficit Hyperactivity Disorder (ADHD) in children and adults. These drugs are also approved for use in Narcolepsy (a sleeping disorder).

Though they are currently not approved for this indication, psychostimulants have been found useful as add-on therapy in the treatment of refractory depression.

The doctor may choose to use this medication for a reason not listed here. If you are not sure why this medication is being prescribed, please ask the doctor.

How quickly will the drug start working?

Some response to psychostimulants is usually noted within the first few days of treatment of ADHD and improvement of symptoms tend to increase over the next 3 weeks.

How does the doctor decide on the dosage?

Psychostimulants come in various preparations including short-acting and long-acting forms (i.e., spansules or extended-release preparations, transdermal patch). The dose is usually based on your age, weight, and how you are responding to the medication. Short-acting forms are usually given several times a day; avoid taking a dose in the late afternoon (e.g., after 4 pm) as this may result in difficulty sleeping. Long-acting preparations are usually taken in the morning, after breakfast. Take the drug exactly as prescribed; **do not increase or decrease the dose without speaking to the doctor.**

How long should you take this medication?

Psychostimulants are usually prescribed for a period of months to years. Some clinicians may prescribe "drug holidays" to individuals on this medication, for short periods of time (e.g., summer holidays, etc.).

Side effects

Side effects occur, to some degree, with all medication. They are usually not serious and do not occur in all individuals. They may sometimes occur before beneficial effects of the medication are noticed. If a side effect continues, speak to the doctor or pharmacist about appropriate treatment.

Common side effects that should be reported to the doctor at the **NEXT APPOINTMENT** include:

- Difficulty sleeping, energizing/agitated feeling, excitability – Some individuals may feel nervous or have difficulty sleeping for a few days after starting this medication. If you are taking the medication in the late afternoon or evening, the physician may decide to prescribe it earlier in the day.
- Loss of appetite, weight loss – Taking the medication after meals, eating smaller meals more frequently or drinking high calorie drinks may help.
- Increased heart rate and blood pressure – Speak to the doctor.
- Headache – This tends to be temporary and can be managed by taking pain medicine (e.g., acetaminophen) when required. Blood pressure may need to be checked.
- Nausea or heartburn – If this happens, take the medication with food or milk.
- Dry mouth – Sour candy, ice chips, popsicles, and sugarless gum help increase saliva in your mouth; try to avoid sweet, calorieladen beverages. Drink water and brush your teeth regularly.
- Feeling dizzy – Get up from a lying or sitting position slowly; dangle your legs over the edge of your bed for a few minutes before getting up. If dizziness persists or you feel faint contact the doctor.
- Respiratory symptoms including sore throat, coughing or sinus pain.
- Skin irritation, rash, redness – can occur at site of application of Daytrana Patch. Inform your doctor immediately if the reaction worsens or if blistering occurs

Rare side effects you should report to the doctor **IMMEDIATELY** include:
- Fast or irregular heart beat
- Muscle twitches, tics or movement problems
- Persistent throbbing headache
- Soreness of the mouth, gums, or throat

- Skin rash or itching, swelling of the face
- Any unusual bruising or bleeding, appearance of splotchy purplish darkening of the skin
- Tiredness, weakness, fever, or feeling like you have the flu, associated with nausea, vomiting, loss of appetite
- Yellow tinge in the eyes or to the skin; dark-colored urine
- Severe agitation or restlessness
- **A switch in mood to an unusual state of happiness or irritability; fluctuations in mood**

Let the doctor know **as soon as possible** if you miss your period, suspect you may be **pregnant** or are trying to get pregnant.

What should you do if you forget to take a dose of your medication?

If you take the psychostimulant 2–3 times a day and forget to take a dose by more than 4 hours, skip the missed dose and continue with your regular schedule. **DO NOT DOUBLE THE DOSE**.

If you forget to apply the patch in the morning, you may do so later in the day, however, remove the patch at the usual time in the evening to reduce the possibility of late-day side effects

Is this drug safe to take with other medication?

Because psychostimulants can change the effect of other medication, or may be affected by other medication, always check with the doctor or pharmacist before taking other drugs, including over-the-counter medication such as cold remedies. Always inform any doctor or dentist that you see that you are taking a psycho-stimulant drug.

Precautions/Considerations

1) This medication should not be used in patients who have high blood pressure, heart disease or abnormalities, hardening of the arteries or an overactive thyroid gland
2) Report to the doctor any changes in sleeping or eating habits or changes in mood or behavior.
3) Do not increase or decrease your dose without consulting the doctor.
4) Do not chew or crush the tablets or capsules unless told to do so by the doctor.
5) Use caution while performing tasks requiring alertness as these drugs can mask symptoms of fatigue.
6) Do not stop your drug suddenly as this may result in withdrawal symptoms such as insomnia and changes in mood and behavior.
7) Do not use alcohol while on this medication.
8) This drug may interact with medication prescribed by your dentist, so let him/her know the name of the drug you are taking.
9) If you are on Concerta you may notice that the tablet shell does not dissolve and you may sometimes see it in the toilet when you have a bowel movement.
10) Store your medication in a clean, dry area at room temperature. Keep all medication out of the reach of children.
11) If you are using Daytrana patches please be aware of the following:
    i) Apply the patch immediately upon removal of the protective pouch (sticky side down) to a clean, dry area on your hip. Do not place it upon inflamed skin. Wash your hands.
    ii) Keep track of the time you apply the patch each morning and make sure you remove it after 9 h (or sooner, if so advised by your doctor).
    iii) When removing the patch, peel it off slowly, fold the sticky side together, and flush it down the toilet. Wash your hands.
    iv) When wearing the patch, DO NOT apply heat (e.g., heat pads, electric blankets) near or on the area of the patch.
    v) Should the patch accidentally fall off, a new patch can be re-applied, however, it should be removed at the usual time in the evening.

If you have any questions regarding this medication, do not hesitate to contact the doctor, pharmacist, or nurse.

PATIENT AND CAREGIVER INFORMATION
on ATOMOXETINE

Atomoxetine is used primarily in the treatment of Attention Deficit Hyperactivity Disorder (ADHD) in children and adults.

How quickly will the drug start working?

Some response to atomoxetine is usually noted within the first 3–4 weeks of treatment of ADHD.

How does the doctor decide on the dosage?

Atomoxetine comes in a capsule; the dose is based on your body weight and how well it works for you. The capsule is usually given once or twice a day, with or without food. Do not increase or decrease the dose without speaking to the doctor.

How long should you take this medication?

Atomoxetine is usually prescribed for a period of several months to years.

Side effects

Side effects occur, to some degree, with all medication. They are usually not serious and do not occur in all individuals. They may sometimes occur before beneficial effects of medication are noticed. If a side effect continues, speak to the doctor or pharmacist about appropriate treatment.

Common side effects that should be reported to the doctor at the **NEXT APPOINTMENT** include:

- Increased anxiety, agitation or excitability – Some individuals may feel nervous or have difficulty sleeping for a few days after starting this medication.
- Headache – This tends to be temporary and can be managed by taking analgesics (e.g., acetaminophen) when required.
- Nausea, abdominal pain, vomiting – try taking your medication with food; if symptoms persist, speak to the doctor.
- Loss of appetite, weight loss – Try eating small meals several times a day.
- Drowsiness and fatigue – The problem goes away with time, however, your doctor may suggest you take your medication at bedtime. Use of other drugs that make you drowsy will worsen the problem. Avoid operating machinery if drowsiness persist.
- Dry mouth – Sour candy, ice chips, popsicles, and sugarless gum help increase saliva in your mouth; try to avoid sweet, calorie laden beverages. Drink water and brush your teeth regularly.
- Dizziness – Get up from a lying or sitting position slowly; dangle your legs over the edge of the bed for a few minutes before getting up. Sit or lie down if dizziness persists or if you feel faint, then contact the doctor.
- Difficulty remembering things – Speak to the doctor.

Rare side effects you should report to the doctor **IMMEDIATELY** include:

- Fast or irregular heart beat.
- Skin rash with swelling, itching.
- Soreness of the mouth, gums or throat.
- Any unusual bruising or bleeding, appearance of splotchy purplish darkening of the skin.
- Fatigue, weakness, fever or flu-like symptoms accompanied by nausea, vomiting, loss of appetite.
- Tenderness on the right side of your abdomen
- Yellow tinge in the eyes or to the skin; dark-colored urine.
- Severe agitation, restlessness or irritability.
- **Switch in mood to an unusual state of happiness, excitement, irritability, or a marked disturbance in sleep.**

Let the doctor know **as soon as possible** if you miss your period or suspect you may be **pregnant**

What should you do if you forget to take a dose of your medication?

If you take atomoxetine more than once a day and you forget to take a dose by more than 6 hours, skip the missed dose and continue with your regular schedule. **DO NOT DOUBLE THE DOSE.**

Is this drug safe to take with other medication?

Because atomoxetine can change the effect of other medication, or may be affected by other medication, always check with the doctor or pharmacist before taking other drugs, including over-the-counter medication such as cold remedies and herbal preparations. Always inform any doctor or dentist that you see that you are taking atomoxetine.

Precautions/Considerations

1) This medication should not be used in patients who have high blood pressure, heart disease or abnormalities, hardening of the arteries or an overactive thyroid gland.
2) Report to the doctor any changes in sleeping or eating habits or changes in mood or behavior.
3) Do not increase or decrease your dose without consulting the doctor.
4) Use caution while performing tasks requiring alertness as atomoxetine can mask fatigue
5) Do not use alcohol while on this medication.
6) This drug may interact with medication prescribed by your dentist, so let him/her know the name of the drug you are taking.
7) Store your medication in a clean dry area at room temperature. Keep all medication out of reach of children.

If you have any questions regarding this medication, do not hesitate to contact the doctor, pharmacist, or nurse.

PATIENT AND CAREGIVER INFORMATION on CLONIDINE

Clonidine is used in the treatment of Attention Deficit Hyperactivity Disorder (ADHD) and tic disorders in children and adolescents. It has also been found effective for controlling some problematic behaviors in children and adolescents with autism and has been used to treat aggression in conduct disorder.

The doctor may choose to use this medication for a reason not listed here. If you are not sure why this medication is being prescribed, please ask the doctor.

How quickly will the drug start working

Some response to clonidine is usually noted within the first week of treatment of ADHD and tends to increase over the next 3 weeks.

How does the doctor decide on the dosage?

Clonidine comes in both a tablet and a transdermal patch (in the USA). The dose is based on the body weight. The tablet is usually given several times a day, while the patch is applied to the upper arm or chest and is left there for a period of one week.

Do not increase or decrease the dose without speaking to the doctor. Do not take off the patch mid-week unless you have been told to do so by the doctor.

How long should you take this medication?

Clonidine is usually prescribed for a period of several months to years.

Side effects

Side effects occur, to some degree, with all medication. They are usually not serious and do not occur in all individuals. They may sometimes occur before beneficial effects of medication are noticed. If a side effect continues, speak to the doctor or pharmacist about appropriate treatment.

Common side effects that should be reported to the doctor at the **NEXT APPOINTMENT** include:

- Feeling sleepy and tired – The problem goes away with time. Use of other drugs that make you drowsy will worsen the problem. Avoid operating machinery if drowsiness persist.
- Dry mouth – Sour candy, ice chips, popsicles, and sugarless gum help increase saliva in your mouth; try to avoid sweet, calorieladen beverages. Drink water and brush your teeth regularly.
- Dizziness – Get up from a lying or sitting position slowly; dangle your legs over the edge of the bed for a few minutes before getting up. Sit or lie down if dizziness persists or if you feel faint, then contact the doctor.
- Headache – This tends to be temporary and can be managed by taking pain medicine (e.g., acetaminophen) when required.
- Increased anxiety, agitation or excitability – Some individuals may feel nervous or have difficulty sleeping for a few days after starting this medication.
- Difficulty remembering things – Speak to the doctor.

Rare side effects you should report to the doctor IMMEDIATELY include:

- Fast or irregular heart beat
- Skin rash with swelling, itching
- Soreness of the mouth, gums or throat
- Any unusual bruising or bleeding, appearance of splotchy purplish darkening of the skin
- Nausea, vomiting, loss of appetite, feeling tired, weak, or like you have the flu
- Yellow tinge in the eyes or to the skin; dark-colored urine
- Severe agitation, restlessness or irritability

Let the doctor know **as soon as possible** if you miss your period or suspect you may be **pregnant**.

What should you do if you forget to take a dose of your medication?

If you take clonidine more than once a day and you forget to take a dose by more than 6 hours, skip the missed dose and continue with your regular schedule. **DO NOT DOUBLE THE DOSE.**

Is this drug safe to take with other medication?

Because clonidine can change the effect of other medication, or may be affected by other medication, always check with the doctor or pharmacist before taking other drugs, including over-the-counter medication such as cold remedies and herbal preparations. Always inform any doctor or dentist that you see that you are taking clonidine.

Precautions/Considerations

1) Report to the doctor any changes in sleeping or eating habits or changes in mood or behavior.

2) Do not increase or decrease your dose without consulting the doctor.
3) Use caution while performing tasks requiring alertness (e.g., operating heavy machinery) as clonidine can cause fatigue
4) Do not use alcohol while on this medication.
5) Do not stop clonidine suddenly as it may result in withdrawal symptoms including insomnia and changes in blood pressure.
6) If taking transdermal clonidine and it begins to loosen from the skin after application, apply adhesive tape directly over the patch to make sure it stays on for the rest of the week.
7) Take off the used patch before applying a new patch to the skin. Handle used transdermal patches carefully; fold the patch in half with the sticky sides together, and place inside a baggie prior to discarding. Keep out of reach of children.
8) Store your medication in a clean dry area at room temperature. Keep all medication out of reach of children.

If you have any questions regarding this medication, do not hesitate to contact the doctor, pharmacist, or nurse.

PATIENT AND CAREGIVER INFORMATION on GUANFACINE

Though not approved for this indication, guanfacine is used in the treatment of Attention Deficit Hyperactivity Disorder (ADHD) in children and adults. It has also been found effective for controlling some problematic behaviors in children with pervasive developmental disorders.

How quickly will the drug start working?

Some response to guanfacine is usually noted within the first few week of treatment of ADHD

How does the doctor decide on the dosage?

Guanfacine is available as an oral tablet and is usually given twice a day. The dose is based on the body weight.

Do not increase or decrease the dose without speaking to your doctor.

How long should you take this medication?

Guanfacine is usually prescribed for a period of several years.

Side effects

Side effects occur, to some degree, with all medication. They are usually not serious and do not occur in all individuals. They may sometimes occur before beneficial effects of medication are noticed. If a side effect continues, speak to your doctor about appropriate treatment.

Common side effects that should be reported to your doctor at the **NEXT APPOINTMENT** include:

- Feeling sleepy and tired – The problem goes away with time. Use of other drugs that make you drowsy will worsen the problem. Avoid operating machinery if drowsiness persists.
- Dizziness – Get up from a lying or sitting position slowly; dangle your legs over the edge of the bed for a few minutes before getting up. Sit or lie down if dizziness persists or if you feel faint, then contact your doctor.
- Headache – This tends to be temporary and can be managed by taking analgesics (e.g., acetaminophen) when required.

- Insomnia, increased irritability – Some individuals may feel more nervous or irritable, or have difficulty sleeping for a few days after starting this medication.
- Loss of appetite – Eating smaller portions more frequently may be of help

Rare side effects you should report to your doctor **IMMEDIATELY** include:

- Severe agitation or elevation in mood (mania)
- Skin rash with swelling, itching
- Soreness of the mouth, gums or throat
- Let your doctor know **as soon as possible** if you miss your period or suspect you may be **pregnant**

What should you do if you forget to take a dose of your medication?

If you take guanfacine twice a day and you forget to take a dose by more than 6 hours, skip the missed dose and continue with your regular schedule. **DO NOT DOUBLE THE DOSE.**

Is this drug safe to take with other medication?

Because guanfacine can change the effect of other medication, or may be affected by other medication, always check with your doctor or pharmacist before taking other drugs, including over-the-counter medication such as cold remedies. Always inform any doctor or dentist that you see that you are taking clonidine.

Precautions

1) Report to your doctor any changes in sleeping or eating habits or changes in mood or behavior.
2) Do not increase or decrease your dose without consulting your doctor.
3) Use caution while performing tasks requiring alertness as guanfacine can cause fatigue
4) Do not stop guanfacine suddenly as it may result in withdrawal symptoms including insomnia and changes in blood pressure.
5) Store your medication in a clean dry area at room temperature. Keep all medication out of reach of children.

If you have any questions regarding this medication, do not hesitate to contact your doctor, pharmacist, or nurse.

PATIENT AND CAREGIVER INFORMATION on SELECTIVE SEROTONIN REUPTAKE INHIBITOR (SSRI) ANTIDEPRESSANTS

The name of your medication is _____.

Use

Certain SSRI antidepressants have been approved for use (in some countries) for the treatment of the following disorders in children and adolescents:

- Major depressive disorder
- Obsessive compulsive disorder
- Though approved only in adults, they have however been fooun useful in the treatment of other conditions in children and adolescents, including:
  - Panic disorder
  - Generalized anxiety disorder
  - Bipolar depression
  - Eating disorders
  - Social phobia
  - Posttraumatic stress disorder
  - Premenstrual changes in mood

These drugs may also be effective in several other disorders, such as separation anxiety disorder and selective mutism.

The doctor may choose to use this medication for a reason not listed here. If you are not sure why this medication is being prescribed, please ask the doctor.

How well do these drugs work in children and adolescents?

Though there is research and data supporting the use of SSRI's in children and adolescents, some studies suggest these drugs are only marginally more effective than placebo in treating depression and anxiety disorders. It is therefore recommended that, whenever possible, psychotneraphy (talk therapy or cognitive behavior therapy) be used together with medication to increase the potential for benefit.

How quickly will the drug start working?

Antidepressants begin to improve sleep and appetite and to increase energy within about 1 week; but feelings of depression may take 4 to 6 weeks to improve. Because antidepressants take time to work, **do not decrease or increase the dose or stop the medication** without discussing this with the doctor.

Improvement in symptoms of obsessive compulsive disorder, panic or generalized anxiety disorder and eating disorders also occur gradually.

These drugs do not work for everyone; if you are not feeling better after several weeks the doctor may recommend you take a different antidepressant

How long should you take this medication?

This depends on what type of illness you have and how well you do.

Following the first episode of depression it is recommended that antidepressants be continued for a minimum of 6–12 months; this decreases the chance of being ill again. The doctor may then decrease the drug slowly and monitor for any symptoms of depression; if none occur, the drug can gradually be stopped. For individuals who have had several episodes of depression, antidepressant medication should be continued indefinitely. DO NOT STOP taking your medication if you are feeling better, without first discussing this with the doctor. Long-term treatment is generally recommended for obsessive compulsive disorder, panic or generalized anxiety disorder and eating disorders.

Side effects

Side effects occur, to some degree, with all medication. They are usually not serious and do not occur in all individuals. They may sometimes occur before beneficial effects of the medication are noticed. If a side effect continues, speak to the doctor about appropriate treatment.

Common side effects that should be reported to the doctor at the **NEXT APPOINTMENT** include:
- Feeling sleepy and tired – This problem goes away with time. Use of other drugs that make you drowsy will worsen the problem. Avoid operating machinery if drowsiness persists.
- Energizing/agitated feeling – Some individuals may feel nervous or have difficulty sleeping for a few days after starting this medication. Report this to the doctor; he/she may advise you to take the medication in the morning.
- Headache – This tends to be temporary and can be managed by taking pain medicine (e.g., acetaminophen) when required.
- Nausea or heartburn – If this happens, take the medication with food.
- Muscle tremor, twitching – Speak to the doctor as this may require a change in your dosage.
- Changes in sex drive or sexual performance – Discuss this with the doctor.
- Blurred vision – This usually occurs at start of treatment and tends to be temporary. Reading under a bright light or at a distance may help; a magnifying glass can be of temporary use. If the problem continues, advise the doctor.
- Dry mouth – Sour candy, ice chips, popsicles, and sugarless gum help increase saliva in your mouth; do not drink sweet, calorie-laden drinks like colas. Drink water and brush your teeth regularly.
- Constipation – Drink plenty of water and try to increase the amount of fibre in your diet (like fruit, vegetables or bran). Some individuals find a bulk laxative (e.g., Metamucil, Fibyrax) or a stool softener (Colace, Surfak) helps regulate their bowels. If these remedies are not effective, speak to your doctor or pharmacist.
- Nightmares – May be managed by changing the time you take your drug.
- Loss of appetite.

Rare side effects you should report to the doctor **IMMEDIATELY** include:
- **Switch in mood to an unusual state of happiness, excitement, irritability, or a marked disturbance in sleep**
- Soreness of the mouth, gums, or throat
- Skin rash or itching, swelling of the face
- Any unusual bruising or bleeding
- Nausea, vomiting, loss of appetite, fatigue, weakness, fever, or flu-like symptoms
- Yellow tinge in the eyes or to the skin; dark-colored urine
- Tingling in the hands and feet, severe muscle twitching
- Severe agitation irritability, or restlessness, or an increase in thoughts of suicide
- Thoughts of suicide or hostility (in rare instances this medication has been associated with having some suicidal or hostile thoughts. Although these thoughts may be seen as a part of the disorder, you should definitely discuss these kinds of thoughts with your doctor)

Let the doctor know **as soon as possible** if you miss your period, suspect you may be **pregnant** or are trying to get pregnant.

What should you do if you forget to take a dose of your medication?

If you take your total dose of antidepressant in the morning and you forget to take it for more than 6 hours, skip the missed dose and continue with your schedule the next day. **DO NOT DOUBLE THE DOSE**. If you take the drug several times a day, take the missed dose when you remember (unless it is within 4 h of your next dose), then continue with your regular schedule.

Is this drug safe to take with other medication?

Because SSRI antidepressant drugs can change the effect of other medication, or may be affected by other medication, always check with the doctor or pharmacist before taking other drugs, including over-the-counter medication such as cold remedies. Always inform any doctor or dentist that you see that you are taking an antidepressant drug.

Precautions/Considerations

1) Do not increase or decrease your dose without consulting the doctor.
2) Take your drug with meals or with water, milk, orange or apple juice; avoid grapefruit juice as it may change the effect of the drug in your body.
3) This drug may impair the mental and physical abilities required for driving a car or operating machinery. Avoid these activities if you feel drowsy or slowed down.

4) This drug may increase the effects of alcohol, making you more sleepy, dizzy and lightheaded.

5) Do not stop your drug suddenly as this may result in withdrawal symptoms such as muscle aches, chills, tingling in your hands or feet, nausea, vomiting, and dizziness.

6) Report any changes in mood or behavior to the physician, including an increase in thoughts of self-harm or suicide

7) This drug may interact with medication prescribed by your dentist, so let him/her know the name of the drug you are taking.

8) Store your medication in a clean, dry area at room temperature. Keep all medication out of the reach of children.

If you have any questions regarding this medication, do not hesitate to contact the doctor, pharmacist, or nurse.

PATIENT AND CAREGIVER INFORMATION on the ANTIDEPRESSANT BUPROPION

Bupropion belongs to a class of antidepressants called Selective Norepinephrine Dopamine Reuptake Inhibitors (NDRI).

Use

Bupropion has not been approved for use in children and adolescents

Bupropion is primarily used in the treatment of Major Depressive Disorders and depression associated with Bipolar Disorder. It has also been approved in the management of smoking cessation.

Bupropion has also been found useful in children and adults with Attention Deficit Hyperactivity Disorder, and has been used as an add-on treatment to increase the effects of other classes of antidepressants.

The doctor may choose to use this medication for a reason not listed here. If you are not sure why this medication is being prescribed, please ask the doctor.

How quickly will the drug start working?

Bupropion is usually prescribed twice a day, morning and evening. It begins to improve sleep and appetite and to increase energy within about one week; however, feelings of depression may take from 4–6 weeks to improve. Because antidepressants take time to work, **do not decrease or increase the dose or stop the medication** without discussing this with the doctor. Improvement in smoking cessation/withdrawal also occurs over a period of 6 weeks.

These drugs do not work for everyone; if you are not feeling better after several weeks, the doctor may recommend you take a different antidepressant.

How long should you take this medication?

This depends on what type of illness you have and how well you do.

Following the first episode of depression it is recommended that antidepressants be continued for a minimum of 6–12 months; this decreases the chance of being ill again.

The doctor may then decrease the drug slowly and monitor for any symptoms of depression; if none occur, the drug can gradually be stopped.

For individuals who have had several episodes of depression, antidepressant medication should be continued indefinitely.

DO NOT STOP taking your medication if you are feeling better, without first discussing this with the doctor.

Use of bupropion for smoking cessation is recommended as a one-time treatment for a period of 6 weeks.

Side effects

Side effects occur, to some degree, with all medication. They are usually not serious and do not occur in all individuals. They may sometimes occur before beneficial effects of the medication are noticed. If a side effect continues, speak to the doctor about appropriate treatment.

Common side effects that should be reported to the doctor at the **NEXT APPOINTMENT** include:

- Energizing/agitated feeling – Some individuals may feel nervous or have difficulty sleeping for a few days after starting this medication. Report this to the doctor; he/she may advise you to take the medication in the morning.
- Vivid dreams or nightmares – This can occur at the start of treatment.
- Headache – This can be managed by taking pain relievers (e.g., acetaminophen) as required. If the headache persists or is "troubling" contact the doctor.
- Muscle tremor, twitching – Speak to the doctor as this may require a change in your dose.
- Nausea or heartburn – If this happens, take the medication with food.
- Loss of appetite.
- Dry mouth – Sour candy, ice chips, popsicles, and sugarless gum help increase saliva in your mouth; try to avoid sweet, calorie-laden beverages. Drink water and brush your teeth regularly.
- Sweating – You may sweat more than usual; use of deodorants and talcum powder may help.

- Blood pressure – A slight increase in blood pressure can occur with this drug. If you are taking medication for high blood pressure, tell the doctor, as this medication may have to be adjusted.

Rare side effects you should report to the doctor **IMMEDIATELY** include:
- Severe agitation, irritability, or restlessness or an increase in thoughts of suicide
- Persistent, troubling headache
- Seizures; these usually occur with high doses – should you have a seizure, stop taking bupropion and contact the physician
- Chest pain, shortness of breath
- Soreness of the mouth, gums, or throat
- Skin rash or itching, swelling of the face
- Nausea, vomiting, loss of appetite, fatigue, weakness, fever, or flu-like symptoms
- Muscle pain and tenderness or joint pain accompanied by fever and rash
- Yellow tinge in the eyes or to the skin; dark-colored urine
- Tingling in the hands and feet, severe muscle twitching
- **Switch in mood to an unusual state of happiness, excitement, irritability, or problems sleeping**

Let the doctor know **as soon as possible** if you miss your period, suspect you may be **pregnant** or are trying to get pregnant.

What should you do if you forget to take a dose of your medication?

If you forget to take the morning dose of antidepressant by more than 4 hours, skip the missed dose and continue with your schedule for the evening dose.

DO NOT DOUBLE THE DOSE as seizures may occur.

Is this drug safe to take with other medication?

Because antidepressant drugs can change the effect of other medication, or may be affected by other medication, always check with the doctor or pharmacist before taking other drugs, including over-the-counter medication such as cold remedies. Always inform any doctor or dentist that you see that you are taking an antidepressant drug.

Precautions/Considerations

1) Do not increase or decrease your dose without consulting the doctor.
2) Do not chew or crush the tablet, but swallow it whole.
3) If you have been advised by the doctor to break a bupropion sustained release tablet in half, do so just prior to taking your medication; throw out the second half unless you can use it within 24 hours (store the half tablet in a tightly-closed container away from light).
4) Do not stop your drug suddenly as this may result in withdrawal symptoms such as muscle aches, chills, tingling in your hands or feet, nausea, vomiting, and dizziness.
5) Report any changes in mood or behavior to the physician. including an increase in thoughts of self-harm or suicide.
6) This drug may interact with medication prescribed by your dentist, so let him/her know the name of the drug you are taking.
7) Store your medication in a clean, dry area at room temperature and away from high humidity. Keep all medication out of the reach of children.

If you have any questions regarding this medication, do not hesitate to contact the doctor, pharmacist, or nurse.

PATIENT AND CAREGIVER INFORMATION on SELECTIVE SEROTONIN NOREPINEPHRINE REUPTAKE INHIBITOR (SNRI) ANTIDEPRESSANTS

The name of your medication is _____.

Use

SNRI antidepressants have not been approved for use in children and adolescents.

These drugs are primarily used in the treatment of Major Depressive Disorders, depression associated with Bipolar Disorders and Generalized Anxiety Disorder in adults.

Venlafaxine has also been found effective in several other disorders including Attention Deficit Hyper-activity Disorder in children and adults, and can improve behavior in children and adolescents with autistic disorders.

The doctor may choose to use this medication for a reason not listed here. If you are not sure why this medication is being prescribed, please ask the doctor.

How quickly will the drug start working?

SNRIs begin to improve sleep and appetite and to increase energy within about one week; however, feelings of depression may take from 4 to 6 weeks to improve. Because antidepressants take time to work, **do not decrease or increase the dose or stop the medication** without discussing this with the doctor.

These drugs do not work for everyone, if you are not feeling better after several weeks, the doctor may recommend you take a different anidepressant.

How long should you take this medication?

This depends on what type of illness you have and how well you do.

Following the first episode of depression it is recommended that antidepressants be continued for a minimum of 6–12 months; this decreases the chance of being ill again. The doctor may then decrease the drug slowly and monitor for any symptoms of depression; if none occur, the drug can gradually be stopped. For individuals who have had several episodes of depression, antidepressant medication should be continued indefinitely.

DO NOT STOP taking your medication if you are feeling better, without first discussing this with the doctor.

Long-term treatment is generally recommended for obsessive compulsive disorder, panic disorder, and social phobia.

Side effects

Side effects occur, to some degree, with all medication. They are usually not serious and do not occur in all individuals. They may sometimes occur before beneficial effects of the medication are noticed. If a side effect continues, speak to the doctor about appropriate treatment.

Common side effects that should be reported to the doctor at the **NEXT APPOINTMENT** include:

- Energizing/agitated feeling – Some individuals may feel nervous or have difficulty sleeping for a few days after starting this medication. Report this to the doctor; he/she may advise you to take the medication in the morning.
- Headache – This can be managed by taking pain relievers (e.g., aspirin, acetaminophen) as required. If the headache persists or is "troubling" contact the doctor.
- Nausea or heartburn – If this happens, take the medication with food.
- Dry mouth – Sour candy, ice chips, popsicles, and sugarless gum help increase saliva in your mouth; try to avoid sweet, calorie-laden beverages. Drink water and brush your teeth regularly.
- Constipation – Increase bulk foods in your diet (e.g., salads, bran) and drink plenty of fluids. Some individuals find a bulk laxative (e.g., Metamucil, Fibyrax) or a stool softener (Colace, Surfak) helps regulate their bowels. If these remedies are not effective, consult the doctor or pharmacist.
- Sweating – You may sweat more than usual; frequent showering, use of deodorants and talcum powder may help.

- Blood pressure – A slight increase in blood pressure can occur with this drug.
- Changes in sex drive or sexual performance – Discuss this with the doctor.

Rare side effects you should report to the doctor **IMMEDIATELY** include:
- Severe agitation, irritability, or restlessness, or an increase in thoughts of suicide
- Persistent, troubling headache
- Soreness of the mouth, gums, or throat
- Skin rash or itching, swelling of the face
- Nausea, vomiting, diarrhea, loss of appetite, fatigue, weakness, fever, or flu-like symptoms
- Yellow tinge in the eyes or to the skin; dark-colored urine
- Tingling in the hands and feet, severe muscle twitching, tremor, shivering
- Racing heart/pulse.
- **Switch in mood to an unusual state of happiness, excitement, irritability, or problems sleeping**

Let the doctor know **as soon as possible** if you miss your period, suspect you may be **pregnant** or are trying to get pregnant.

What should you do if you forget to take a dose of your medication?

If you take your total dose of antidepressant in the morning and you forget to take it for more than 6 hours, skip the missed dose and continue with your schedule the next day. **DO NOT DOUBLE THE DOSE**. If you take the drug several times a day, take the missed dose when you remember (unless it is within 4 h of your next dose), then continue with your regular schedule.

Is this drug safe to take with other medication?

Because antidepressant drugs can change the effect of other medication, or may be affected by other medication, always check with the doctor or pharmacist before taking other drugs, including over-the-counter medication such as cold remedies. Always inform any doctor or dentist that you see that you are taking an antidepressant drug.

Precautions/Considerations

1) Do not increase or decrease your dose without consulting the doctor.
2) Do not chew or crush the sustained-release tablet (Effexor XR or Cymbalta), but swallow it whole.
3) This drug may impair the mental and physical abilities required for driving a car or operating machinery. Avoid these activities if you feel drowsy or slowed down.
4) This drug may increase the effects of alcohol, making you more sleepy, dizzy and lightheaded.
5) Do not stop your drug suddenly as this may result in withdrawal symptoms such as muscle aches, chills, tingling in your hands or feet, nausea, vomiting, and dizziness.
6) Report any changes in mood or behavior to the physician, including an increase in thoughts of self-harm or suicide.
7) This drug may interact with medication prescribed by your dentist, so let him/her know the name of the drug you are taking.
8) Store your medication in a clean, dry area at room temperature. Keep all medication out of the reach of children.

If you have any questions regarding this medication, do not hesitate to contact the doctor, pharmacist, or nurse.

PATIENT AND CAREGIVER INFORMATION on SEROTONIN-2 ANTAGONIST/REUPTAKE INHIBITOR (SARI) ANTIDEPRESSANTS

The name of your medication is _____.

Use

SARI antidepressants are used in the treatment of Major Depressive Disorder and depression associated with Bipolar Disorder. Though not approved for these indication, these drugs have also been found effective in several other disorders including social phobia, posttraumatic stress disorder, acute and chronic insomnia, as well as disruptive behavior.

The doctor may choose to use this medication for a reason not listed here. If you are not sure why this medication is being prescribed, please ask the doctor.

How quickly will the drug start working?

Antidepressants begin to improve sleep and appetite and to increase energy within about one week; however, feelings of depression may take from 4–6 weeks to improve. Because antidepressants take time to work, **do not decrease or increase the dose or stop the medication** without discussing this with the doctor. Improvement in symptoms of other disorder or behaviors also occur gradually.

These drugs do not work for everyone; if you are not feeling better after several weeks, the doctor may recommend you take a different antidepressant.

How long should you take this medication?

This depends on what type of illness you have and how well you do.

Following the first episode of depression it is recommended that antidepressants be continued for a minimum of 6–12 months; this decreases the chance of being ill again. The doctor may then decrease the drug slowly and monitor for any symptoms of depression; if none occur, the drug can gradually be stopped. For individuals who have had several episodes of depression, antidepressant medication should be continued indefinitely.

DO NOT STOP taking your medication if you are feeling better, without first discussing this with the doctor.

Side effects

Side effects occur, to some degree, with all medication. They are usually not serious and do not occur in all individuals. They may sometimes occur before beneficial effects of the medication are noticed. If a side effect continues, speak to the doctor about appropriate treatment.

Common side effects that should be reported to the doctor at the **NEXT APPOINTMENT** include:
- Feeling sleepy and tired – This problem goes away with time. Use of other drugs that make you drowsy will worsen the problem. Avoid operating machinery if drowsiness persists.
- Energizing/agitated feeling – Some individuals may feel nervous or have difficulty sleeping for a few days after starting this medication.
- Headache – This tends to be temporary and can be managed by taking analgesics (e.g., acetaminophen) when required.
- Nausea or heartburn – If this happens, take the medication with food.
- Muscle tremor, twitching – Speak to the doctor as this may require an adjustment in your dosage.
- Changes in sex drive or sexual performance – Discuss this with the doctor.
- Dry mouth – Sour candy, ice chips, popsicles, and sugarless gum help increase saliva in your mouth; try to avoid sweet, calorie laden beverages. Drink water and brush your teeth regularly.
- Loss of appetite.

Rare side effects you should report to the doctor **IMMEDIATELY** include:
- Severe agitation, irritability or restlessness, including an increase in thoughts of suicide
- Soreness of the mouth, gums, or throat

- Skin rash or itching, swelling of the face
- Any unusual bruising or bleeding
- Nausea, vomiting, loss of appetite, fatigue, weakness, fever, or flu-like symptoms (rare cases of liver toxicity have occurred)
- Persistent abdominal pain, pale stools
- Yellow tinge in the eyes or to the skin; dark-colored urine
- Tingling in the hands and feet, severe muscle twitching
- **Switch in mood to an unusual state of happiness, excitement, irritability, or problems sleeping**

Let the doctor know **as soon as possible** if you miss your period, suspect you may be **pregnant** or are trying to get pregnant.

What should you do if you forget to take a dose of your medication?

If you take your total dose of antidepressant in the morning and you forget to take it for more than 6 hours, skip the missed dose and continue with your schedule the next day. **DO NOT DOUBLE THE DOSE**. If you take the drug several times a day, take the missed dose when you remember (unless it is within 4 h of your next dose), then continue with your regular schedule.

Is this drug safe to take with other medication?

Because SARI antidepressant drugs can change the effect of other medication, or may be affected by other medication, always check with the doctor or pharma- cist before taking other drugs, including over-the-counter medication such as cold remedies. Always inform any doctor or dentist that you see that you are taking an antidepressant drug.

Precautions/Considerations

1) Do not increase or decrease your dose without consulting the doctor.
2) Take your drug with meals or with water, milk, orange or apple juice; avoid grapefruit juice as it may interfere with the effect of the drug.
3) This drug may impair the mental and physical abilities required for driving a car or operating machinery. Avoid these activities if you feel drowsy or slowed down.
4) This drug may increase the effects of alcohol, making you more sleepy, dizzy and lightheaded.
5) Do not stop your drug suddenly as this may result in withdrawal symptoms such as muscle aches, chills, tingling in your hands or feet, nausea, vomiting, and dizziness.
6) Report any changes in mood or behavior to the physician including an increase in thoughts of self-harm or suicide.
7) This drug may interact with medication prescribed by your dentist, so let him/her know the name of the drug you are taking.
8) Store your medication in a clean, dry area at room temperature. Keep all medication out of the reach of children.

If you have any questions regarding this medication, do not hesitate to contact the doctor, pharmacist, or nurse.

Mirtazapine belongs to a class of antidepressants called Noradrenergic/Specific Serotonergic Antidepressants (NaSSA)

Use

Mirtazapine has not been approved for use in children and adolescents.

Mirtazapine is primarily used in the treatment of Major Depressive Disorders, depression associated with Bipolar Disorder.

Mirtazapine has also been found effective in several anxiety disorders including panic disorder and post-traumatic stress disorder.

The doctor may choose to use this medication for a reason not listed here. If you are not sure why this medication is being prescribed, please ask the doctor.

How quickly will the drug start working?

Mirtazapine begins to improve sleep and appetite and to increase energy within about one week; however, feelings of depression may take from 4 to 6 weeks to improve. Because antidepressants take time to work, **do not decrease or increase the dose or stop the medication** without discussing this with the doctor.

Improvement in symptoms of anxiety disorder also occur gradually over several weeks.

This drug does not work for everyone; if you are not feeling better after several weeks, the doctor may recommend you take a different antidepressant.

How long should you take this medication?

This depends on what type of illness you have and how well you do.

Following the first episode of depression it is recommended that antidepressants be continued for a minimum of 6–12 months; this decreases the chance of being ill again. The doctor may then decrease the drug slowly and monitor for any symptoms of depression; if none occur, the drug can gradually be stopped. For individuals who have had several episodes of depression, antidepressant medication should be continued indefinitely.

DO NOT STOP taking your medication if you are feeling better, without first discussing this with the doctor.

Long-term treatment is generally recommended for anxiety disorders.

Side effects

Side effects occur, to some degree, with all medication. They are usually not serious and do not occur in all individuals. They may sometimes occur before beneficial effects of the medication are noticed. If a side effect continues, speak to the doctor about appropriate treatment.

Common side effects that should be reported to the doctor at the **NEXT APPOINTMENT** include:

- Feeling sleepy and tired – This problem goes away with time, and with an increase in dose. Use of other drugs that make you drowsy will worsen the problem. Avoid driving a car or operating machinery if drowsiness persists.
- Dry mouth – Sour candy, ice chips, popsicles, and sugarless gum help increase saliva in your mouth; try to avoid sweet, calorieladen beverages. Drink water and brush your teeth regularly.
- Constipation – Increase bulk foods in your diet (e.g., salads, bran) and drink plenty of fluids. Some individuals find a bulk laxative (e.g., Metamucil, Fibyrax) or a stool softener (Colace, Surfak) helps regulate their bowels. If these remedies are not effective, consult the doctor or pharmacist.
- Dizziness – Get up from a lying or sitting position slowly; dangle your legs over the edge of the bed for a few minutes before getting up. Sit or lie down if dizziness persists or if you feel faint, then contact the doctor.
- Increased appetite and weight gain – Monitor your food intake and try to avoid foods with a high fat content (e.g., cakes and pastry).

Rare side effects you should report to the doctor **IMMEDIATELY** include:

- Severe agitation, irritability or restlessness, including an increase in thoughts of suicide
- Soreness of the mouth, gums, or throat
- Skin rash or itching, swelling of the face
- Nausea, vomiting, loss of appetite, fatigue, weakness, fever, or flu-like symptoms
- Yellow tinge in the eyes or to the skin; dark-colored urine
- **Switch in mood to an unusual state of happiness, excitement, irritability, or problems sleeping**

Let the doctor know **as soon as possible** if you miss your period, suspect you may be **pregnant** or are trying to get pregnant.

What should you do if you forget to take a dose of your medication?

If you take your total dose of antidepressant at bedtime and you forget to take your medication, skip the missed dose and continue with your schedule the next day. **DO NOT DOUBLE THE DOSE**. If you take the drug several times a day, take the missed dose when you remember (unless it is within 4 h of your next dose), then continue with your regular schedule.

Is this drug safe to take with other medication?

Because antidepressant drugs can change the effect of other medication, or may be affected by other medication, always check with the doctor or pharmacist before taking other drugs, including over-the-counter medication such as cold remedies. Always inform any doctor or dentist that you see that you are taking an antidepressant drug.

Precautions/Considerations

1) Do not increase or decrease your dose without consulting the doctor.
2) This drug may impair the mental and physical abilities required for driving a car or operating machinery. Avoid these activities if you feel drowsy or slowed down.
3) This drug may increase the effects of alcohol, making you more sleepy, dizzy and lightheaded.
4) Do not stop your drug suddenly as this may result in withdrawal symptoms such as muscle aches, chills, tingling in your hands or feet, nausea, vomiting, and dizziness.
5) Report any changes in mood or behavior to the physician, including an increase in thoughts of self-harm or suicide.
6) This drug may interact with medication prescribed by your dentist, so let him/her know the name of the drug you are taking.
7) Store your medication in a clean, dry area at room temperature. Keep all medication out of the reach of children.

If you have any questions regarding this medication, do not hesitate to contact the doctor, pharmacist, or nurse.

The name of your medication is _____.

Use

Certain tricyclic antidepressants have been approved for the following indications in children and adolescents:
- obsessive-compulsive disorder
- bedwetting

In adults, cyclic antidepressants are primarily used in the treatment of major depressive disorders and depression associated with Bipolar Disorder. Though not approved for these indications, certain cyclic antidepressants have also been found effective in other disorders including Attention Deficit Hyperactivity Disorder not responsive to other therapies, school phobias, separation anxiety disorder, eating disorders, premenstrual mood disorders, behavioral symptoms associated with autistic disorder and the management of chronic pain conditions (e.g., migraines).

The doctor may choose to use this medication for a reason not listed here. If you are not sure why this medication is being prescribed, please ask the doctor.

How quickly will the drug start working?

Antidepressants begin to improve sleep and appetite and to increase energy within about one week; however, feelings of depression may take from 4 to 6 weeks to improve. Because antidepressants take time to work, **do not decrease or increase the dose or stop the medication** without discussing this with the doctor.

Improvement in symptoms of obsessive compulsive disorder, eating disorders, pain management, enuresis and other disorders also occur gradually.

These drugs do not work for everyone; if you are not feeling better after several weeks, the doctor may recommend you take a different antidepressant.

How long should you take this medication?

This depends on what type of illness you have and how well you do.

Following the first episode of depression it is recommended that antidepressants be continued for a minimum of 6–12 months; this decreases the chance of being ill again. The doctor may then decrease the drug slowly and monitor for any symptoms of depression; if none occur, the drug can gradually be stopped. For individuals who have had several episodes of depression, antidepressant medication should be continued indefinitely. Long-term treatment is generally recommended for obsessive compulsive disorder, eating disorders, pain management, enuresis and other disorders.

DO NOT STOP taking your medication if you are feeling better, without first discussing this with the doctor.

Side effects

Side effects occur, to some degree, with all medication. They are usually not serious and do not occur in all individuals. They may sometimes occur before beneficial effects of the medication are noticed. If a side effect continues, speak to the doctor about appropriate treatment.

Common side effects that should be reported to the doctor at the **NEXT APPOINTMENT** include:
- Feeling sleepy and tired – This problem goes away with time. Use of other drugs that make you drowsy will worsen the problem. Avoid operating machinery if drowsiness persists.
- Energizing/agitated feeling – Some individuals may feel nervous or have difficulty sleeping for a few days after starting this medication. Report this to the doctor; he/she may advise you to take the medication in the morning.
- Blurred vision – This usually occurs at the start of treatment and tends to be temporary. Reading under a bright light or at a distance may help; a magnifying glass can be of temporary use. If the problem continues, advise the doctor.
- Dry mouth – Sour candy, ice chips, popsicles, and sugarless gum help increase saliva in your mouth; try to avoid sweet, calorieladen beverages. Drink water and brush your teeth regularly.
- Constipation – Increase bulk foods in your diet (e.g., salads, bran) and drink plenty of fluids. Some individuals find a bulk laxative (e.g., Metamucil, Fibyrax) or a stool

softener (Colace, Surfak) helps regulate their bowels. If these remedies are not effective, consult the doctor or pharmacist.
- Headache – This tends to be temporary and can be managed by taking pain medicine (aspirin, acetaminophen) when required.
- Nausea or heartburn – If this happens, take the medication with food.
- Dizziness – Get up from a lying or sitting position slowly; dangle your legs over the edge of the bed for a few minutes before getting up. Sit or lie down if dizziness persists or if you feel faint, then contact the doctor.
- Sweating – You may sweat more than usual; frequent showering, use of deodorants and talcum powder may help.
- Muscle tremor, twitching – Speak to the doctor as this may require a change in your dosage.
- Changes in sex drive or sexual performance – Discuss this with the doctor.
- Nightmares – Can be managed by changing the time you take your drug.

Rare side effects you should report to the doctor **IMMEDIATELY** include:
- Severe agitation, irritability or restlessness, or an increase in thoughts of suicide
- Soreness of the mouth, gums, or throat.
- Skin rash or itching, swelling of the face.
- Nausea, vomiting, loss of appetite, fatigue, weakness, fever, or flu-like symptoms
- Yellow tinge in the eyes or to the skin; dark-colored urine
- Going 24 hours or more without peeing
- Inability to have a bowel movement (more than 3 days)
- Tingling in the hands and feet, severe muscle twitching
- **Switch in mood to an unusual state of happiness, excitement, irritability, or problems sleeping**

Let the doctor know **as soon as possible** if you miss your period, suspect you may be **pregnant** or are trying to get pregnant.

What should you do if you forget to take a dose of your medication?

If you take your total dose of antidepressant in the morning and you forget to take it for more than 6 hours, skip the missed dose and continue with your schedule the next day. **DO NOT DOUBLE THE DOSE.** If you take the drug several times a day, take the missed dose when you remember (unless it is within 4 h of your next dose), then continue with your regular schedule.

Is this drug safe to take with other medication?

Because antidepressant drugs can change the effect of other medication, or may be affected by other medication, always check with the doctor or pharmacist before taking other drugs, including over-the-counter medication such as cold remedies. Always inform any doctor or dentist that you see that you are taking an antidepressant drug.

Precautions/Considerations

1) Do not increase or decrease your dose without consulting the doctor.
2) Take your drug with meals or with water, milk, orange or apple juice; avoid grapefruit juice as it may interfere with the effect of the drug.
3) Avoid taking high-fiber foods (e.g., bran) or laxatives (e.g., psyllium) together with your medication, as this may reduce the antidepressant effect.
4) This drug may impair the mental and physical abilities required for driving a car or operating machinery. Avoid these activities if you feel drowsy or slowed down.
5) This drug may increase the effects of alcohol, making you more sleepy, dizzy and lightheaded.
6) Avoid exposure to extreme heat and humidity since this drug may affect your body's ability to regulate temperature.
7) Do not stop your drug suddenly as this may result in withdrawal symptoms such as muscle aches, chills, tingling in your hands or feet, nausea, vomiting, and dizziness.
8) Report any changes in mood or behavior to the physician, including an increase in thoughts of self-harm or suicide.
9) This drug may interact with medication prescribed by your dentist, so let him/her know the name of the drug you are taking.
10) Store your medication in a clean, dry area at room temperature. Keep all medication out of the reach of children.

If you have any questions regarding this medication, do not hesitate to contact the doctor, pharmacist, or nurse.

PATIENT AND CAREGIVER INFORMATION on the ANTIDEPRESSANT MOCLOBEMIDE

The name of your medication is moclobemide. It belongs to a class of antidepressants called RIMA (Reversible Inhibitor of Monoamine Oxidase-A).

Use

Moclobemide has not been approved for use in children and adolescents.

Moclobemide is primarily used in the treatment of major depressive disorders and depression associated with Bipolar Disorder. It has been approved in the management of chronic mild depression in adults.

Moclobemide may improve attention and concentration in children with Attention Deficit Hyperactivity Disorder not responsive to other agents, and may be effective in social phobia.

The doctor may choose to use this medication for a reason not listed here. If you are not sure why this medication is being prescribed, please ask the doctor.

How quickly will the drug start working?

Moclobemide begins to improve sleep and appetite and to increase energy within about one week; however, feelings of depression may take from 4–6 weeks to improve. Because antidepressants take time to work, **do not decrease or increase the dose or stop the medication** without discussing this with the doctor. Improvement in symptoms of social phobia and Attention Deficit Hyperactivity Disorder also occur gradually.

This drug does not work for everyone; if you are not feeling better after several weeks the doctor may recommend you take a different antidepressant.

When should I take this medication?

Moclobemide is usually prescribed to be taken twice daily, morning and evening. Take this drug after meals to minimize side effects. If a meal is missed, the drug should still be taken, but a large meal should not be eaten for at least 1 hour.

How long should you take this medication?

This depends on what type of illness you have and how well you do.

Following the first episode of depression it is recommended that antidepressants be continued for a minimum of 6–12 months; this decreases the chance of being ill again. The doctor may then decrease the drug slowly and monitor for any symptoms of depression; if none occur, the drug can gradually be stopped. For individuals who have had several episodes of depression, antidepressant medication should be continued indefinitely.

DO NOT STOP taking your medication if you are feeling better, without first discussing this with the doctor.

Long-term treatment is generally recommended for social phobia and Attention Deficit Hyperactivity Disorder.

Side effects

Side effects occur, to some degree, with all medication. They are usually not serious and do not occur in all individuals. They may sometimes occur before beneficial effects of the medication are noticed. If a side effect continues, speak to the doctor about appropriate treatment.

Common side effects that should be reported to the doctor at the **NEXT APPOINTMENT** include:
- Energizing/agitated feeling – Some individuals may feel nervous or have difficulty sleeping for a few days after starting this medication. Report this to the doctor; he/she may advise you to take the medication in the morning and afternoon (rather than the evening).
- Headache – This can be managed by taking pain medicine (e.g., aspirin, acetaminophen) as required. If the headache persists or is "troubling" contact the doctor.
- Dizziness – Get up from a lying or sitting position slowly; dangle your legs over the edge of the bed for a few minutes before getting up. Sit or lie down if dizziness persists or if you feel faint, – then call the doctor.

- Nausea or heartburn – If this happens, take the medication with food.
- Sweating – You may sweat more than usual; use of deodorants and talcum powder may help.

Rare side effects you should report to the doctor **IMMEDIATELY** include:
- Severe agitation, irritability or restlessness, or an increase in thoughts of suicide
- Persistent, throbbing headache
- Soreness of the mouth, gums, or throat
- Skin rash or itching, swelling of the face
- nausea, vomiting, loss of appetite, fatigue, weakness, fever, or flu-like symptoms
- Yellow tinge in the eyes or to the skin; dark-colored urine
- **Switch in mood to an unusual state of happiness, excitement, irritability, or problems sleeping**

Let the doctor know **as soon as possible** if you miss your period, suspect you may be **pregnant** or are trying to get pregnant.

Treatment with moclobemide does NOT require special diet restrictions as with other MAOI's. However, you should avoid eating excessive amounts of aged, overripe cheeses or yeast extracts. If a **hypertensive reaction** should occur, the symptoms usually come on suddenly, so be alert for these signs:
- Severe, throbbing headache which starts at the back of the head and move towards the front. Often nausea and vomiting occur at the same time
- Neck stiffness
- Heart palpitations, fast heart beat, chest pain
- Sweating, cold and clammy skin
- Enlarged (dilated) pupils of the eyes
- Sudden unexplained nose bleeds

If a combination of these symptoms does occur, **contact the doctor IMMEDIATELY**; if you are unable to do so, go to the Emergency Department of your nearest hospital.

Moclobemide should always be taken after meals to avoid any food-related side effects (e.g., headaches).

What should you do if you forget to take a dose of your medication?

If you take your total dose of antidepressant in the morning and you forget to take it for more than 6 hours, skip the missed dose and continue with your schedule the next day. **DO NOT DOUBLE THE DOSE**. If you take the drug several times a day, take the missed dose when you remember (unless it is within 4 h of your next dose), then continue with your regular schedule.

Is this drug safe to take with other medication?

Because antidepressant drugs can change the effect of other medication, or may be affected by other medication, always check with the doctor or pharmacist before taking other drugs, including over-the-counter medication such as cold remedies. Always inform any doctor or dentist that you see that you are taking the antidepressant drug moclobemide.

Precautions/Considerations

1) Do not increase or decrease your dose without consulting the doctor.
2) Do not stop your drug suddenly as this may result in withdrawal symptoms such as muscle aches, chills, tingling in your hands or feet, nausea, vomiting, and dizziness.
3) Report any changes in mood or behavior to the physician including an increase in thoughts of self-harm or suicide
4) This drug may interact with medication prescribed by your dentist, so let him/her know the name of the drug you are taking.
5) Take no other medication (including over-the-counter or herbal products) without consulting with the doctor or pharmacist. Avoid all products containing dextromethorphan.
6) Store your medication in a clean, dry area at room temperature. Keep all medication out of the reach of children.

If you have any questions regarding this medication, do not hesitate to contact the doctor, pharmacist, or nurse.

The name of your medication is _____.

Use

This medication is primarily used in the treatment of major depressive disorders and depression associated with Manic Depressive Illness (Bipolar Disorder). It has also been approved in the management of atypical depression, phobic anxiety states or social phobia in adults.

Though not approved for these indications in children and adolescents, MAOIs have also been found effective in mild depression, panic disorder, posttraumatic stress disorder, separation anxiety, selective mutism, eating disorders and Attention Deficit Hyperactivity Disorder not responsive to other agents.

The doctor may choose to use this medication for a reason not listed here. If you are not sure why this medication is being prescribed, please ask the doctor.

How quickly will the drug start working?

MAOIs begin to improve sleep and appetite and to increase energy within about one week; however, feelings of depression may take from 4 to 6 weeks to improve. Because antidepressants take time to work, **do not decrease or increase the dose or stop the medication** without discussing this with the doctor.

Improvement in symptoms of other conditions also occur gradually.

These drugs do not work for everyone; if you are not feeling better after several weeks, the doctor may recommend you take a different antidepressant.

How long should you take this medication?

This depends on what type of illness you have and how well you do.

Following the first episode of depression it is recommended that antidepressants be continued for a minimum of 6–12 months; this decreases the chance of being ill again.

The doctor may then decrease the drug slowly and monitor for any symptoms of depression; if none occur, the drug can gradually be stopped. For individuals who have had several episodes of depression, antidepressant medication should be continued indefinitely.

DO NOT STOP taking your medication if you are feeling better, without first discussing this with the doctor.

Long-term treatment is generally recommended for conditions for which this medication is prescribed.

Side effects

Side effects occur, to some degree, with all medication. They are usually not serious and do not occur in all individuals. They may sometimes occur before beneficial effects of the medication are noticed. If a side effect continues, speak to the doctor about appropriate treatment.

Common side effects that should be reported to the doctor at the **NEXT APPOINTMENT** include:

- Feeling sleepy and tired – This problem goes away with time. Use of other drugs that make you drowsy will worsen the problem. Avoid operating machinery if drowsiness persists.
- Energizing/agitated feeling – Some individuals may feel nervous or have difficulty sleeping for a few days after starting this medication. Report this to the doctor; he/she may advise you to take the medication in the morning and afternoon (rather than the evening).
- Headache – This can be managed by taking pain medicine (e.g., acetaminophen) as required. If the headache persists or is "troubling" contact the doctor.
- Dizziness – Get up from a lying or sitting position slowly; dangle your legs over the edge of the bed for a few minutes before getting up. Sit or lie down if dizziness persists or if you feel faint – then call the doctor.
- Nausea or heartburn – If this happens, take the medication with food.
- Dry mouth – Sour candy, ice chips, popsicles, and sugarless gum help increase saliva in your mouth; try to avoid sweet, calorie–laden beverages. Drink water and brush your teeth regularly.

- Blurred vision – This usually occurs at start of treatment and tends to be temporary. Reading under a bright light or at a distance may help; a magnifying glass can be of temporary use. If the problem continues, advise the doctor.
- Constipation – Increase bulk foods in your diet (e.g., salads, bran) and drink plenty of fluids. Some individuals find a bulk laxative (e.g., Metamucil, Fibyrax) or a stool softener (Colace, Surfak) helps regulate their bowels. If these remedies are not effective, consult the doctor or pharmacist.
- Muscle tremor, twitching, jerking – Speak to the doctor as this may require a change in your dosage.
- Sweating – You may sweat more than usual; frequent showering, use of deodorants and talcum powder may help.
- Loss of appetite.

Rare side effects you should report to the doctor **IMMEDIATELY** include:
- Severe agitation, irritability or restlessness or an increase in thoughts of suicide
- Persistent, throbbing headache
- Soreness of the mouth, gums, or throat
- Skin rash or itching, swelling of the face
- Nausea, vomiting, loss of appetite, fatigue, weakness, fever, or flu-like symptoms
- Yellow tinge in the eyes or to the skin; dark-colored urine
- Going 24 hours or more without peeing
- **Switch in mood to an unusual state of happiness, excitement, irritability, or problems sleeping**

Let the doctor know **as soon as possible** if you miss your period, suspect you may be **pregnant** or are trying to get pregnant.

Caution

Certain foods and drugs contain chemicals which are broken down by the enzyme monoamine oxidase. Since this drug inhibits this enzyme, these chemicals increase in the body and may raise the blood pressure and cause a severe reaction called a **hypertensive crisis**.

Listed below are the foods and drugs which should be **avoided** while taking this drug.

Do not eat the following foods:
- All matured or aged cheeses (Cheddar, Brick, Blue, Stilton, Camembert, Roquefort)
- Broad bean pods (e.g., Fava Beans)
- Concentrated yeast extracts ("Marmite")

- Sausage (if aged, especially salami, mortadella, pastrami, summer sausage), other unrefrigerated fermented meats, game meat that has been hung, aged liver
- Dried salted fish, pickled herring
- Sauerkraut
- Soya sauce or soybean condiments, tofu
- Packet soup (especially miso)
- Tap (draft) beer, alcohol-free beer
- Improperly stored or spoiled meat, poultry, or fish

Wait for 14 days after stopping a MAOI drug before restarting to eat the above foods.

Hypertensive reactions have been reported, by some individuals, with the following foods; try small portions to determine if these foods will cause a reaction:
- Smoked fish, caviar, snails, tinned fish, shrimp paste
- Yogurt
- Meat tenderizers
- Meat extract ("Bovril," "Oxo")
- Homemade red wine, Chianti, canned/bottled beer, sherry, champagne
- Cheeses (e.g., Parmesan, Muenster, Swiss, Gruyere, Mozzarella, Feta)
- Pepperoni
- Overripe fruit, avocados, raspberries, bananas, plums, canned figs and raisins, orange pulp, tomatos
- Oriental foods
- Spinach, eggplant

It is SAFE to use the following foods, in moderate amounts (only if fresh):
- Cottage cheese, cream cheese, farmer's cheese, processed cheese, Cheez Whiz, ricotta, Havarti, Boursin, Brie without rind, Gorgonzola
- Liver (as long as it is fresh), fresh or processed meats, poultry or fish (e.g., hot dogs, bologna)
- Spirits, liquor (in moderation)
- Soy milk
- Sour cream
- Salad dressings
- Worcestershire sauce
- Yeast-leavened bread

Make sure all food is fresh, stored properly, and eaten soon after being purchased. Never touch food that is fermented or possibly "off" (spoiled). Avoid restaurant sauces, gravy and soup.

Do not use the following over-the-counter drugs without prior consultation with the doctor or pharmacist:

- Cold remedies, decongestants (including nasal sprays and drops), some antihistamines and cough medicine
- Narcotic painkillers (e.g., products containing codeine)
- All stimulants including pep-pills (Wake-ups, Nodoz), or appetite suppressants
- Anti-asthma drugs (Primatine P)
- Sleep aids and Sedatives (Sominex, Nytol)
- Yeast, dietary supplements (e.g., Ultrafast, Optifast)

It is SAFE to use:

- Plain ASA (aspirin), acetaminophen (e.g., Tylenol), or ibuprofen (e.g., Motrin, Advil)
- Antacids (e.g., Tums, Maalox)
- Throat lozenges

If a **hypertensive reaction** should occur, the symptoms usually come on suddenly, so be alert for these signs:

- Severe, throbbing headache which starts at the back of the head and radiates forward; often the headache is accompanied by nausea and vomiting
- Stiff neck
- Heart palpitations, fast heart beat, chest pain
- Sweating, cold and clammy skin
- Enlarged (dilated) pupils of the eyes
- Sudden unexplained nose bleeds

If a combination of these symptoms does occur, **contact the doctor IMMEDIATELY**; if you are unable to do so, go to the Emergency Department of your nearest hospital.

What should you do if you forget to take a dose of your medication?

If you take your total dose of antidepressant in the morning and you forget to take it for more than 6 hours, skip the missed dose and continue with your schedule the next day. **DO NOT DOUBLE THE DOSE**. If you take the drug several times a day, take the missed dose when you remember (unless it is within 4 h of your next dose), then continue with your regular schedule.

Is this drug safe to take with other medication?

Because antidepressant drugs can change the effect of other medication, or may be affected by other medication, always check with the doctor or pharmacist before taking other drugs, including over-the-counter medication such as cold remedies. Always inform any doctor or dentist that you see that you are taking an antidepressant drug.

Precautions/Considerations

1) Do not increase or decrease your dose without consulting the doctor.
2) Be aware of foods to avoid with this medication.
3) Take no other medication (including over-the-counter or herbal products) without consulting with the doctor or pharmacist. Avoid all products containing dextromethorphan.
4) This drug may interact with medication prescribed by your dentist, so let him/her know the name of the drug you are taking.
5) This drug may impair the mental and physical abilities required for driving a car or operating other machinery. Avoid these activities if you feel drowsy or slowed down.
6) Do not stop your drug suddenly as this may result in withdrawal symptoms such as muscle aches, chills, tingling in your hands or feet, nausea, vomiting, and dizziness.
7) Report any changes in mood or behavior to the physician, including an increase in thoughts of self-harm or suicide.
8) Store your medication in a clean, dry area at room temperature. Keep all medication out of the reach of children.

If you have any questions regarding this medication, do not hesitate to contact the doctor, pharmacist, or nurse.

PATIENT AND CAREGIVER INFORMATION on ELECTROCONVULSIVE TREATMENT (ECT)

Use

ECT is a procedure used primarily to treat patients with severe Depression. It has also been found effective in the manic phase of Bipolar Disorder, and in some patients with treatment-refractory schizophrenia.

What is the ECT procedure?

ECT is given to the patient while he/she is under an anesthetic which has put them to sleep; a muscle relaxant is also given to relax the muscles, bones and joints.

ECT involves passing a small, controlled electric current between two metal discs (electrodes) which are applied on the surface of the scalp. The two electrodes may be placed on one side of the head for unilateral ECT or on both sides of the forehead for bilateral ECT. The electric current passes between the two electrodes and through part of the brain in order to stimulate the brain; that electrical stimulation induces a convulsion or seizure which usually lasts from 20 to 90 seconds.

The procedure takes approximately 10 minutes from the time the anesthetic is given until its effect wears off. Oxygen is given throughout this time and the patient is monitored continuously by the physician. The treatment is not painful and the electric current and seizure are not felt by the patient.

How does ECT work?

As is the case with many medical treatments, the actual way that ECT relieves symptoms of illness is not totally understood. It is believed that ECT affects some of the chemicals which transfer impulses or messages between nerve cells in the brain, perhaps more strongly and quickly than some medications. The treatment may correct some of the biochemical changes which accompany the illness.

How effective is ECT?

Studies comparing the effectiveness of ECT and drug therapy in depression have consistently shown that ECT is the most effective treatment of depression, especially in patients whose illness does not respond adequately to drug treatment.

The total number of treatments required to get the full benefit from ECT may range from 6 to 20, depending on the patient's diagnosis and response to treatment. In some patients, a response may be seen after 3 treatments, however, a full course is generally recommended to obtain a full response. Some patients require periodic treatments to maintain their improvement.

How safe is ECT and what are the potential side effects?

ECT is considered a safe treatment, when given according to modern standards. It has been shown to be safe when given to children and adolescents as well as during pregnancy, with proper monitoring. Side effects that can occur include the following:

- Nausea following ECT – If severe, an antinauseant can be prescribed
- Memory – The most common side effect seen following ECT is some degree of memory loss. Recovery from that memory loss begins a few weeks after treatment and is usually complete in most patients after 6 to 9 months. There may be a permanent loss of memory for details of some events, particularly those which occurred some time before and during the weeks the treatment was given. Also, there may be some difficulty learning and remembering new information for a short period after ECT. However, the ability to acquire new memories recovers completely, usually a few months after treatment. A very small number of patients report severe problems with memory that remain for months or years.
- Confusion – Some patients experience a brief period of confusion after waking from the anesthetic.

- Headache – Common, but not usually severe.
- Muscle aches – Usually temporary.
- Increased heart rate and blood pressure – This can occur during treatment and last for several minutes. Monitoring of patients during and following ECT includes temperature, pulse, blood pressure and electrocardiogram (ECG).
- Prolonged seizure – Occurs rarely; seizure activity is monitored during the procedure by an electroencephalogram (EEG). Rarely a patient may have a spontaneous seizure following the ECT.
- Dental injury (e.g., broken teeth) or bone fractures – Occur very rarely.

The risk of death is very rare (2 to 4 per 100,000 treatments) and is similar to that seen with any treatment given under a general anesthetic.

What else do I need to know about the ECT procedure?

1) Make sure that you understand the information that has been provided to you by the doctor or nurse regarding ECT; ask them to explain anything about the treatment which you do not understand.
2) Do not eat or drink anything for approximately 8 hours before each treatment (and nothing after midnight).
3) Any essential medication (e.g., for high blood pressure) which the physician has told you must be taken before ECT, should be swallowed only with a very small sip of water.
4) Any other medication which you usually take in the morning should not be taken until after the ECT procedure.

If you have any questions regarding this procedure, do not hesitate to contact the doctor or nurse.

PATIENT AND CAREGIVER INFORMATION on ANTIPSYCHOTIC (NEUROLEPTIC) DRUGS

Antipsychotics have been classified as being either conventional (typical or first generation antipsychotics) or atypical (second or third generation antipsychotics)

The name of your medication is _____.

It is classified as a _____ agent.

Use

The main use of this drug is to **treat symptoms of acute or chronic psychosis**, including schizophrenia, mania, psychotic depression, delusional disorders and organic disorders. There are several other uses for these drugs (including Tourette's Syndrome, impulsive/aggressive behavior, obsessive-compulsive disorder, autism, Asperger's syndrome, and conduct disorder)

The doctor may choose to use this medication for a reason not listed here. If you are not sure why this medication is being prescribed, please ask the doctor.

What symptoms will this drug help control?

Symptoms of psychosis differ in children and adolescents, both as to the type of symptom and severity. Some common symptoms which antipsychotics have been found to help include:

- Hallucinations (e.g., hearing voices, seeing things, smelling odors, feeling unusual body sensations)
- Fixed beliefs, often of a paranoid nature (i.e., someone is persecuting or following you; people are talking about you) or of a grandiose nature (i.e., you are a special or famous person)
- Disorganized thoughts (difficulty in focusing on a thought), or speeded-up thoughts
- Irritability, agitation, hyperexcitement, over-elated mood
- They may also help decrease aggressive or repetitive behaviors seen in autism

Some atypical antipsychotics may also help symptoms of social withdrawal, lack of interest in oneself and in others, and poor motivation.

How quickly will the drug start working?

Antipsychotics begin to relieve agitation and sleep disturbances in about 1 week, help control mood changes in about 2 weeks, and help difficulties in thoughts and awareness in 6–8 weeks; voices (hallucinations) will decrease in intensity and frequency over 2–8 weeks. Feelings of apathy and lack of motivation may decrease gradually over 3–6 months. Improvements in behaviors can be seen in 2–6 weeks.

Because antipsychotics require time to work, **do not decrease or increase the dose or stop the medication** without discussing this with the doctor.

How long should you take this medication?

This depends on what type of illness you have and how well you do. Following the first episode of psychosis, it is recommended that antipsychotic medication be continued for at least 1–2 years; this decreases the chance of being ill again.

For individuals who have had a psychotic illness for several years or repeated psychotic episodes, antipsychotic medication should be continued indefinitely. The physician may adjust the dose from time to time.

Preparations of antipsychotics

Antipsychotics are available in different forms:
- Fast-acting injection – To help control symptoms quickly, when the patient is in distress
- Oral liquid
- Oral tablets – The usual, most common form, e.g., pills, capsules, sublingual tablets
- Quick dissolving tablets
- Long-acting (depot) injection – Convenient for patients who have been stabilized on an oral antipsychotic. This eliminates the need for the patient to remember to take his/her medication daily, helps in compliance with treatment and has been shown to lower the risk of relapse.

How should you take your medication?

Oral tablets or liquid are usually taken once or twice a day (at the same time each day). All antipsychotic tablets can be taken with or without food, except for ziprasidone, which must be taken with meals.

Liquid risperidone is usually taken once or twice a day (at the same time each day) with water, orange juice, coffee, or low-fat milk. Do not take it with tea or cola

When taking fast-dissolving tablets (Risperdal M-tabs, Zyprexa Zydis, or Fazaclo ODT), use dry hands and peel back the foil before removing the tablet (rather than pushing it through the foil); place the tablet on the tongue – do not chew it. The tablet will quickly dissolve and may be swallowed with or without water.

A long-acting injection is given every 1 to 4 weeks by a nurse.

Side effects

Side effects occur, to some degree, with all medication. They are usually not serious and do not occur in all individuals. Most will decrease or disappear with time. If a side effect continues, speak to the doctor about appropriate treatment.

Common side effects to some antipsychotic medication that should be reported to the doctor **IMMEDIATELY** include:

- Muscle spasms, excessive rigidity, shaking, or restlessness. These symptoms can be controlled with other agents (less common with atypicals)

Common side effects that should be reported to the doctor at the **NEXT APPOINTMENT** include:

- Feeling sleepy and tired – This problem usually goes away with time. Use of other drugs that make you drowsy will worsen the problem. Avoid operating machinery if drowsiness persists.
- Dizziness – Get up from a lying or sitting position slowly; dangle your legs over the edge of the bed for a few minutes before getting up. Sit or lie down if dizziness persists or if you feel faint, then contact the doctor.
- Dry mouth – Sour candy, ice chips, popsicles, and sugarless gum help increase saliva in your mouth; try to avoid sweet, calorie-laden drinks like colas, as they may give you cavities and help put on weight. Drink water and brush your teeth regularly.
- Blurred vision – This usually occurs at start of treatment and may last 1–2 weeks. Reading under a bright light or at a distance may help; a magnifying glass can be of temporary assistance.
- Constipation – Increase bulk foods in your diet (e.g., salads, bran), drink plenty of fluids, and exercise regularly. Some individuals find a bulk laxative (e.g., Metamucil, Fibyrax) or a stool softener (Colace, Surfak) helps regulate their bowels. If these remedies are not effective, consult the doctor or pharmacist.
- Increased thirst and/or frequent urinating or loss of bladder control
- Stuffy nose – Increase humidity. Temporary use of a decongestant nose spray (e.g., Otrivin) may help.
- Weight changes – Monitor your food intake; you may notice a craving for carbohydrates (e.g., sweets, potatoes, rice, pasta), but try to avoid foods with high fat content (e.g., cakes and pastry). Let your doctor know if you notice a rapid increase in your weight or in your waist measurement
- Nausea or heartburn – If this happens, take the medication with food.
- Breast tenderness, liquid discharge from breasts, or missed periods.
- **Tardive dyskinesia** can occur in some patients who have been treated with some antipsychotics, (mostly conventional agents) usually for many years. It involves involuntary movements of certain muscles, usually those of the lips and tongue, and sometimes those of the hands, neck, and other parts of the body. Movements initially tend to increase over several years, but then stabilize and in some patients will decrease with time; in a few patients symptoms worsen. Withdrawal of the antipsychotic at the first signs of tardive dyskinesia, or switching to a "second generation" class of drug, improves the chance that this adverse effect with disappear with time. This has to be balanced against the risk of recurrent illness.

Rare side effects you should report to the doctor **IMMEDIATELY** include:

- Skin rash or itching
- Unusual headache
- Persistent dizziness, lightheadedness or fainting, heart palpitations
- Nausea, vomiting, loss of appetite, fatigue, weakness, fever, or flu-like symptoms
- Soreness of the mouth, gums, or throat
- Yellow tinge in the eyes or to the skin; dark colored urine
- Inability to pass urine (more than 24 hours)
- Inability to have a bowel movement (more than 2–3 days)
- Fever (high temperature) with muscle stiffness/rigidity

Let the doctor know **as soon as possible** if you miss your menstrual period, suspect you may be **pregnant** or are trying to get pregnant.

What should you do if you forget to take a dose of medication?

If you take your total dose of antipsychotic at bedtime and you forget to take it, DO NOT take the dose in the morning, but continue with your schedule the next evening. If you take the drug several times a day, take the missed dose when you remember (unless it is within 4 h of your next dose), then continue with your regular schedule.

Is this drug safe to take with other medication?

Because antipsychotic drugs can change the effect of other medication, or may be affected by other medication, always check with the doctor or pharmacist before taking other drugs, including over-the-counter medication such as cold remedies. Always inform any doctor or dentist that you see that you are taking an antipsychotic medication.

Precautions/Considerations

1) Do not increase or decrease your dose without consulting the doctor.
2) Take your drug with meals or with water, milk or orange juice; avoid grapefruit juice as it may interfere with the effect of the drug. Avoid apple juice if taking liquid preparations as it may precipitate the drug.
3) Do not break or crush your medication unless you have been advised to do so by the doctor or pharmacist.
4) If you are taking ziprasidone (Geodon), make sure you take your tablets with meals; if you are prescribed risperidone (Risperdal) solution, do not take it with tea or colas.
5) This drug may impair the mental and physical abilities required for driving a car or operating machinery. Avoid these activities if you feel drowsy or slowed down.
6) This drug may increase the effects of alcohol, making you more sleepy, dizzy and lightheaded.
7) Avoid exposure to extreme heat and humidity (e.g., saunas) since this drug may affect your body's ability to regulate temperature changes and blood pressure.
8) Antacids (e.g., Maalox, Amphogel, etc.) interfere with absorption of these drugs in your stomach and therefore may decrease their effect. To avoid this, take the antacid at least 2 h before or 1 hour after taking your antipsychotic drug.
9) Some patients may get a serious sunburn with little exposure to sunlight. Avoid direct sun, wear protective clothing and use a sunscreen preparation on exposed areas.
10) Excessive use of caffeinated beverages (coffee, tea, colas, etc.) can cause anxiety, agitation and restlessness and counteract some of the beneficial effects of your medication.
11) Cigarette smoking can change the amount of antipsychotic that remains in your bloodstream; inform the doctor if you make any changes to your current smoking habit.
12) Do not stop your drug suddenly as this may result in withdrawal symptoms such as nausea, dizziness, sweating, headache, sleeping problems, agitation and tremor, and also result in the return of psychotic symptoms.
13) Store your medication in a clean, dry area at room temperature. Keep all medication out of the reach of children.

If you have any questions regarding this medication, do not hesitate to contact the doctor, pharmacist, or nurse.

PATIENT AND CAREGIVER INFORMATION on CLOZAPINE

Clozapine belongs to the class of drugs called **Atypical Antipsychotics**.

Use

The primary use of this medication is to **treat symptoms of acute or chronic schizophrenia**; it is used in patients who have not had an adequate response to other antipsychotic drugs. Clozapine has been found effective in other psychotic disorders, including psychosis, Bipolar Disorder and organic brain disorders. Though not approved for this indication, it has also been used in the treatment of impulsive/aggressive behaviors associated with childhood psychiatric disorders.

The doctor may choose to use this medication for a reason not listed here. If you are not sure why this medication is being prescribed, please ask the doctor.

What symptoms will this drug help control?

Symptoms of psychosis differ in children and adolescents, both as to the type of symptom and severity. Some common symptoms which clozapine has been found to help include:
- Hallucinations (e.g., hearing voices, seeing things, smelling odors, feeling unusual body sensations)
- Fixed beliefs, often of a paranoid nature (i.e., someone is persecuting or following you; people are talking about you)
- Disorganized thoughts (difficulty in focusing on a thought), or speeded-up thoughts
- Irritability, agitation, hyperexcitement, overelated mood

Clozapine may also help symptoms of social withdrawal, lack of interest in oneself and in others and poor motivation.

How quickly will the drug start working?

Clozapine begins to relieve agitation within a few days, helps control mood changes in about 2 weeks, and helps difficulties in thoughts and awareness in 6–8 weeks; voices (hallucinations) will decrease in intensity and frequency over 2–8 weeks. Some patients respond to clozapine gradually over a period of months. Because antipsychotics require time to work, **do not decrease or increase the dose or stop the medication** without discussing this with the doctor.

How long should you take this medication?

For individuals who have had a psychotic illness for several years or repeated psychotic episodes, clozapine should be continued indefinitely. The physician may adjust the dose, from time to time, based on results of blood levels of clozapine and response to treatment.

DO NOT STOP taking your medication if you are feeling better, without first discussing this with the doctor.

Why are blood tests necessary with clozapine, and why is medication given for a week at a time?

A rare side effect (affects less than 1% of people) has been reported with clozapine; it is called **agranulocytosis.** With this side effect, the white cells in the blood decrease in quantity, which makes it difficult for the body to fight off any infections. Because this can result in a serious problem, if identified early, agranulocytosis can be reversed by stopping clozapine. It is therefore necessary to measure the amount of white blood cells in the body on a weekly basis to identify those individuals who may be at risk for agranulocytosis.

After taking clozapine for 6 months, individuals are at a decreased risk for agranulocytosis and may have their bloodwork done, and be given prescriptions every 2 weeks.

Side effects

Side effects occur, to some degree, with all medication. They are usually not serious and do not occur in all individuals. Most will decrease or disappear with time. If a side effect continues, speak to the doctor about appropriate treatment.

Common side effects that should be reported to the doctor at the **NEXT APPOINTMENT** include:

- Feeling sleepy and tired – This problem often goes away with time. Use of other drugs that make you drowsy will worsen the problem. Avoid operating machinery if drowsiness persists.
- Dizziness – Get up from a lying or sitting position slowly; dangle your legs over the edge of the bed for a few minutes before getting up. Sit or lie down if dizziness persists or if you feel faint, then contact the doctor.
- Dry mouth – Sour candy, ice chips, popsicles, and sugarless gum help increase saliva in your mouth; try to avoid sweet, calorieladen beverages. Drink water and brush your teeth regularly.
- Blurred vision – This usually occurs at start of treatment and may last 1–2 weeks. Reading under a bright light or at a distance may help; a magnifying glass can be of temporary use. If the problem continues, advise the doctor.
- Constipation – Increase bulk foods in your diet (e.g., salads, bran), drink plenty of fluids, and exercise regularly. Some individuals find a bulk laxative (e.g., Metamucil, Fibyrax) or a stool softener (Colace, Surfak) helps regulate their bowels. If these remedies are not effective, consult the doctor or pharmacist.
- Excess salivation or drooling – This often occurs at night. Use a towel on the pillow when sleeping. If this also occurs during waking hours or causes choking, speak to the doctor about other remedies.
- Weight gain – Monitor your food intake; you may notice a craving for carbohydrates (e.g., sweets, potatoes, rice, pasta), but try to avoid foods with high fat content (e.g., cakes and pastry). Let your doctor know if you notice a rapid increase in your weight or in your waist measurement.
- Nausea or heartburn – If this happens, take the medication with food.
- Increased thirst and/or frequent urinating or loss of bladder control

Rare side effects you should report to the doctor **IMMEDIATELY** include:
- **Soreness of the mouth, gums, or throat**
- **Fatigue, weakness, fever or flu-like symptoms or other signs of infections**
- **Rapid heart beat, chest pain and shortness of breath**
- **Periods of blackouts or seizures**
- Skin rash or itching
- Unusual headache
- Severe or persistent dizziness or fainting
- Yellow tinge in the eyes or to the skin; dark-colored urine
- Inability to have a bowel movement (more than 2–3 days)
- Worsening of repetitive behavior or obsessional symptoms

Tardive dyskinesia is an adverse effect that has been recognized in some patients who have been treated with antipsychotics, usually for many years. The risk of this adverse effect with clozapine is considered to be very low, and clozapine may help in treating this problem. Tardive dyskinesia describes involuntary movements of certain muscles – usually those of the lips and tongue, and sometimes those of the hands, neck and other parts of the body.

Let the doctor know **as soon as possible** if you miss your menstrual period, suspect you may be **pregnant** or are trying to get pregnant.

What should you do if you forget to take a dose of your medication?

If you take your total dose of antipsychotic at bedtime and you forget to take it, DO NOT take the dose in the morning, but continue with your schedule in the evening. If you take the drug several times a day, take the missed dose when you remember (unless it is within 4 h of your next dose), then continue with your regular schedule.

Is this drug safe to take with other medication?

Because clozapine can change the effect of other medication, or may be affected by other medication, always check with the doctor or pharmacist before taking other drugs, including over-the-counter medication such as cold remedies. Always inform any doctor or dentist that you see that you are taking an antipsychotic medication.

Precautions/Considerations

1) Do not increase or decrease your dose without consulting the doctor.
2) Take your drug with meals or with water, milk or orange juice; avoid grapefruit juice as it may interfere with the effect of the drug.
3) This drug may impair the mental and physical abilities required for driving a car or operating machinery. Avoid these activities if you feel drowsy or slowed down.
4) This drug may increase the effects of alcohol, making you more sleepy, dizzy and lightheaded.
5) Avoid exposure to extreme heat and humidity (e.g., saunas) since this drug may affect your body's ability to regulate temperature changes.

6) Antacids (e.g., Maalox, Amphogel, etc.) interfere with absorption of these drugs in your stomach and therefore may decrease their effect. To avoid this, take the antacid at least 2 hours before or 1 hour after taking your antipsychotic drug.

7) Excessive use of caffeinated beverages (coffee, tea, colas, etc.) can cause anxiety, agitation and restlessness and may affect the blood level of your medication.

8) Cigarette smoking can change the amount of antipsychotic that remains in your bloodstream; inform the doctor if you make any changes to your current smoking habit.

9) Do not stop your drug suddenly as this may result in withdrawal symptoms such as nausea, dizziness, sweating, headache, sleeping problems, agitation and tremor, and also result in the return of psychotic symptoms.

10) Store your medication in a clean, dry area at room temperature. Keep all medication out of the reach of children.

If you have any questions regarding this medication, do not hesitate to contact the doctor, pharmacist, or nurse.

PATIENT AND CAREGIVER INFORMATION on ANTIPARKINSONIAN DRUGS (for Treating Extrapyramidal Side Effects)

The name of your medication is _____.

Use

This medication is used to **treat muscle side effects** that some individuals experience when they are being treated with antipsychotic drugs. These muscle side effects can include:

- Muscle spasms or contractions (e.g., in the neck, eyes or tongue)
- Muscle stiffness, tremor, or a shuffling walk
- Feeling restless, unable to sit still, having a need to pace
- Muscle weakness or a slowing of movement

How quickly will the drug start working?

"Antiparkinsonian" drugs can reduce or stop the above side effects, usually within an hour. Sometimes they have to be given by injection for a quicker effect.

How long should you take this medication?

Some patients take antiparkinsonian drugs for 2–3 weeks, usually when first prescribed an antipsychotic drug, and while its dose is being stabilized. The doctor may reduce the dose of this drug to see if the muscle symptoms return; if not, you may be advised to stop using this medication. **Do not increase the dose or stop the drug without consulting with the doctor.**

Some patients require an antiparkinsonian drug for longer time periods, because they are more sensitive to muscle side effects from the antipsychotic drug they are receiving. Others require it only from time to time, i.e., as needed (e.g., for 1 week after receiving an injection of an antipsychotic).

Side effects

Side effects occur, to some degree, with all medication. They are usually not serious and do not occur in all individuals. Most will decrease or disappear with time. If a side effect continues, speak to the doctor about appropriate treatment.

Common side effects that should be reported to the doctor at the **NEXT APPOINTMENT** include:

- Dry mouth – Sour candy, ice chips, popsicles, and sugarless gum help increase saliva in your mouth; try to avoid sweet, calorie-laden drinks such as colas, as they may give you cavities and help put on weight. Drink water and brush your teeth regularly.
- Blurred vision – This usually occurs at the start of treatment and may last 1–2 weeks. Reading under a bright light or at a distance may help; a magnifying glass can be of temporary use. If the problem continues, advise the doctor.
- Constipation – Increase bulk foods in your diet (e.g., salads, bran) and drink plenty of fluids. Some individuals find a bulk laxative (e.g., Metamucil, Fibyrax) or a stool softener (Colace, Surfak) helps regulate their bowels. If these remedies are not effective, consult the doctor or pharmacist.
- Feeling sleepy and tired – This problem goes away with time. Use of other drugs that make you drowsy will worsen the problem. Avoid operating machinery if drowsiness persists.
- Nausea or heartburn – If this happens, take the medication with food.

Less common side effects that you should report to the physician **IMMEDIATELY** include:

- Disorientation, confusion, worsening of your memory, increase in psychotic symptoms
- Inability to have a bowel movement (more than 2–3 days)
- Inability to pass urine (more than 24 hours)
- Skin rash

Let the doctor know **as soon as possible** if you miss your menstrual period, suspect you may be **pregnant** or are trying to get pregnant.

Precautions/Considerations

1) Do not increase your dose without consulting the doctor
2) Check with the doctor or pharmacist before taking other drugs, including over-the-counter medication such as cold remedies
3) This drug may impair the mental and physical abilities required for driving a car or operating machinery. Avoid these activities if you feel drowsy or slowed down.
4) This drug may increase the effects of alcohol, making you more sleepy, dizzy and lightheaded
5) Avoid exposure to extreme heat and humidity (e.g., saunas) since this drug may affect your body's ability to regulate temperature changes.
6) Store your medication in a clean, dry area at room temperature. Keep all medication out of the reach of children.

If you have any questions regarding this medication, do not hesitate to contact the doctor, pharmacist, or nurse.

PATIENT AND CAREGIVER INFORMATION on BENZODIAZEPINE ANTIANXIETY DRUGS (ANXIOLYTICS)

The name of your medication is _____.

Use

This medication is used to **treat symptoms of anxiety.** Anxiety is a normal human response to stress and is considered necessary for effective functioning and coping with daily activities. It may, however, be a symptom of many other disorders, both medical and psychiatric. There are different types of anxiety and different approaches to treating it. Anxiolytics can help relieve the symptoms of anxiety but will not alter its cause. In usually prescribed doses, they help to calm and sedate the individual; in high doses these drugs may be used to induce sleep.

Benzodiazepines may also be used as a muscle relaxant, to treat agitation, to suppress seizures, and prior to some diagnostic procedures or surgery.

The doctor may choose to use this medication for a reason not listed here. If you are not sure why this medication is being prescribed, please ask the doctor.

How quickly will the drug start working?

Anxiolytic drugs can reduce agitation and induce calm or sedation usually within an hour. Sometimes they have to be given by injection, or dissolved under the tongue, for a quicker effect.

How long should you take this medication?

Anxiety is usually self-limiting; often when the cause of anxiety is treated or eliminated, symptoms of anxiety will decrease. Therefore, anxiolytics are usually prescribed for a limited period of time. Many individuals take the medication only when needed (during periods of excessive stress) rather than on a daily basis. Tolerance or loss of effectiveness can occur in some individuals if they are used continuously beyond 4 months. If you have been taking the medication for a continuous period of time, the physician may

try to reduce the dose of this drug slowly to see if the anxiety symptoms return; if not, the dosage may be further reduced and you may be advised to stop using this medication. **Do not increase the dose or stop the drug without consulting with the doctor.** Some patients need to use an anxiolytic drug for longer time periods, because of the type of anxiety they may be experiencing. Others require it only from time to time, i.e., as needed.

Side effects

Side effects occur, to some degree, with all medication. They are usually not serious and do not occur in all individuals. Most will decrease or disappear with time. If a side effect continues, speak to the doctor or pharmacist about appropriate treatment.

Common side effects that should be reported to the doctor at the **NEXT APPOINTMENT** include:

- Feeling sleepy and tired – This problem goes away with time, or when the dose is reduced. Use of other drugs that make you drowsy will worsen the problem. Avoid operating machinery if drowsiness persists.
- Muscle incoordination, weakness or dizziness – Inform the doctor; an adjustment in your dosage may be needed.
- Forgetfulness, memory lapses – Inform the doctor.
- Slurred speech – An adjustment in your dosage may be needed.
- Nausea or heartburn – If this happens, take the medication with food.

Less common side effects that you should report to the physician **IMMEDIATELY** include:

- Disorientation, confusion, worsening of memory, difficulty learning new things, blackouts, or amnesia
- Nervousness, restlessness, excitement, or any behavior changes
- Incoordination leading to falls
- Skin rash

Let the doctor know **as soon as possible** if you miss your period, suspect you may be **pregnant** or are trying to get pregnant.

Precautions/Considerations

1) Do not increase your dose without consulting the doctor
2) Take your medication with meals or with water, milk, orange or apple juice. Avoid grapefruit juice as it may change the effects of the drug in your body.
3) Check with the doctor or pharmacist before taking other drugs, including over-the-counter medication such as cold remedies
4) If you are taking the extended-release alprazolam (Xanax XR) do not cut, crush or chew the tablet, but swallow it whole. Take this drug at the same time in relation to meals (preferably in the morning).
5) This drug may impair the mental and physical abilities required for driving a car or operating machinery. Avoid these activities if you feel drowsy or slowed down.
6) This drug may increase the effects of alcohol, making you more sleepy, dizzy and lightheaded
7) Do not stop taking the drug suddenly, especially if you have been on the medication for a number of months or have been taking high doses. Anxiolytics need to be withdrawn gradually to prevent withdrawal reactions.
8) Avoid excessive consumption of caffeinated beverages (i.e., more than 2 cups of coffee, 3 cups of tea or cola) as it may counteract the beneficial effects of the anxiolytic.
9) Store your medication in a clean, dry area at room temperature. Keep all medication out of the reach of children.

If you have any questions regarding this medication, do not hesitate to contact the doctor, pharmacist, or nurse.

PATIENT AND CAREGIVER INFORMATION
on BUSPIRONE

Buspirone is an anti-anxiety drug (anxiolytic).

Use

Buspirone is used to **treat symptoms of chronic anxiety.** Anxiety is a normal human response to stress and is considered necessary for effective functioning and coping with daily activities. It may, however, be a symptom of many other disorders, both medical and psychiatric. There are different types of anxiety and there are different approaches to treating it.

Though not approved for these indications, buspirone has also been used to treat irritability and hyperactivity seen in autism.

The doctor may choose to use this medication for a reason not listed here. If you are not sure why this medication is being prescribed, please ask the doctor.

How quickly will the drug start working?

Buspirone causes a gradual improvement in symptoms of anxiety and can reduce agitation and induce calm usually within 1 to 2 weeks. The maximum effect is seen in 3–4 weeks.

How long should you take this medication?

This depends on what type of illness you have and how well you do.

Anxiety is usually self-limiting; often when the cause of anxiety is treated or eliminated, symptoms of anxiety will decrease. Therefore, anxiolytics are usually prescribed for a limited period of time. To maintain effectiveness, buspirone cannot be taken only when needed (during periods of excessive stress), but needs to be taken on a daily basis. The physician may try to reduce the dose of this drug to see if the anxiety symptoms return; if not, the dosage may be further reduced and you may be advised to stop using this medication. **Do not increase the dose or stop the drug without consulting with the doctor.** Some patients need to use an anxiolytic drug for longer time periods, because of the type of anxiety they may be experiencing.

Side effects

Side effects occur, to some degree, with all medication. They are usually not serious and do not occur in all individuals. Most will decrease or disappear with time. If a side effect continues, speak to the doctor or pharmacist about appropriate treatment.

Common side effects that should be reported to the doctor at the **NEXT APPOINTMENT** include:
- Feeling sleepy and tired – This problem goes away with time, or when the dose is reduced. Avoid operating machinery if drowsiness persists.
- Headache – tends to be temporary and can be managed by taking pain medicine (e.g., acetaminophen) when required.
- Nausea or heartburn – If this happens, take the medication with food.
- Dizziness, lightheadedness – sit or lie down; if symptoms persist, contact the doctor.
- Energized/agitated feeling – some individuals may feel nervous for a few days after starting this medication. Report this to the doctor.
- Tingling or numbing in fingers or toes – report this to the doctor.

Less common side effects that you should report to the physician **IMMEDIATELY** include:
- Severe agitation, excitement or any changes in behavior.

Let the doctor know **as soon as possible** if you miss your period, suspect you may be **pregnant** or are trying to get pregnant.

What should you do if you forget to take a dose of medication?

If you take your total dose of antipsychotic at bedtime and you forget to take it, DO NOT take the dose in the morning, but continue with your schedule the next evening. If you take the drug several times a day, take the missed dose when you remember (unless it is within 4 h of your next dose), then continue with your regular schedule.

Is this drug safe to take with other medication?

Because antipsychotic drugs can change the effect of other medication, or may be affected by other medication, always check with the doctor or pharmacist before taking other drugs, including over-the-counter medication such as cold remedies. Always inform any doctor or dentist that you see that you are taking an antipsychotic medication.

Precautions/Considerations

1) Do not increase your dose without consulting the doctor
2) Take your medication at the same time each day, with meals or with water, milk, orange or apple juice. Avoid grapefruit juice as it may change the effects of the drug in your body.
3) Avoid excessive consumption of caffeinated beverages (i.e., more than 2 cups of coffee, 3 cups of tea or cola) as it may counteract the beneficial effects of buspirone.
4) Check with the doctor or pharmacist before taking other drugs, including over-the-counter medication or herbal remedies.
5) Store your medication in a clean, dry area at room temperature. Keep all medication out of the reach of children.

If you have any questions regarding this medication, do not hesitate to contact the doctor, pharmacist, or nurse.

PATIENT AND CAREGIVER INFORMATION on HYPNOTICS/SEDATIVES

The name of your medication is _____.

Use

This medication is used to **treat sleep problems,** such as problems falling asleep or remaining asleep for a reasonable number of hours or waking up often during the night. Sleeping problems occur in most individuals from time to time. If, however, sleeping problems persist, this may be a symptom of some other disorder, either medical and psychiatric.

A person may have difficulty in falling asleep because of stress or anxiety felt during the day, pain, physical discomfort or changes in daily routine. Any disease that causes pain (e.g., ulcers) or breathing difficulties (e.g., asthma or a cold) can interfere with continuous sleep. Stimulant drugs, including caffeine, may also contribute to problems falling asleep; other medications may change sleep patterns when they are stopped (e.g., antidepressants, antipsychotics). Sleep will improve when these causes have been identified, corrected, or treated. Certain disorders, including depression, may also affect sleep.

Hypnotic/sedatives are similar to antianxiety drugs, but tend to cause more drowsiness and incoordination; therefore, sometimes antianxiety drugs are given to treat sleep problems.

These drugs may also be given to sedate and relax children prior to diagnostic procedures or surgery.

How quickly will the drug start working?

Hypnotics/sedatives can induce calm or sedation usually within an hour. As some drugs act quickly, take the medication just prior to going to bed and relax in bed until the drug takes effect.

How long should you take this medication?

Sleep problems are usually self-limiting; often when the cause of sleep difficulties is treated or eliminated, sleep will improve. Therefore, hypnotic/sedatives are usually prescribed for a limited period of time. Many individuals take the medication only when needed (during periods of insomnia) rather than on a daily basis. It is suggested that once you have slept well for 2 or 3 nights in a row, try to get to sleep without taking the sedative/hypnotic. Tolerance or loss of effectiveness can occur in some individuals if they are used every day beyond 4 months. Individuals taking hypnotics for long periods of time have a risk of developing dependence – they may have difficulty stopping the medication and may experience withdrawal symptoms.

If you have been taking the medication every day for a period of time, the physician may try to reduce the dose of this drug slowly to see if sleeping problems persist; if not, the dosage may be further reduced and you may be advised to stop using this medication. **Do not increase the dose or stop the drug without consulting with the doctor.**

Some patients need to use a sedative/hypnotic drug for longer time periods, because of the type of problems they may be experiencing. Others require it only from time to time, i.e., PRN.

Side effects

Side effects occur, to some degree, with all medication. They are usually not serious and do not occur in all individuals. Most will decrease or disappear with time. If a side effect continues, speak to the doctor or pharmacist about appropriate treatment.

Common side effects that should be reported to the doctor at the **NEXT APPOINTMENT** include:
- Morning hangover, feeling sleepy and tired – This problem may lessen with time; inform the doctor. Use of other drugs that make you drowsy will worsen the problem. Avoid operating machinery if drowsiness persists.
- Muscle incoordination, weakness, lightheadedness or dizziness – Inform the doctor; a change in your dosage may be needed.
- Forgetfulness, memory lapses – Inform the doctor.
- Slurred speech – A change in your dosage may be needed.
- Nausea or heartburn – If this happens, take the medication with food.
- Bitter taste – Can occur with certain drugs (e.g., zopiclone). Avoid milk in the morning to lessen this effect.

Less common side effects that you should report to the physician **IMMEDIATELY** include:

- Disorientation, confusion, worsening of your memory, periods of blackouts, or amnesia
- Nervousness, excitement, agitation, hallucinations or any behavior changes
- Incoordination leading to falls
- Skin rash

Let the doctor know **as soon as possible** if you miss your period, suspect you may be **pregnant** or are trying to get pregnant.

Precautions/Considerations

1) Do not increase your dose without consulting the doctor
2) Check with the doctor or pharmacist before taking other drugs, including over-the-counter medication such as cold remedies
3) Speak to the doctor if you begin having sleeping problems after starting any new medication (e.g., for a medical condition)
4) This drug may impair the mental and physical abilities required for driving a car or operating machinery. Avoid these activities if you feel drowsy or slowed down.
5) This drug may increase the effects of alcohol, making you more sleepy, dizzy and lightheaded
6) Take your medication about half an hour before bedtime; do not smoke in bed afterwards.
7) Do not stop taking the drug suddenly, especially if you have been on the medication for a number of months or have been taking high doses. Hypnotics/sedatives need to be withdrawn gradually to prevent withdrawal reactions.
8) Avoid excessive consumption of caffeinated beverages (i.e., more than 2 cups of coffee, 3 cups of tea or cola) as it may counteract the beneficial effects of the anxiolytic.
9) Store your medication in a clean, dry area at room temperature. Keep all medication out of the reach of children.

10) If you are precribed Ambien CR, do not split, crush or chew the tablet, but swallow it whole

Nondrug methods to help you sleep include:

1) Avoid taking caffeine-containing drinks or foods (e.g., chocolate) after 6 pm and avoid heavy meals several hours before bedtime. A warm glass of milk is effective for some people.
2) Napping and sleeping during the day will make restful sleep at night difficult. Keep active during the day and exercise regularly.
3) Engage in relaxing activities prior to bedtime such a reading, listening to music or taking a warm bath. Strenuous exercise (e.g., jogging) immediately before bedtime may make it difficult to get to sleep.
4) Establish a routine or normal pattern of sleeping and waking.
5) Use the bed and bedroom only for sleep and sexual activity.
6) Minimize external stimulation which might disturb sleep. If necessary, use dark shades over windows or wear ear plugs.
7) Once in bed, make sure you are comfortable (i.e., not too hot or cold); use a firm mattress.
8) Relaxation techniques (e.g., muscle relaxation exercises) may be helpful in decreasing anxiety and promoting sleep
9) If you have problems getting to sleep, rather than toss and turn in bed, get up, have some warm milk, read a book, listen to music, or try relaxation techniques until you again begin to feel tired.
10) Don't worry about the amount of sleep you are getting as the amount will vary from day to day. The more you worry the more anxious you will get and this may make it harder for you to fall asleep.

If you have any questions regarding this medication, do not hesitate to contact the doctor, pharmacist, or nurse.

PATIENT AND CAREGIVER INFORMATION on LITHIUM

Lithium is classified as a mood stabilizer. It is an element, found in nature, and is also present in small amounts in the human body.

Uses

Lithium is used primarily to treat symptoms of acute mania and in the long-term control or prevention of Bipolar Disorder.

Though not approved for these indications, lithium has also been found to add to the effects of antidepressants in depression and may be useful in the treatment of aggression or impulsivity.

The doctor may choose to use this medication for a reason not listed here. If you are not sure why this medication is being prescribed, please ask the doctor.

How does the doctor decide what dose (how many milligrams) to prescribe?

The dose of lithium is different for every patient and is based on how much lithium is in the blood, as well as the response to treatment. The doctor will measure the lithium level in the blood on a regular basis during the first few months. The lithium level that is usually found to be effective for most patients is between 0.6 and 1.2 mmol/L (mEq/L).

You may initially take your medication several times a day (2 or 3); after several weeks, the doctor may tell you to take it only once daily. It is important to drink 8–12 cups of fluid daily when on lithium (e.g., water, juice, milk, etc. – try to avoid sugar-filled drinks like soda pop or colas).

On the morning of your lithium blood test, take the morning dose of lithium **after** the test to avoid inaccurate results.

How quickly will the drug start working?

Control of manic symptoms may require 7 to 14 days of treatment. Because lithium takes time to work, **do not decrease or increase the dose or stop the medication** without discussing this with the doctor.

Improvement in symptoms of depression and aggression/impulsivity also occur gradually.

DO NOT STOP taking your medication if you are feeling better, without first discussing this with the doctor.

How long should you take this medication?

This depends on what type of illness you have and how well you do.

Following the first episode of mania it is recommended that lithium be continued for a minimum of 6–12 months; this decreases the chance of being ill again. The doctor may then decrease the drug slowly and monitor for any symptoms; if none occur, the drug can gradually be stopped.

For individuals who have had several episodes of mania or depression, lithium should be continued indefinitely.

Long-term treatment is generally recommended for recurring depression or aggression/impulsivity.

DO NOT STOP taking your medication if you are feeling better, without first discussing this with the doctor.

Side effects

Side effects occur, to some degree, with all medication. They are usually not serious and do not occur in all individuals. They may sometimes occur before beneficial effects of the medication are noticed. If a side effect continues, speak to the doctor or pharmacist about appropriate treatment.

Common side effects that should be reported to the doctor at the **NEXT APPOINTMENT** include:

- Feeling tired and sleepy or having difficulty concentrating – This problem usually goes away with time. Use of other drugs that make you drowsy will worsen the problem. Avoid operating machinery if drowsiness persists.
- Nausea or heartburn – If this happens, take the medication with food. If vomiting or diarrhea occur and persist for more than 24 hours, call the doctor.

- Muscle tremor, weakness, shakiness, stiffness – Speak to the doctor as this may require an adjustment in your dosage.
- Changes in sex drive – Discuss this with the doctor.
- Weight changes – Watch the type of food you eat; avoid foods with high fat content (e.g., cakes and pastry).
- Increased thirst and increase in frequency of urination – Discuss this with the doctor.
- Skin changes, e.g., dry skin, acne, rashes.

Side effects you should report IMMEDIATELY, as they may indicate the amount of lithium in the body is higher than it should be, include:
- Loss of balance
- Slurred speech
- Visual disturbances (e.g., double-vision)
- Nausea, vomiting, stomach ache
- Watery stools, diarrhea (more than twice a day)
- Abnormal general weakness or drowsiness
- Marked trembling (e.g., shaking that interferes with holding a cup), muscle twitches, jaw shaking

IF THESE OCCUR CALL THE DOCTOR RIGHT AWAY. If you cannot reach the doctor, stop taking the lithium until you get in touch with him. Drink plenty of fluids and snack on salty foods (e.g., chips, crackers). If symptoms continue to get worse, or if they do not clear within 12 hours, go to the Emergency Department of the nearest hospital. A clinical check-up and a blood test may show the cause of the problem.

Rare side effects you should report to the doctor **IMMEDIATELY** include:
- Soreness of the mouth, gums, or throat
- Skin rash or itching, swelling of the face
- Vomiting, loss of appetite, fatigue, weakness, fever, or flu-like symptoms
- Swelling of the neck (goiter)
- Abnormally frequent urination and increased thirst (e.g., having to get up in the night several times to pass urine)

Let the doctor know **as soon as possible** if you miss your period, suspect you may be **pregnant** or are trying to get pregnant.

What should you do if you forget to take a dose of your medication?

If you take your total dose of lithium in the morning or evening and you forget to take it for more than 6 hours, skip the missed dose and continue with your schedule the next day. **DO NOT DOUBLE THE DOSE.** If you take the drug several times a day, take the missed dose when you remember (unless it is within 4 h of your next dose), then continue with your regular schedule.

Is this drug safe to take with other medication?

Because lithium can change the effect of other medication, or may be affected by other medication, always check with the doctor or pharmacist before taking other drugs, including over-the-counter medication such as cold remedies. Always inform any doctor or dentist that you see that you are taking lithium.

Precautions/Considerations

1) Do not increase or decrease your dose without consulting the doctor.
2) This drug may impair the mental and physical abilities and reaction time required for driving a car or operating other machinery. Avoid these activities if you feel drowsy or slowed down and until you know how lithium affects you.
3) Do not stop your drug suddenly as this may result in withdrawal symptoms such as anxiety, irritability and change in mood.
4) Report any changes in mood or behavior to the physician.
5) It is important to drink 8–12 cups of fluids daily (e.g., water, juice, milk, etc.)
6) Limit the number of caffeinated beverages you drink (pop, coffee, tea) and avoid excessive alcohol (> 3 drinks/week).
7) Do not change your salt intake during your treatment, without first speaking to the doctor (e.g., avoid no-salt or low-salt diets).
8) To treat occasional pain, avoid the use of nonsteroidal anti-inflammatory drugs (e.g., ibuprofen or Mortin, Advil) as they can affect the blood level of lithium and may result in toxicity. Acetaminophen is a safer alternative.
9) If you have the flu, especially if vomiting or diarrhea occur, check with the doctor regarding your lithium dose.
10) Use extra care in hot weather and during activities that cause you to sweat heavily (e.g., hot baths, saunas, exercising). The loss of too much water and salt from your body may lead to changes in the level of lithium in your body.
11) Tablets or capsules of lithium should be swallowed whole; do not crush them.
12) Store your medication in a clean, dry area at room temperature. Keep all medication out of the reach of children.

If you have any questions regarding this medication, do not hesitate to contact the doctor, pharmacist, or nurse.

PATIENT AND CAREGIVER INFORMATION on ANTICONVULSANT MOOD STABILIZERS

The name of your medication is _____.

Uses

Anticonvulsant medication can be used to treat symptoms of mania and in the long-term control or prevention of Bipolar Disorder.

They are also used to treat and prevent seizure disorders as well as certain pain syndromes (e.g., trigeminal neuralgia – carbamazepine; migraines – valproate; neuropathic pain – gabapentin).

Though not approved for these indications, these drugs have been found useful in the treatment of several other conditions, including: adding to the effects of antidepressants in the treatment of depression and of antipsychotics in the treatment of schizophrenia, and in decreasing behavior disturbances, such as chronic aggression or impulsivity.

The doctor may choose to use this medication for a reason not listed here. If you are not sure why this medication is being prescribed, please ask the doctor.

How does the doctor decide what dose (how many milligrams) to prescribe?

The dose (amount in milligrams) of the medication is different for every patient and is based on the amount of drug in the blood as well as your response to treatment. You may initially take your medication several times a day (2 or 3); after several weeks, the doctor may decide to prescribe the drug once daily.

How often will you need to have blood levels done with carbamazepine and valproate?

The doctor may measure the drug level in the blood on a regular basis during the first few months until the dose is stable. Thereafter, drug levels will be done at least once a year or whenever there is a change in drug therapy.

What do the blood levels mean?

The carbamazepine level that is usually found to be effective for most patients is between 17 and 50 umol/L (4–12 µg/ml). The valproate level that is usually found to be effective for most patients is between 350 and 700 umol/L (50–100 µg/ml).

On the morning of your blood test, take the morning dose of your medication **after** the test to avoid inaccurate results.

Blood levels do not need to be done with either lamotrigine, gabapentin, or topiramate.

How quickly will the drug start working?

Control of manic symptoms or stabilization of mood may require up to 14 days of treatment. Because these medications need time to work, **do not decrease or increase the dose or stop the medication** without discussing this with the doctor.

Improvement in seizures, pain symptoms, as well as aggression/impulsivity also occur gradually.

How long should you take this medication?

This depends on what type of illness you have and how well you do.

Following the first episode of mania it is recommended that these drugs be continued for a minimum of 6–12 months; this decreases the chance of being ill again. The doctor may then decrease the drug slowly and monitor for any symptoms; if none occur, the drug can gradually be stopped. For individuals who have had several or severe episodes of mania or depression, medication may need to be continued indefinitely.

Long-term treatment is generally recommended for recurring depression, seizure disorder and aggression/impulsivity.

Side effects

Side effects occur, to some degree, with all medication. They are usually not serious and do not occur in all individuals. They may sometimes occur before beneficial effects of the medication are noticed. If a side effect continues, speak to the doctor about appropriate treatment.

Common side effects that should be reported to the doctor at the **NEXT APPOINTMENT** include:

- Feeling sleepy and tired or having difficulty concentrating – This problem usually goes away with time. Use of other drugs that make you drowsy will worsen the problem. Avoid operating machinery if drowsiness persists.
- Dizziness – Get up from a lying or sitting position slowly; dangle your legs over the edge of the bed for a few minutes before getting up. Sit or lie down if dizziness persists or if you feel faint – then call the doctor.
- Incoordination or unsteadiness – Discuss this with the doctor as this may require an adjustment in your dosage.
- Blurred vision – This may occur at the start of treatment and tends to be temporary. Reading under a bright light or at a distance may help; a magnifying glass can be of temporary use. If the problem continues, advise the doctor.
- Dry mouth – Sour candy, ice chips, popsicles, and sugarless gum help increase saliva in your mouth; try to avoid sweet, calorie-laden beverages (like colas). Drink water and brush your teeth regularly.
- Nausea or heartburn – If this happens, take the medication with food. If vomiting or diarrhea occur and last for more than 24 hours, call the doctor.
- Muscle tremor – Speak to the doctor as this may require a change in your dosage.
- Changes in hair texture, hair loss (valproate).
- Changes in the menstrual cycle (valproate).
- Changes in sex drive – Discuss this with the doctor. ·
- Weight changes – Watch the type of food you eat; avoid foods with high fat content (e.g., cakes and pastry).
- Periods of hyperventilation or rapid breathing

Rare side effects you should report to the doctor **IMMEDIATELY** include:

- Fatigue, weakness, fever, or flu-like symptom
- Soreness of the mouth, gums, or throat, mouth ulcers or sores
- Skin rash or itching, swelling of the face, skin blistering or crusting (especially with carbamazepine, oxcarbazepine, and lamotrigine)
- Severe stomach pain, nausea, vomiting, loss of appetite, lethargy
- Confusion or disorientation
- Easy bruising, bleeding, appearance of splotchy purplish darkening of the skin
- Yellowing of the skin or eyes, darkening of urine
- Unusual eye movements
- Sudden blurring of vision and/or painful or red eyes
- Feeling very dizzy or falling/fainting
- Sudden rise in body temperature and decreased sweating when exposed to warm temperatures and/or exercise

Let the doctor know **as soon as possible** if you miss your period, suspect you may be **pregnant** or are trying to get pregnant.

What should you do if you forget to take a dose of your medication?

If you take your total dose of medication in the morning or at bedtime and you forget to take it for more than 6 hours, skip the missed dose and continue with your schedule the next day. **DO NOT DOUBLE THE DOSE**. If you take the drug several times a day, take the missed dose when you remember (unless it is within 4 h of your next dose), then continue with your regular schedule.

Is this drug safe to take with other medication?

Because these drugs can change the effect of other medication, or may be affected by other medication, always check with the doctor or pharmacist before taking other drugs, including over-the-counter medication such as cold remedies. Always inform any doctor or dentist that you see that you are taking this drug.

Precautions/Considerations

1) Do not increase or decrease your dose without consulting the doctor.
2) Avoid drinking grapefruit juice while on *carbamazepine* as it can affect the level of carbamazepine in your body.
3) If your are on *liquid carbamazepine*, do not mix it with any other liquid medication. The liquid form of valproic acid should not be mixed with carbonated beverages, such as soda pop. This may cause an unpleasant taste or mouth irritation.
4) Unless you are prescribed a chewable tablet, capsules or tablets should be swallowed whole; do not break or crush them.

5) These drugs may impair the mental and physical abilities and reaction time required for driving a car or operating other machinery. Avoid these activities if you feel drowsy or slowed down or until you know how this medication affects you.

6) Do not stop your drug suddenly as this may result in withdrawal symptoms such as anxiety, irritability and changes in mood.

7) To treat occasional pain, avoid the use of ASA (aspirin and related products) if you are taking divalproex or valproic acid, as it can affect the amount of this drug in your body; acetaminophen (Tylenol) or ibuprofen (Motrin, Advil) are safer alternatives.

8) *Gabapentin* should not be taken within 2 hours of an antacid (Maalox, Tums)

9) If you are taking *topiramate*, drink plenty of fluids before and during activities such as exercise or exposure to warm temperatures. Avoid the regular use of antacids. (e.g., Tums, Maalox)

10) Report any changes in mood or behavior to the physician.

11) Store your medication in a clean, dry area at room temperature. Keep all medication out of the reach of children.

If you have any questions regarding this medication, do not hesitate to contact the doctor, pharmacist, or nurse.

Use

Disulfiram is primarily used as a **deterrent to alcohol use/abuse.**

How quickly will the drug start working?

Disulfiram inhibits the breakdown of alcohol in the body, resulting in a buildup of a chemical called acetaldehyde; this results in an unpleasant reaction when alcohol is consumed. The reaction can occur 10–20 minutes after drinking alcohol and may last up to 2 hours.

The reaction consists of: flushing, choking, nausea, vomiting, increased heart rate and decreased blood pressure (dizziness).

How long should you take this medication?

Disulfiram is usually prescribed for a set period of time to help the individual stop the use of alcohol. **Do not decrease or increase the dose** without discussing this with the doctor.

Side effects

Side effects occur, to some degree, with all medication. They are usually not serious and do not occur in all individuals. They may sometimes occur before beneficial effects of the medication are noticed. If a side effect continues, speak to the doctor or pharmacist about appropriate treatment.

Common side effects that should be reported to the doctor at the **NEXT APPOINTMENT** include:

- Feeling sleepy, tired or depressed – This problem goes away with time. Use of other drugs that make you drowsy will worsen the problem. Avoid driving a car or operating machinery if drowsiness persists.
- Energizing/agitated feeling – Some individuals may feel nervous or have difficulty sleeping for a few days after starting this medication.

- Headache – Temporary use of pain medicine (e.g., acetaminophen, ASA).
- Skin rash – Contact the doctor.
- Garlic-like taste

Rare side effects you should report to the doctor **IMMEDIATELY** include:
- Yellow tinge in the eyes or to the skin; dark-colored urine
- Soreness of the mouth, gums, or throat
- Skin rash or itching, swelling of the face
- Feeling tired, weak, feverish, or like you have the flu, associated with nausea, vomiting, loss of appetite

Let the doctor know **as soon as possible** if you miss your period, suspect you may be **pregnant** or are trying to get pregnant.

What should you do if you forget to take a dose of your medication?

If you take your total dose of the drug in the morning and you forget to take it for more than 6 hours, skip the missed dose and continue with your schedule the next day. **DO NOT DOUBLE THE DOSE**.

Is this drug safe to take with other medication?

Because disulfiram can change the effect of other medication, or may be affected by other medication, always check with the doctor or pharmacist before taking other drugs, including over-the-counter medication such as cold remedies and herbal preparations. Always inform any doctor or dentist that you see that you are taking this medication.

Precautions/Considerations

1) Do not increase or decrease your dose without consulting the doctor.
2) Report to the doctor any changes in sleeping or eating habits or changes in mood

3) Avoid all products (food and drugs) containing alcohol, including tonics, cough syrups, mouth washes and alcohol-based sauces. A delay in the reaction may be as long as 24 hours.

4) Exposure to alcohol-containing rubs or solvents (e.g., after-shave) may trigger a reaction.

5) Carry an identification card stating the name of the drug you are taking.

6) Store your medication in a clean, dry area at room temperature. Keep all medication out of the reach of children.

If you have any questions regarding this medication, do not hesitate to contact the doctor, pharmacist, or nurse.

PATIENT INFORMATION on ACAMPROSATE

Use

Acamprosate has not been approved for use in children and adolescents. In adults, acamprosate is primarily used in the treatment of alcohol dependence, where it reduces alcohol cravings and can prevent relapse

How quickly will the drug start working?

Acamprosate is usually prescribed after an individual has been withdrawn from alcohol use. It is not effective if the person is actively drinking, nor will it treat withdrawal symptoms. It reduces cravings to alcohol.

Acamprosate has been shown to maintain abstinence if taken, as directed, as part of a treatment program that includes counseling and support.

How long should you take this medication?

Acamprosate is usually prescribed for a set period of time (months) to help the individual remain alcohol-free. Do not increase or decrease your dose of medication without discussing this with your physician.

Side effects

Side effects occur, to some degree, with all medication. They are usually not serious and do not occur in all individuals. They may sometimes occur before beneficial effects of the medication are noticed. If a side effect continues, speak to your doctor about appropriate treatment.

Common side effect that should be reported to your doctor at the **NEXT APPOINTMENT** include:
- Upset stomach, nausea, gas, diarrhea – if these symptoms continue, the doctor may need to re-evaluate the dose

- Headache – this tends to be temporary and can be managed by taking pain medicine (Aspirin, acetaminophen, ibuprofen)
- Increased anxiety, sleeping difficulties – some individuals may feel nervous or have difficulty sleeping for a few days after starting this medication
- Itching, skin rash

Rare side effects you should report to your doctor **IMMEDIATELY** include:
- Severe anxiety, change in your mood or behavior, suicidal thoughts

Let your doctor know **as soon as possible** if you miss your period, think that you may be pregnant, or are planning to become pregnant during therapy.

What should you do if you forget to take a dose of your medication?

If you are taking the medication 3 times a day with meals, and miss taking your dose by more than 2 hours, skip the missed dose and continue with your next scheduled dose.

Is this drug safe to take with other medication?

Because acamprosate can change the effect of other medication, or may be affected by other medication, always check with your doctor or pharmacist before taking other drugs, including over-the-counter medication such as cold remedies and herbal preparations. Always inform any doctor or dentist that you see that are taking acamprosate.

Precautions/Considerations

1) This drug may impair the mental and physical abilities and reaction time required for driving or operating other machinery. Avoid these activities if you feel drowsy or slowed down.

2) Do not increase or decrease your dose, or stop the drug suddenly without discussing this with your physician

3) Should you restart drinking during treatment, continue taking the acamprosate but notify your physician as soon as possible.

4) Report any changes in mood or behavior to your physician.

5) Store your medication in a clean, dry area at room temperature. Keep all medication out of reach of children.

If you have any questions regarding this medication, do not hesitate to contact your doctor, pharmacist, or nurse.

PATIENT INFORMATION on NALTREXONE

Use

Naltrexone has not been approved for use in children and adolescents. In adults, naltrexone is mainly used as an aid in the treatment of alcohol dependence or addiction to opiates. Though not approved for this indication, naltrexone has also been used in the treatment of self-injurious behavior and impulse-control disorders as well as obsessive-compulsive disorder.

How quickly will the drug start working?

Naltrexone blocks the "craving" for alcohol and opiates. It does not suppress withdrawal symptoms that can occur in opiate users and should not be used in anyone using narcotics in the previous 10 days; these individuals must undergo detoxification programs before starting naltrexone. Naltrexone is started at a low dose and increased gradually based on effectiveness. Onset of response is quick (within the hour).

How long should you take this medication?

Naltrexone is usually prescribed for a set period of time to help the individual discontinue the use of alcohol or opiates. Naltrexone is used for a prolonged period of time in the treatment of behavior and impulse-control problems and obsessive-compulsive disorder. Do not decrease or increase the dose without discussing this with the doctor.

Side effects

Side effects occur, to some degree, with all medication. They are usually not serious and do not occur in all individuals. They may sometimes occur before beneficial effects of the medication are noticed. If a side effect continues, speak to your doctor about appropriate treatment.

Common side effects that should be reported to your doctor at the **NEXT APPOINT-MENT** include:
- Feeling tired, confused, depressed – This problem goes away with time. Use of other drugs that make you drowsy will worsen the problem. Avoid driving a car or operating machinery if drowsiness persists.
- Nervousness, anxiety, problem sleeping – Some individuals may feel nervous or have difficulty sleeping for a few days after starting this medication.
- Headache – Temporary use of pain medicine (e.g., acetaminophen, ASA).
- Joint and muscle pain, stiffness – Temporary use of pain medicine
- Abdominal pain, cramps, nausea and vomiting – If this happens take the medication with food or milk.
- Weight loss.

Rare side effects you should report to your doctor **IMMEDIATELY** include:
- Yellow tinge in the eyes or to the skin; dark-colored urine
- Soreness of the mouth, gums, or throat
- Skin rash or itching, swelling of the face
- Nausea, vomiting, loss of appetite, fatigue, weakness, fever, or flu-like symptoms
- Shortness of breath, persistent coughing, wheezing

Let your doctor know **as soon as possible** if you miss your period, think that you may be **pregnant,** or are planning to become pregnant during therapy.

What should you do if you forget to take a dose of your medication?

If you take your total dose of the drug in the morning and you forget to take it for more than 6 h, skip the missed dose and continue with your schedule the next day. **DO NOT DOUBLE THE DOSE**. If you take the drug several times a day, take the missed dose when you remember, then continue with your regular schedule.

Interactions with other medication

Because naltrexone can change the effect of other medication, or may be affected by other medication, always check with your doctor or pharmacist before taking other drugs, including over-the-counter medication such as cold remedies and herbal preparations. Always inform any doctor or dentist that you see that you are taking this medication.

Precautions/Considerations

1) Do not increase or decrease your dose without consulting your doctor.

2) Report to your doctor any changes in sleeping or eating habits or changes in mood or behavior.
3) Carry an identification card stating the name of the drug you are taking.
4) Store your medication in a clean, dry area at room temperature. Keep all medication out of the reach of children.
5) DO NOT use narcotic preparations while taking naltrexone as this may cause serious adverse effects including coma and death.
6) Limit the use of over-the-counter pain medicines such as aspirin, acetaminophen or non-steroidal anti-inflammatory drugs (e.g., Motrin).

If you have any questions regarding this medication, do not hesitate to contact your doctor, pharmacist, or nurse.

PATIENT AND CAREGIVER INFORMATION on METHADONE

Use

Methadone has not been approved for use in children and adolesents. Methadone is primarily used as a substitute drug in the treatment of narcotic (opiate) dependent patients who desire maintenance therapy. It suppresses withdrawal symptoms as well as the craving for narcotics. It is part of a complete addiction treatment program that also includes behavior therapy and counseling.

How quickly will the drug start working?

Methadone blocks the "craving" and withdrawal reactions from narcotics/opiates immediately. Methadone is started at a low dose and increased gradually, based on effectiveness, to a maintenance dose. It is then prescribed once daily.

Why is methadone given on a daily basis?

Methadone is a narcotic and its dispensing and usage is governed by Federal regulations. It is prepared as a liquid, mixed with orange juice. Most patients receive their methadone, on a daily basis, from the Pharmacy and are required to drink the contents of the bottle in the presence of the pharmacist.

Some patients (who are stable on their medication) are permitted to carry several days' supply of methadone to use at home.

How long should you take this medication?

The length of time methadone is prescribed varies among individuals and depends on a number of factors, including their progress in therapy; most patients receive methadone for several months, while others may require it for several years. Any decreases in dose should be done very gradually under the direction of the physician. It has been demonstrated that methadone is beneficial in helping patients avoid illicit narcotic use and helps them attain social stability.

Side effects

Side effects occur, to some degree, with all medication. They are usually not serious and do not occur in all individuals. They may sometimes occur before beneficial effects of the medication are noticed. If a side effect continues, speak to the doctor or pharmacist about appropriate treatment.

Common side effects that should be reported to the doctor at the **NEXT APPOINTMENT** include:

- Feeling tired, confused, depressed – This problem goes away with time. Use of other drugs that make you drowsy will worsen the problem. Avoid operating machinery if drowsiness persists.
- Energized feeling, insomnia – Some individuals may feel nervous or have difficulty sleeping for a few days after starting this medication.
- Dizziness, lightheadedness, weakness – This should go away with time.
- Joint and muscle pain – Temporary use of non-narcotic pain medicines may help (e.g., acetaminophen, aspirin).
- Nausea and vomiting – If this happens take the medication after eating.
- Loss of appetite, weight loss – Taking the medication after meals, eating smaller meals more frequently or drinking high calorie drinks may help.
- Changes in sex drive or sexual performance – Though rare, should this problem occur, discuss it with the doctor.
- Sweating, flushing – You may sweat more than usual; use of deodorants and talcum powder may help.
- Constipation – Increase bulk foods in your diet (e.g., salads, bran) and drink plenty of fluids. Some individuals find a bulk laxative (e.g., Metamucil, Fibyrax) or a stool softener (Colace, Surfak) helps regulate their bowels. If these remedies are not effective, consult the doctor or pharmacist.

Rare side effects you should report to the doctor **IMMEDIATELY** include:
- Yellow tinge in the eyes or to the skin; dark-colored urine
- Soreness of the mouth, gums, or throat
- Skin rash or itching, swelling of the face
- Feeling tired, weak, feverish, or like you have the flu, associated with nausea, vomiting, loss of appetite

Let your doctor know **as soon as possible** if you miss your period, think that you may be **pregnant,** or are planning to become pregnant during therapy.

What should you do if you forget to take a dose of your medication?

It is important to take this medication at approximately the same time, on a daily basis. Missing a dose can result in a withdrawal reaction, consisting of restlessness, insomnia, nausea, vomiting, headache, increased perspiration, congestion, "gooseflesh," abdominal cramps, muscle and bone pain.

Is this drug safe to take with other medication?

Because methadone an change the effect of other medication, or may be affected by other medication, always check with the doctor or pharmacist before taking other drugs, including over-the-counter medication such as cold remedies. Always inform any doctor or dentist that you see that you are taking this medication.

Precautions/Considerations

1) Do not share this medication with anyone. If you receive "carries" of methadone, store them out of the reach of children (preferably in a lockable compartment in the refrigerator); methadone can be poisonous to individuals who do not take opiates
2) Report to the doctor any changes in sleeping or eating habits or changes in mood or behavior.
3) This drug may impair the mental and physical abilities and reaction time required for driving or operating other machinery. Avoid these activities if you feel drowsy or slowed down.
4) Carry an identification card stating the name of the drug you are taking.

If you have any questions regarding this medication, do not hesitate to contact the doctor, pharmacist, or nurse.

*Page numbers in **bold type** indicate main entries.

Index of Drugs (cont.)

Cocaine 99, 153, 166, 210, 231, 233, **234–236**, 240, 241, 246, 247, 257, 259

Cocoethylene 235, 246

Codeine 51, 80, 90, 140, 193, 246, **247–249**, 264, 309

Cogentin *see* Benztropine

Concerta *see* Methylphenidate

Corticosteroids 50, 57, 193, 224

Coumarins 259

Crack 234, 236

Cyclic antidepressant 48, 77, 79, 90

Cyclizine 248

Cyclobenzaprine 50

Cyclophosphamide 57

Cyclosporin *see* Immunosuppressants

Cyclosporin A *see* Immunosuppressants

Cyproheptadine 45, 47, 50, 153, 164

D

d-Amphetamine *see* Dextroamphetamine

Dalmane *see* Flurazepam

Danazol 224

Dantrolene 122, 136

Darvon *see* Propoxyphene

DDAVP *see* Desmopressin

Debrisoquin 67, 79

Decongestants 313

Delavirdine 29

Demeclocycline 121, 135

Demerol *see* Meperidine

Depakene *see* Valproate

Depakote *see* Valproate

Depakote ER *see* Valproate

Depakote sprinkle *see* Valproate

Desipramine 35, 38, 48, 56, 62, **72–81**, 84, 90, 93, 94, 96, 100, 176, 192, 206, 234, 235, 240, 245, 259, 268

Desmopressin 119, 134, 203, 224

Desoxyephedrine *see* Methamphetamine

Desoxyn *see* Methamphetamine

Desyrel *see* Trazodone

Dexamethasone 193

Dexampex *see* Dextroamphetamine

Dexedrine *see* Dextroamphetamine

Dexfenfluramine 90

Dexmethylphenidate **19–26**, 30–32, 38

Dextroamphetamine **19–26**, 30–32, 38, 57, 62, 71, 158, 192, 236, 273

Dextromethorphan 51, 85, 91, 237, 306, 309

Dextropropoxyphene 85

Dextrostat *see* Dextroamphetamine

Diacetylmorphine 248

Diastat *see* Diazepam

Diazemuls *see* Diazepam

Diazepam 50, 68, 77, 105, 107, 125, 153, 161, 164, 165, 166, **170–180**, 187, 226, 234, 239, 245, 254, 255, 259, 269

Diazepam Intensol *see* Diazepam

Diclofenac 207, 224

Dicumarol 191, 223

Didanosine 268

Diethylpropion 55

Digoxin 51, 68, 165, 177, 187, 228, 277

Dihydrocarbostyril 109, 127

Dihydroergotamine 51

Dihydroindolone 109, 130

Dilantin *see* Phenytoin

Dilaudid *see* Hydromorphone

Diltiazem 50, 80, 126, 140, 176, 187, 192, 206, 224

Dimenhydrinate 76, 105

Dimethyltryptamine 239, 242

Diphenhydramine 26, 49, 79, 90, 153, 161, 162, 163, 164, 165, 166, 188, 191, 192, 193, 309

Diphenoxylate 91

Disopyramide 123, 137, 138, 224

Disulfiram 126, 140, 177, 192, 196, 235, 240, 245, 246, **257–260**, 269, 331

– Interactions 259

Diuretics 67, 79, 203, 207

Divalproex *see* Valproate

DMT *see* Dimethyltryptamine

Docusate 113, 119, 134, 164

Dolophine *see* Methadone

DOM (2,5-dimethoxy-4-methyl-amphetamine 238

Donepezil 126, 140, 272

Dopamine 13, 21, 26, 27, 30, 33, 40, 53, 54, 56, 57, 58, 65, 76, 82, 86, 89, 90, 91, 101, 104, 109, 110, 118, 119, 120, 127, 133, 135, 147, 152, 157, 158, 161, 162, 163, 185, 232, 236, 237, 239, 253, 273, 295

Dopamine agonists 21, 158, 161

Dopaminergic agents 19, 273

Doral *see* Quazepam

Doxepin **72–81**, 93, 94, 96, 223, 248

Doxycycline 191, 206, 223, 245

Doxylamine 188

Droperidol 109, 134, 137

Drysol 46, 75

Duloxetine **58–62**, 92, 94, 97

Duragesic *see* Fentanyl

Duralith *see* Lithium

E

Ecstasy *see* MDA *see* MDMA

ECT *see* Electroconvulsive treatment

Efavirenz 57, 268

Effexor XR *see* Venlafaxine

Elavil *see* Amitriptyline

Electroconvulsive treatment 6, 88, 101, **103–108**, 122, 158, 174, 208, 210, 310, 311

– Interactions 107–108

– Patient Information 310

Enalapril 79, 125, 139, 206

Enflurane 79, 138

Enoxacin 61, 176

Enzyme inducer 213

Ephedra 26, 237

Ephedrine 85, 91, 236, 237, 258

Epinephrine 81, 85, 91, 126, 140

Epival *see* Valproate

Epival ER *see* Valproate

Ergot alkaloids 51, 68

Ergotamine 51, 68

Erythromycin 48, 99, 124, 129, 138, 176, 186, 191, 223, 225, 248

Escitalopram **41–52**, 79, 92, 94, 97

Eskalith *see* Lithium

Eskalith CR *see* Lithium

Estazolam 169, 170, 176, 177, 245

Estrogens 57, 80, 120, 126, 135, 140, 177

Ethanol 50, 177, 235, **243–246**

Ethanolamine 188

Ethopropazine 161

Ethosuximide 223, 226

Etretinate 224

F

Famotidine 129, 177, 211, 224, 246

Felbamate 223, 226

Fenfluramine 15, 90

Fentanyl 51, 248, 249

Fexofenadine 67

Fiorinal-C 249

Flecainide 48, 61

Fluanxol *see* Flupenthixol

Fluanxol Depot *see* Flupenthixol

Fluconazole 79, 125, 139, 176, 224, 268

Flumazenil 174, 193

Flunitrazepam 231, 236, 240, 248, **255–256**

Fluoxetine 29, 40, **41–52**, 56, 60, 61, 66, 67, 71, 77, 79, 84, 90, 92, 94, 97, 98, 101, 107, 115, 125, 129, 139, 164, 176, 186, 191, 198, 206, 223, 226, 227, 235, 240, 244, 247, 248

Flupenthixol **131–145**, 146, 149, 150, 224, 234, 235

Flupenthixol decanoate *see* Flupenthixol

Fluphenazine 49, 113, 114, **130–144**, 146, 148, 150, 192

Fluphenazine decanoate *see* Fluphenazine

Flurazepam 170, 171, 181

Fluvoxamine **41–52**, 61, 67, 71, 79, 84, 92, 94, 97, 125, 129,

Index of Drugs (cont.)

Index of Drugs (cont.)

Index of Drugs (cont.)

Order Forms

I would like to order:		
QTY	**Price**	**Total**
Clinical Handbook...for Children & Adolescents, 2nd edition	US $59.00 / € 49.95	
Clinical Handbook of Psychotropic Drugs, 17th edition	US $64.00 / € 54.95	
Understanding Rett Syndrome	US $34.95 / € 34.95	
Deficit/Hyperactivity Disorder in Children and Adults	US $24.95 / € 24.95	
Childhood Maltreatment	US $24.95 / € 24.95	
Advances in Psychotherapy – Evidence-Based Practice – Series Standing Order (Standing order price for min. 4 successive vols.: US $19.95 each)		
	Subtotal	
WA residents add 8.8% sales tax		
Postage & handling: USA: 1st item US $6.00, each additional item US $1.25 Canada: 1st item US $8.00, each additional item US $2.00 South America: 1st item US $10.00, each additional item US $2.00 Europe: 1st item € 6.00, each additional item € 1.25 Rest of the World: 1st item € 8.00, each additional item € 1.50		
	Total	

- Professor examination copies are available
- We offer discounts on bulk orders of 10 copies or more
  Call (800) 228-3749 for details

Call our order desk on (800) 228-3749 or order online at www.hhpub.com

Shipping and Billing information

❏ Check enclosed ❏ Please bill me   Charge my: ❏ VISA ❏ MC ❏ AmEx

Card # _____

CVV2/CVC2/CID # _____ Exp date _____

Cardholder's name _____

Signature _____

Shipping address:
Name _____

Address _____

City, State, ZIP _____

E-mail _____

Phone / Fax _____

Hogrefe & Huber Publishers · 30 Amberwood Parkway · Ashland, OH 44805 · Tel: (800) 228-3749 · Fax: (419) 281-6883
Hogrefe & Huber Publishers · Rohnsweg 25 · D-37085 Göttingen · Tel: +49 551 49 609-0 · Fax: +49 551 49 609-88
E-Mail: custserv@hogrefe.com

HOGREFE

I would like to order:		
QTY	**Price**	**Total**
Clinical Handbook...for Children & Adolescents, 2nd edition	US $59.00 / € 49.95	
Clinical Handbook of Psychotropic Drugs, 17th edition	US $64.00 / € 54.95	
Understanding Rett Syndrome	US $34.95 / € 34.95	
Deficit/Hyperactivity Disorder in Children and Adults	US $24.95 / € 24.95	
Childhood Maltreatment	US $24.95 / € 24.95	
Advances in Psychotherapy – Evidence-Based Practice – Series Standing Order (Standing order price for min. 4 successive vols.: US $19.95 each)		
	Subtotal	
WA residents add 8.8% sales tax		
Postage & handling: USA: 1st item US $6.00, each additional item US $1.25 Canada: 1st item US $8.00, each additional item US $2.00 South America: 1st item US $10.00, each additional item US $2.00 Europe: 1st item € 6.00, each additional item € 1.25 Rest of the World: 1st item € 8.00, each additional item € 1.50		
	Total	

- Professor examination copies are available
- We offer discounts on bulk orders of 10 copies or more
  Call (800) 228-3749 for details

Call our order desk on (800) 228-3749 or order online at www.hhpub.com

Shipping and Billing information

❏ Check enclosed ❏ Please bill me   Charge my: ❏ VISA ❏ MC ❏ AmEx

Card # _____

CVV2/CVC2/CID # _____ Exp date _____

Cardholder's name _____

Signature _____

Shipping address:
Name _____

Address _____

City, State, ZIP _____

E-mail _____

Phone / Fax _____

Hogrefe & Huber Publishers · 30 Amberwood Parkway · Ashland, OH 44805 · Tel: (800) 228-3749 · Fax: (419) 281-6883
Hogrefe & Huber Publishers · Rohnsweg 25 · D-37085 Göttingen · Tel: +49 551 49 609-0 · Fax: +49 551 49 609-88
E-Mail: custserv@hogrefe.com

HOGREFE

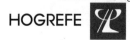

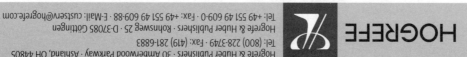

Barbro Lindberg

Understanding Rett Syndrome
A Practical Guide for Parents, Teachers, and Therapists

2nd, completely revised edition 2006, 208 pp., hardcover US $34.95 / € 34.95, ISBN: 978-0-88937-306-8

The brand new edition of this unique book describes the difficulties and challenges of girls and women with Rett Syndrome, and proposes solutions that can help them in everyday life. Written from an educational perspective, and based on extensive practical, real-life experience, it also takes into consideration living conditions as a whole to provide practical and effective help for all those involved in the care of those with Rett Syndrome.

Rett Syndrome is a severe neurological disorder with no cure affecting 1 out of every 10,000–15,000 female births worldwide. It is now known to result from a chromosomal defect that leads to problems such as mental retardation, serious motor handicaps, epileptic seizures, and difficulties with communication. This syndrome is found only in girls, and usually becomes noticeable during their second year of life.

In this new edition, the chapters on intelligence and understanding, learning, and communication have been elucidated and deepened. There are also some new sections on digital pictures, computers, and sensory environments.

Understanding Rett Syndrome is primarily intended for people close to those with Rett Syndrome, including teachers, therapists, and parents, but should be valuable to anyone involved with children with mental and functional disorders.

Table of Contents

Foreword (Andreas Rett)

Introduction: Background; Aim; Sample; Methods

Development and Progress in Rett Syndrome

The Individuals in the Study

Typical Symptoms and Behaviors: Deficiencies in Perception and Sensory Integration; Stereotypical Behaviors; Dyspraxia – "Want of Success"; Severe Motor Disabilities; Difficulties in Coordination; Mental Retardation; Communication Disorders; Emotional Channels; Large Fluctuations in Behavior; Emotional Reactions; Insecure Identity

Guidelines for Treatment and Teaching: Two Principal Teaching Groups; Multi-handicap; Understanding the Environment; Using the Body; Interacting and Communicating with the Environment; Being Active; Expanding One's World

Appendices: Questions Forming a Basis for Interviews with Parents; Questions Forming a Basis for Interviews with Parents/Care Givers; Questions Forming a Basis for Interviews with School Staff

References

From the Reviews:

"...this book delivers useful observations on clinical signs, symptoms, and behaviors in Rett syndrome, and does so in a personal manner with specific examples from patients.

"...the suggestions for the management of problematic behaviors and enrichment of the patients' lives are insightful. Readers approaching the book in this hands-on manner will find it valuable..."

Christopher J. Graver, PhD (Western State Hospital) in *Doody's Book Review*

Order online at: **www.hhpub.com** or call toll-free **(800) 228-3749**

Hogrefe & Huber Publishers · 30 Amberwood Parkway · Ashland, OH 44805
Tel: (800) 228-3749 · Fax: (419) 281-6883

Hogrefe & Huber Publishers · Rohnsweg 25 · D-37085 Göttingen
Tel: +49 551 49 609-0 · Fax: +49 551 49 609-88 · E-Mail: custserv@hogrefe.com

Annette U. Rickel, Ronald T. Brown

Attention-Deficit/Hyperactivity Disorder in Children and Adults

In the series: Advances in Psychotherapy – Evidence-Based Practice , Vol., 7

2007, 96 pages, softcover, US $24.95 / € 24.95 (Series Standing Order US $19.95/ € 19.95), ISBN: 978-0-88937-322-8

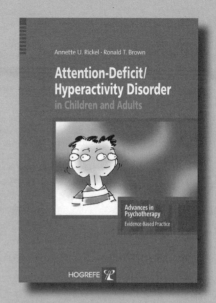

Attention-Deficit/Hyperactivity Disorder is a common condition that affects both children and adults, and can have serious consequences for academic, emotional, social, and occupational functioning. When properly identified and diagnosed, however, there are many interventions for the disorder that have established benefits. This volume in the new series, Advances in Psychotherapy – Evidence-Based Practice, provides therapists with practical, evidence-based guidance on diagnosis and treatment from leading experts – and does so in a uniquely "reader-friendly" manner. Readers will gain an understanding of recent advances in the etiology and symptom presentations of ADHD in children and adults, as well as the use of stimulant medications, other psychopharmacological approaches, and psychotherapeutic interventions. The book is both a compact "how-to" reference, for use by professional clinicians in their daily work, and an ideal educational resource for students and practice-oriented continuing education.

The most important feature of the book is that it is practical and "reader friendly." It has a similar structure to others in the series, and is a compact and easy-to-follow guide covering all aspects of practice that are relevant in real life. Tables, boxed clinical "pearls," and marginal notes assist orientation, while checklists for copying and summary boxes provide tools for use in daily practice.

The series has been developed and is edited with the support of the Society of Clinical Psychology (APA Division 12). The Society is planning a system of home study continuing education courses based on the series that an individual can complete on the web.

1. Description of Attention-Deficit/Hyperactivity Disorder • Terminology • Definition • Epidemiology • Course and Prognosis • Differential Diagnosis • Comorbidities in ADHD Patients • Diagnostic Procedures and Documentation
2. Theories and Models of ADHD • Biological Factors in ADHD • Perinatal Factors in ADHD • Psychological Factors in ADHD • Interactions between Biological and Psychological Factors
3. Diagnosis and Treatment Indications • Assessment Proceedures • Specific Assessment Techniques • The Decision-Making Prosess • Treatment Considerations.
4. Treatment: Methods of Treatment • Mechanisms of Action • Efficacy and Prognosis • Variations and Combinations of Methods • Problems in Carrying out the Treatments
5. Case Vignettes • 6. Further Reading • 7. References • 8. Appendix: Tools and Resources

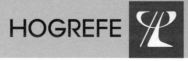

A compact "how-to" reference, and an ideal education resource!

Order online at: **www.hhpub.com** or call toll-free **(800) 228-3749**

Hogrefe & Huber Publishers · 30 Amberwood Parkway · Ashland, OH 44805
Tel: (800) 228-3749 · Fax: (419) 281-6883
Hogrefe & Huber Publishers · Rohnsweg 25 · D-37085 Göttingen
Tel: +49 551 49 609-0 · Fax: +49 551 49 609-88 · E-Mail: custserv@hogrefe.com

HOGREFE

Keep Up with the Advances in Psychotherapy!

Christine Wekerle, Alec L. Miller, David A. Wolfe, Carrie B. Spindel

Childhood Maltreatment

In the series: Advances in Psychotherapy – Evidence-Based Practice , Vol., 4

2007, 98 pages, softcover, US $24.95/ € 24.95 (Series Standing Order US $19.95/ € 19.95), ISBN: 978-0-88937-314-3

The serious consequences of child abuse or maltreatment are among the most challenging things therapists encounter. In recent years there has been a surge of interest, and of both basic and clinical research, concerning early traumatization. This volume in the series *Advances in Psychotherapy – Evidence-Based Practice* integrates results from the latest research showing the importance of early traumatization into a compact and practical guide for practitioners. Advances in biological knowledge have highlighted the potential chronicity of effects of childhood maltreatment, demonstrating particular life challenges in managing emotions, forming and maintaining healthy relationships, healthy coping, and holding a positive outlook of oneself. Despite the resiliency of many maltreated children, adolescent and young adult well-being is often compromised. This text first overviews our current knowledge of the effects of childhood maltreatment on psychiatric and psychological health, then provides diagnostic guidance, and subsequently goes on to profile promising and effective evidence-based interventions. Consistent with the discussions of treatment, prevention programming that is multi-targeted at issues for maltreated individuals is highlighted. This text helps the practitioner or student to know what to look for, what questions need to be asked, how to handle the sensitive ethical implications, and what are promising avenues for effective coping.

Table of Contents

Preface • Acknowledgments • **1 Description** • Terminology • Definition • Epidemiology • **2 Theories and Models of the Effects of Childhood Maltreatment** • PTSD Model • Social Cognitie Processing Models • **3 Diagnosis and Treatment Indications** • Course and Prognosis of Childhood Maltreatment Effects • Psychiatric Impairment and Specific Disorders Associated with Childhood Maltreatment • Asymptomatic Victims • **4 Treatment** • Methods of Treatment • Mechanisms of Action • Efficacy and Prognosis • Variations and Combinations of Methods • Prevention of Childhood Maltreatment and Related Disorders • Problems and Issues in Carrying Out Inteventiion • **5 Case Vignette** • **6 Further Reading** • **7 References** • **8 Appendix: Tools and Resources**

From the Reviews:

"This book provides outstanding suggestions and specific guidelines for mental health practitioners, from students to experienced therapists, in integrating empirically-based approaches into their clinical practice. The book clearly advances the field of intervention and treatment for children who have experienced abuse and neglect."

Barbara L. Bonner, PhD, Professor of Pediatrics, Child Study Center, Oklahoma City, OK

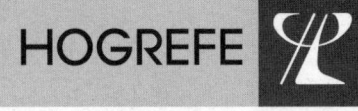

Order online at: www.hhpub.com or call toll-free **(800) 228-3749**

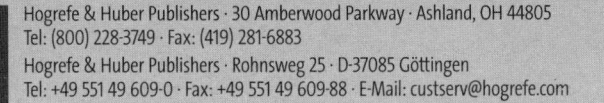

HOGREFE

Hogrefe & Huber Publishers · 30 Amberwood Parkway · Ashland, OH 44805
Tel: (800) 228-3749 · Fax: (419) 281-6883
Hogrefe & Huber Publishers · Rohnsweg 25 · D-37085 Göttingen
Tel: +49 551 49 609-0 · Fax: +49 551 49 609-88 · E-Mail: custserv@hogrefe.com

CINCINNATI STATE LIBRARY